Medication Errors

The inclusion in this book of any drug in respect to which patent or trademark rights may exist shall not be deemed, and is not intended as, a grant of or authority to exercise any right or privilege protected by such patent or trademark. All such rights or trademarks are vested in the patent or trademark owner, and no other person may exercise the same without express permission, authority, or license secured from such patent or trademark owner.

The inclusion of a brand name does not mean the editor, the authors, or the publisher have any particular knowledge that the brand listed has properties different from other brands of the same drug, nor should its inclusion be interpreted as an endorsement by the editor, authors, or publisher. Similarly, the fact that a particular brand has not been included does not indicate the product has been judged to be in any way unsatisfactory or unacceptable. Further, no official support or endorsement of this book by any federal or state agency or pharmaceutical company is intended or inferred.

The nature of drug information is that it is constantly evolving because of ongoing research and clinical experience and is often subject to interpretation. Readers are advised that decisions regarding drug therapy must be based on the independent judgment of the clinician, changing information about a drug (e.g., as reflected in the literature and manufacturers' most current product information), and changing medical practices.

The editor, the authors, and the publisher have made every effort to ensure the accuracy and completeness of the information presented in this book. However, the editor, the authors, and the publisher cannot be held responsible for the continued currency of the information, any inadvertent errors or omissions, or the application of this information.

Therefore, the editor, the authors, and the publisher shall have no liability to any person or entity with regard to claims, loss, or damage caused, or alleged to be caused, directly or indirectly, by the use of information contained herein.

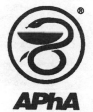

APhA

American Pharmaceutical Association
Washington, D.C.

Medication Errors

Causes, Prevention, and Risk Management

Edited by
Michael R. Cohen, MS, FASHP
President
Institute for Safe Medication Practices
Huntingdon Valley, Pennsylvania

JONES AND BARTLETT PUBLISHERS
Sudbury, Massachusetts
BOSTON   TORONTO   LONDON   SINGAPORE

World Headquarters

Jones and Bartlett Publishers
40 Tall Pine Drive
Sudbury, MA 01776
978-443-5000
info@jbpub.com
www.jbpub.com

Jones and Bartlett Publishers Canada
2100 Bloor Street West
Suite 6-272
Toronto, ON M6S 5A5
CANADA

Jones and Bartlett Publishers International
Barb House, Barb Mews
London W6 7PA
UK

American Phamaceutical Association Staff

Acquiring Editor: Julian I. Graubart
Substantive Editor: Linda R. Harteker
Managing Editor: Vicki Meade, Meade
  Communications
Copyeditor: Deborah J. Shuman
Proofreader: L. Luan Corrigan
Indexer: Mary E. Coe
Layout and Graphic Artist: Cynthia Tourison,
  Modified Concepts
Cover Designer: Jonathan Pennell

Jones and Bartlett Staff

Senior Acquisitions Editor: Greg Vis
Production Editor: Linda S. DeBruyn
Manufacturing Director: Therese Bräuer

Editorial development of *Medication Errors* was underwritten by the American Pharmaceutical Association Foundation, William M. Ellis, Executive Director

This title is a rerelease of a volume originally published in 1999 by the American Pharmaceutical Association, 2215 Constitution Avenue, N.W., Washington, DC 20037-2985 (http://www.aphanet.org). ISBN 0-917330-89-7

Library of Congress Cataloging-in-Publication Data
Medication Errors/edited by Michael R. Cohen.

       p.   cm.
       Includes index.
       ISBN 0-7637-1271-X
       1. Medication Errors.   I. Cohen, Michael R. (Michael Richard).
       1944-   .   II. American Pharmaceutical Association.
       [DNLM: 1. Medication Errors.   QZ 42 M489 1999]
       RM146.M415   1999
       615, 5'8—dc21
       DNLM/DLC
       for Library of Congress

       99-31972
       CIP

Printed in the United States of America
07 06 05 04   10 9 8 7 6 5 4

Dedication

To Hedy

Errors are everywhere and it seems that everyone makes them. Just ask my wife, Hedy, to whom this book is dedicated. No one ever gets her name right. This collection of misnomers was compiled by me, without her knowledge, from envelopes mailed to her at the Institute for Safe Medication Practices, where she works as a registered nurse. Since no one ever gets her name right, it's safe to assume that, from now on, when "Hedy" is spelled correctly on an envelope, we'll know that the sender read this book.

Betti, Betty, Hatti, Hatty, Hazzy, Headi, Heady, Heaty, Heavy, Heday, Heddi, Heddy, Hedt, Heidi, Heidy, Heini, Henny, Henrietta, Hette, Hetti, Hetty, Hezy, Hilda, Hildy, Holly, Hootie, Hyde, Medy

Contents

Back in 1974, during my transition from being a "real physician" to on-the-job training as an academic health center administrator, I recall receiving a report on medication errors in the university hospital. It was many pages long but spanned only a one-week period. Thumbing through the report, and others that I would occasionally receive over time, I could see that most of these errors were trivial—of no consequence or harm to patients. But I wondered whether there were also serious medication errors—those that caused temporary or permanent impairment in patients, or even death. Maybe these were in separate reports that I, as the senior clinical administrator of the university hospital, was not supposed to see. Or maybe these errors were not being reported... to anyone.

Publication of *Medication Errors* would not have been possible 25 years ago. We didn't talk about medication errors then. There seemed to be a certain fatalism that medication errors were an inevitable by-product of patient care. No one had added the numbers up; no one had begun to categorize the types of errors; no one had recognized the immense learning and improvement opportunities that stood to be harvested from the endless array of organization performance shortfalls. *Medication Errors* is about the courage and intellectual curiosity of individuals who have cared enough to count, catalogue, harvest, and share; who don't accept medication errors as inevitabilities and believe that improved systems and individual caregiver support can produce safer patient care.

Medication Errors is more than the rich content it contains. It is a ringing symbol of a new willingness to tell the truth—to begin educating the public about the significant imperfections in patient care and engaging patients and their families in becoming part of the solution. We need to recalibrate public expectations and expectations of ourselves, and then set and achieve ambitious improvement goals over time. This book will be a principal blueprint for that process.

Timing does matter, and for *Medication Errors*, the timing could not be better. It emerges in the midst of growing public policy concerns about medical errors, adverse events, and what can be done to enhance patient safety. This arena is of course broader than medication errors, but many believe, as do I, that medication errors make up the lion's share of what we will progressively find ourselves dealing with. For this reason and others, *Medication Errors* is likely to become an important reference source in the coming public policy debates.

Even more to the point, however, medication errors graphically illustrate the depth of the problem we must confront. Medication errors, even those resulting in patient impairment or death, are relatively easy to hide. However, there is usually no purposeful intent to hide. Rather, no other viable alternative is apparent. As catastrophic as adverse events are for patients, they are also devastating for the caregivers involved. You—the caregiver—are most commonly left to deal with your own imperfections. There are no support systems and certainly no incentives for you to report the event to anyone. If you do choose to report, you are at great risk of vilification and even loss of your job. You may also be sued.

As is well described in this book, we face the imposing challenge of overcoming the mind set of a blame- and punishment-oriented society, of which health care professionals and managers are but a microcosm. Some days, the broad understanding that most human errors are, in the end, solvable systems errors seems light years away. Yet, if we are to succeed in creating safer environments for patients, we must create environments in which it is safe for caregivers to report, and learn from, medication and other errors.

Now, almost at the end of the 20th century, we understand remarkably little about what makes America's health care organizations tick—why what happens happens. The advent of planned performance measurement, much of which will focus on medication usage, will begin to open the door to systems analysis and the eventual ability to literally manage patient outcomes. But unplanned occurrences, especially medication errors, constitute perhaps an even richer treasure trove of opportunities to learn about and improve organization systems. We owe it to the public and to ourselves to capitalize on these opportunities.

Dennis S. O'Leary, M.D.
President
Joint Commission on Accreditation of Healthcare Organizations
Oak Brook Terrace, Ill.
March 1999

No matter how long I work in pharmacy, I'll never get over the fact that medications are an unbelievable blessing. From the "wonder drugs" that we now take for granted to modern miracles like protease inhibitors, drug products reduce suffering, promote healing, and improve health.

Drug therapy is becoming more complex. More than 1000 new prescription drugs have been approved in this country since 1975. As a result, thousands of pages of complex drug information on these and other products are released every month across the United States. Moreover, patients today are older and sometimes sicker. They need more potent, more sophisticated drug therapy.

What does all this mean in terms of errors? The good news is that most errors are not serious. But many are. When results from the New York State Department of Health mandatory reporting program are extrapolated, they show that up to 1000 deaths every year in this country result from medication errors. This is a terrible and avoidable tragedy.

In a study at Brigham and Women's Hospital,[1] 6.5% of nonobstetric patients suffered an adverse drug event (ADE). Of these events, 1% were fatal, 12% were life threatening, and 30% were serious. In another study, ADEs complicated 2.43 of every 100 hospital admissions. The mortality among patients who had experienced an ADE was 3 times higher than that among a matched group of control patients. The mean length of hospital stay attributable to an ADE was almost 2 days, and the excess cost ranged from $2000 to $3000.[2,3] For medication errors, the increase in hospital stay was nearly 5 days; the excess cost was nearly $6000. This translates to an estimated annual cost of nearly $3 million for a 700-bed teaching hospital.[3]

Administering the wrong drug, strength, or dose; confusion over "look-alike" and "sound-alike" drugs; incorrect routes of administration; miscalculations; misuse of medical equipment; errors in prescribing and transcription—despite our efforts, these things happen every day, to every kind of person, in every kind of health care setting. The potential for adverse drug events and medication errors is a reality. Every error is potentially tragic and costly in both human and economic terms, for patient and professional alike.

Fortunately, we've seen a real increase in the focus on medication error prevention in the United States over the past few years. The U.S. Pharmacopeia (USP) Medication Errors Reporting Program (MERP), which is operated in cooperation with the Institute for Safe Medication Practices (ISMP) and for which ISMP provides independent practitioner review, is a good example. A voluntary reporting program with a 24-hour-a-day, toll-free telephone line, USP MERP is a front-line defense against errors.

Reporting is absolutely essential. If errors go unreported, no one benefits. If we learn about errors, we are a giant step closer to preventing them. Because health care professionals are increasingly recognizing that they can report medication errors with confidentiality, the number of errors reported to USP MERP and the quality of the information reported are improving.

Collaborative efforts involving practitioners, the pharmaceutical industry, and the Food and Drug Administration (FDA) are making a difference in improving medication safety. One example is the interdisciplinary effort that ISMP has spearheaded to reduce accidents related to potassium chloride concentrate for injection. One focus of this program was to encourage regulatory authorities and manufacturers to use special labeling (e.g., black caps, special closures, and warning statements) to make these products look as different as possible from other pharmaceuticals. For years FDA received scattered reports of deaths associated with the accidental direct injection of potassium. Vials of the drug, which is one of the most commonly used replacement electrolytes in hospitals, were always stored for rapid access, just like sodium chloride injection 0.9% (saline), which was also needed quickly for reconstituting medications or flushing intravenous catheters. In many cases, the vials were very hard to tell apart. Not only were they stored alongside one another, the vials were also manufactured by the same company, were of similar sizes and shapes, had identical coloring, and shared the word "chloride."

The pattern of errors was always similar. A nurse or doctor, usually working in a hurry, picked up a vial from a bin labeled "sodium chloride 0.9%," but the contents were used without actually reading the vial label. During or immediately after injection, the patient would cry out from the pain of the potassium being accidentally injected, have a seizure, gasp for a breath, and then stop breathing altogether—in full cardiac arrest.

Finally, in 1988, we heard from the father of a new graduate nurse. His daughter was devastated by having recently injected a newborn infant with an antibiotic that she'd accidentally reconstituted with potassium chloride instead of saline. The father, also shattered by the event and the effect it had on the baby's family as well as on his daughter, wrote an emotional letter to me, pleading that we do something to make these vials look different so that they would never be confused with saline. In 1989 in Nashville, Neil M. Davis and I, cofounders of ISMP, held a meeting on this subject. We were joined by over 50 health care practitioners, representatives from professional organizations and the pharmaceutical industry, FDA, and USP in recommending changes to drug labeling and packaging. The changes noted above were approved by USP and drug manufacturers in 1991 and are now enforced by FDA.

Unfortunately, the problem did not end there. Although the potassium labeling changes did help to reduce the number of error reports, it also became clear that some of the potassium errors had a more cognitive basis. When doctors order diuretics, serum potassium levels are monitored because potassium is lost from the body along with water. A typical order might state: "furosemide 80 mg iv now. Serum potassium." Then, in preparing the furosemide injection, the nurse, now with potassium in mind, might actually prepare 80 mEq of potassium instead of 80 mg of furosemide! In fact, we have received numerous reports describing just such a slip.

We realized that labeling changes alone were not going to be enough to prevent errors with potassium, so we also began to focus on encouraging health professionals to correct dangerous practices associated with the storage of this drug. We were joined in this effort by Dr. Lucian Leape of the Harvard School of Public Health and by Dr. Donald Berwick of the Institute for Healthcare Improvement (IHI) in Boston. Through constant publication and educational programs by Dr. Leape, IHI, and ISMP, combined with the efforts of the pharmaceutical industry in preparing premixed commercial forms of potassium chloride solutions and pharmacy practitioners who provide extemporaneously prepared potassium solutions, it is now possible to totally eliminate dangerous potassium containers and make potassium accidents a thing of the past. In fact, in 1998, the Joint Commission on Accreditation of Healthcare Organizations announced that their surveyors would ask probing questions about potassium error prevention during accreditation visits. In addition, Dr. Kenneth Kizer, Undersecretary of Health for the U.S. Veterans Health Administration, served as a model for administrators when he notified all Veterans Administration hospitals of the need to remove potassium chloride concentrate from patient care areas. A 1998 ISMP survey in which responses were received from more than 400 U.S. hospitals (see Chapter 5, page 5.32) showed that more than 75% of U.S. hospitals have removed the drug from patient care areas. It is now rare for a report of a potassium-related incident to reach us. Because of such collaborative efforts, health care professionals today can learn much more about drug errors and how to prevent them than at any time in the past.

If we're going to prevent errors, we have to start by acknowledging some basic realities. The first is that human beings make mistakes. Second, medication errors are not typically made or prevented by one person in isolation. For this reason, fail-safe systems are at the heart of prevention. Finally, it is important for us to get away from the idea of blame, because punishment and blame simply are not productive ways to solve the problem. It is far more important to search for the complex factors that may have led to an error in the first place. In Chapter 2, Dr. Lucian Leape gives the reader a basis for understanding the role of systems failures in health care and how they can be addressed.

Within the health care community, ISMP has promoted the use of an error prevention technique called *failure mode and effects analysis* (FMEA). FMEA has been used for many years in the space, airline, and automobile industries. Using FMEA, we can look at medication therapy as a process and can pinpoint the areas in which people and systems are most likely to fail. By using this approach, the possible effects of failures can be predicted before the errors even occur. Effective preventive safeguards can then be developed and put in place. FMEA has been so effective that the FDA is considering making it a requirement in the pharmaceutical industry's review process for all naming, packaging, and labeling decisions. In Chapter 3, Drs. John Senders and Stefan Senders explain systems theory in general. In Chapter 4, I provide an example of one institution's application of this principle.

To reduce the number of medication errors, it is helpful to know which drug products, medication categories, and work circumstances have most often been associated with errors. It is especially important to be aware of which precautions should be taken with those "high-alert" drugs that seem to be associated with errors most often. ISMP and others have developed a good base of research in these areas. In Chapter 5, Dr. Charles Kilo of IHI and I provide recommendations for preventing errors with high-alert medications.

In Chapter 6, Drs. Elizabeth Flynn and Kenneth Barker bring the reader up to date on the substantive studies conducted in the field of medication error research. The authors tell us how often medication errors occur and what changes in the medication distribution system can decrease errors and can provide new information about medication errors with automated dispensing equipment.

Dr. Zane Wolf, noted researcher in the field of medication errors and an expert on the effects of medication errors on the practitioners who make them, discusses this often overlooked aspect. The impact of the "blame game," punitive reporting systems, and perceptions by colleagues are just some of the areas that Dr. Wolf and I cover in Chapter 7, in the hope that health system managers will have a much clearer understanding of the absolute need for creating an environment that fosters open and honest discussion about errors. People who make errors that adversely affect patients are often devastated and frequently need psychological support.

As already stated, medication errors usually happen because of breakdowns in the systems that have been developed for handling and processing drugs, from prescribing and ordering to distribution and administration. These systems don't exist as neat little packages in just one professional area, like the pharmacy. The systems associated with drug therapy cross every discipline and spread beyond arbitrary boundaries of responsibility. That's where teamwork comes in. In Chapters 8, 9, and 11, on drug prescribing, dispensing, and administration, respectively, I discuss errors and prevention methods that require interdisciplinary cooperation. These chapters are illustrated with examples of actual errors that have come to ISMP's attention over the years. It is imperative that pharmacists cooperate with nurses, physicians, risk managers, hospital executives, and patients. Teamwork is fundamental to effective medication error prevention systems.

Related to the dispensing aspect is the growing use of automation in drug distribution systems. We foresee a day when computerization and automation of the drug distribution process will save us from even the slightest possibility of an unintended adverse drug event. However, automation can be a double-edged sword when human factors aren't taken into account, and poorly designed or improperly used systems are the result. No one has more experience and knowledge in this particular area than Mark Neuenschwander. His Chapter 10, on effective use of dispensing automation, should be required reading for all, especially the engineers who are developing this equipment.

The need for teamwork also extends to the pharmaceutical industry and regulatory agencies. The chapters on drug product characteristics call attention to product-related factors such as labeling, packaging, nomenclature, marketing, and advertising that can contribute to, or help prevent, errors. In Chapter 12, trademark experts Dr. Dan Boring of FDA and George Di Domizio of ISMP join me in presenting information about the complicated process of developing trademarks and official names for pharmaceuticals. In Chapter 13, I discuss the role of drug labeling and packaging in medication errors.

The patient also has a role in medication safety. In Chapter 14, Dr. Stacy Wiegman, an ISMP staff member, and I describe the role that communicating with and educating patients can play in preventing errors.

Some areas of drug therapy are especially fraught with risk when dosing is inaccurate. Among them are cancer chemotherapy (Chapter 15) and pediatric drug therapy (Chapter 16). An entire chapter is devoted to each of these areas. Also included is a chapter on errors with immunologic products (Chapter 17). A somewhat confusing array of vaccine products is now available for prophylaxis against a wide variety of diseases. It is helpful to consider this group of drugs separately because certain types of errors with these products may affect thousands of people.

When we began our error prevention efforts in 1975, our purpose was to establish a system whereby health care practitioners and others could learn from the experiences of others. This requires the willingness to share our mistakes. Based on the response of practitioners who are given the opportunity of reporting medication errors to a national program, it is obvious that health professionals are willing to do so. Diane Cousins and Rita Calnan discuss these issues in Chapter 18, focusing on USP MERP and the FDA's MedWatch Program.

Error prevention must be based on two foundations: sound, interdisciplinary processes and full information. Therefore, we must spearhead the development and implementation of formal review processes that have the broadest possible interdisciplinary participation. This can be done most effectively by developing programs that not only explore all internal medication error incidents but also keep abreast of errors reported outside our own facility. A discussion of risk management is presented in Chapter 19 by risk managers Judy Smetzer and Charles Milazzo.

Although a variety of error prevention strategies are being used across the nation, every successful prevention program I have ever studied or helped develop is distinguished by excellent systems in key areas. Among the most important of these areas are communication of drug orders; patient education; information about the drug; drug naming, packaging, and labeling; drug preparation; and quality assurance. Using the case study format, Judy Smetzer and I review these and additional systems in Chapter 20, showing how risk managers can apply them to an analysis of the root causes of medication errors.

I hope that this book will help each of us redouble our efforts to prevent medication errors. We must work together, harder and longer than ever before, and apply all our knowledge and all our skill to ensure that medications are used safely. We have the expertise; we have only to exercise the leadership. Our professional future, and the safety of every patient, depend on it.

Michael R. Cohen
June 1999

•••• References

1. Bates DW, Cullen DJ, Laird N, et al. Incidence of adverse drug events and potential adverse drug events. Implications for prevention. *JAMA.* 1995; 274: 29–34.

2. Classen DC, Pestotnik SL, Evans S, et al. Adverse drug events in hospitalized patients. *JAMA.* 1997; 277: 301–06.

3. Bates DW, Spell N, Cullen DJ, et al. The costs of adverse drug events in hospitalized patients. *JAMA.* 1997; 277: 307–11.

Institute for Safe Medication Practices

The Institute for Safe Medication Practices (ISMP) was established in January 1994 as a nonprofit organization that works closely with practitioners, regulatory agencies, health care institutions, professional organizations, and the pharmaceutical industry to provide education about adverse drug events. ISMP is governed by a board of trustees representing a cross-section of the health care community, including medicine, community pharmacy, health system pharmacy, consultant pharmacy, academia, nursing, the pharmaceutical industry, professional health care organizations, managed care, health care consumers, and health care administration and medical communication. Under an agreement with the U.S. Pharmacopeia (USP) in Rockville, Md., the multidisciplinary ISMP provides independent review of all reports submitted to the USP Medication Errors Reporting Program. Reports are also reviewed that are retrieved from the Food and Drug Administration (FDA) under the Freedom of Information Act.

Information about medication errors and other adverse drug events, along with prevention recommendations, is shared with the medical community through its publication *ISMP Medication Safety Alert!* and through publications and communications with regulatory authorities and pharmaceutical manufacturers. The following journals and newsletters regularly publish ISMP error advisories and safety alerts:

- *ASHP Newsletter* (American Society of Health-System Pharmacists)
- *ASHP Homecare Newsletter* (American Society of Health-System Pharmacists)
- *Hospital Pharmacy* (Lippincott)
- *ISMP Medication Safety Alert!* (ISMP)
- *International Pharmaceutical Federation Journal* (FIP)
- *Family Practice News* (International Medical News Group)
- *INS Newsline* (Intravenous Nurse Society)
- *Internal Medicine News* (International Medical News Group)
- *Nursing 2000* (Springhouse)
- *Nurse Practitioner Journal* (Springhouse)
- *Oncology Times* (Lippincott)
- *Pharmacy Today* (American Pharmaceutical Association)
- *Physician Assistant* (Springhouse)
- *US Pharmacist* (Jobson Healthcare Group)
- *WHO Pharmaceuticals Newsletter* (World Health Organization)

ISMP is an FDA MedWatch partner.

Institute for Safe Medication Practices
1800 Byberry Road
Huntingdon Valley, PA 19006

Phone: 215-947-7797   E-mail: ismpinfo@ismp.org   Web site: www.ismp.org

Acknowledgments

Since the publication of my first column in *Hospital Pharmacy* in March 1975, I have devoted my professional life as a pharmacist to the prevention of medication errors. I have never pretended to do this alone. My work at the Institute for Safe Medication Practices (ISMP), and any success derived from it, are shared with many.

First, it is shared with my wife, Hedy, a registered nurse and, as a full-time staffer at ISMP, an active participant in our work. Hedy's selfless attitude and caring about patient safety has been an inspiration to all of us. The other members of my family, each in their own way, have also been unfailingly helpful and supportive. Thanks to Mom, Rachel, Jennifer, Neil, Mitch, Brett, Rosanne, Paul, Lauren, and Chad for the sacrifices you have had to endure.

I would like to thank ISMP's board of trustees, especially George Di Domizio, who has been responsible for much of the progress we have made. I would also like to acknowledge other ISMP staff members—Susan Proulx, PharmD; Stacy Wiegman, PharmD, MS; Judy Smetzer, RN; Rebecca Wilfinger; Larry Dwork, RPh, MS; and Mimi Spiegel. Each of these individuals has proven many times a willingness to make personal sacrifices to advance our cause.

Thanks also to Linda Harteker for editorial assistance in writing and organizing this book, to Vicki Meade for production assistance, and to Julian Graubart at the American Pharmaceutical Association (APhA) for helping me realize that it could be accomplished even while working full time at ISMP. I am also very grateful to Sam Kalman, Bill Ellis, and the board of the APhA Foundation for supporting the effort.

My mentor, Neil Davis, PharmD, has been instrumental in the patient safety movement. His vision of a national medication error prevention effort led to an ongoing feature article that I contribute to *Hospital Pharmacy*, and more recently to the establishment of a program that became the U.S. Pharmacopeia Medication Error Reporting Program. The world owes Neil a debt of gratitude for his work in this area.

I would also like to mention my colleague Leonard Macalush of Hospital Central Services Corporation (HCSC) in Allentown, Pa. Leonard and his colleague Jim Burns of HCSC gave us the support we needed to establish the ISMP in 1994. Their commitment to patient safety is extraordinary.

I must also thank all the concerned professionals and organizations who work now with the ISMP. There are far too many to mention here by name.

Finally, I would like to thank all the pharmacists, nurses, and doctors who are making a real difference in the all-too-human world of medicine. These are the people who take time out from their schedules to report medication errors to the U.S. Pharmacopeia Medication Errors Reporting Program and adverse drug reactions to the Food and Drug Administration's MedWatch Program, so that others can learn from their experiences. They work every day to ensure that the medications our patients trust us to provide do what they are supposed to do—without errors and without harm.

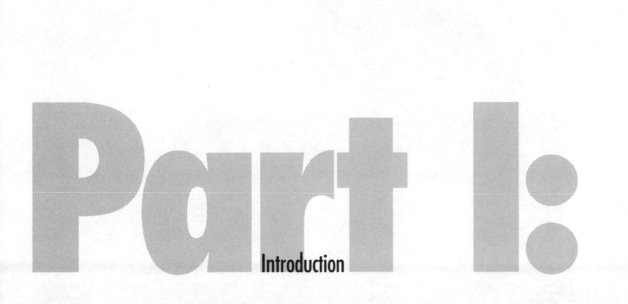

Part I:

Introduction

Causes of Medication Errors

Michael R. Cohen, MS, FASHP

Institute for Safe Medication Practices
Huntingdon Valley, Pa.

To ensure safe medication use, health professionals must be aware of the "five rights" of drug administration: "right patient, right drug, right dose, right route, and right time." Risk managers often turn these "rights" into medication error categories. For example, hospital reporting forms and tracking systems may categorize incidents as "wrong patient" errors, "wrong drug" errors, "wrong dose" errors, and so forth.

Although such categories may be useful for purposes of data collection and management, they do nothing to reveal the true sources of medication errors. Furthermore, they focus on the person who was most directly associated with the error while overlooking other system components, as well as the contributions of prescribers, dispensers, patients, the pharmaceutical industry, regulatory agencies, and health systems managers and administrators.

Where medication errors are concerned, the question of who was involved is of less importance than what went wrong, how, and why. This philosophy is the basis for the approach to education about preventing medication errors that is promoted by the Institute for Safe Medication Practices (ISMP). As part of its involvement with the U.S. Pharmacopeia Medication Errors Reporting Program (USP MERP), and the Food and Drug Administration's (FDA) MedWatch Program, ISMP has reviewed thousands of reports of medication errors and visited hundreds of sites after accidents occurred. In all cases, the causes are multifactorial, cutting across many lines of responsibility. At the same time, they involve similar circumstances.

In their landmark article on systems analysis of adverse drug events, Leape et al.[1] define broad categories, or domains, where the underlying problems that result in medication errors may be found. They then identify the following "proximal causes" of medication errors:

- Lack of knowledge of the drug,
- Lack of information about the patient,
- Violations of rules,
- Slips and memory lapses,
- Transcription errors,
- Faulty identity checking,
- Faulty interaction with other services,
- Faulty dose checking,
- Infusion pump and parenteral delivery problems,
- Inadequate monitoring,
- Drug stocking and delivery problems,
- Preparation errors,
- Lack of standardization.

Other authors have suggested different categorization systems. In many cases, the key differences reside primarily in the nomenclature. This chapter provides an overview of the causes of medication errors on the basis of six categories commonly seen by the ISMP (Table 1–1). More in-depth coverage of these and other issues is provided in other chapters throughout the book.

Failed Communication

Handwriting

Poor handwriting can blur the distinction between two medications that have similar names. Moreover, many drug names sound similar, especially when spoken over the telephone, enunciated poorly, or mispronounced. Problems are compounded when the drugs in question are administered by the same route and are exacerbated when they have similar dosages.

Drugs with Similar Names

Name mix-ups account for more than one-third of the medication errors reported to the USP MERP.[2] Davis and colleagues[3] published the names of more than 1000 products that have been confused with one another. For example, when the gastrointestinal drug Losec® (omeprazole) was first

---

Table 1-1

Some Common Causes of Medication Errors

1. Failed communication
2. Poor drug distribution practices
3. Dose miscalculations
4. Drug- and drug device-related problems
5. Incorrect drug administration
6. Lack of patient education

marketed in the United States, handwritten prescriptions were frequently misread as Lasix® (furosemide). The manufacturer and FDA received so many error reports that FDA eventually mandated a name change.

Examples of "sound-alike" drug names that have caused medication errors include the anticoagulant Coumadin® and Kemadrin®, an anti-Parkinson drug. Taxol® (paclitaxel), an anticancer agent, sounds like Paxil® (paroxetine), an antidepressant. Zebeta®, a beta-blocker antihypertensive, sounds like Diabeta®, a sulfonamide antidiabetic; and Seldane® (terfenadine), a nonsedating antihistamine, withdrawn from the market in 1998, was often confused with Feldene®, a nonsteroidal anti-inflammatory agent.

Generic names can also cause confusion. For example, amrinone (Inocor®), an inotrope used in patients with cardiomyopathy, looks and sounds like amiodarone (Cordarone®), an antiarrhythmic. Finally, problems arise when generic names look or sound like brand names. Ritonavir (Norvir®), a protease inhibitor used in patients with human immunodeficiency virus (HIV) infection, looks similar to Retrovir®, a brand of zidovudine, also for patients with HIV. Errors such as these are predictable. Given the large number of medications available, no practitioner can be expected to keep abreast of them all. Thus, when faced with a new name (e.g., Losec®), the reader may automatically read it as Lasix®, a product with which he or she is already familiar. This natural tendency is called "confirmation bias."

Zeroes and Decimal Points

Hastily written orders can cause problems, even when the name of the medication is clear. An order for "vincristine 2.0 mg" was misread by clinical personnel as "20 mg" because the decimal point fell on a line on the order form. The patient died after receiving a massive overdose. In another case, an infant received 0.17 mg of digoxin instead of 0.017 mg because a decimal point was misplaced during dose calculation.

Trailing zeroes are a frequent cause of 10-fold overdoses. Lack of a zero before a decimal point also leads to substantial dosage errors. For example, an order for "Synthroid® .1 mg" has been misread as "1 mg."

Metric and Apothecary Systems

When the metric system is not enforced as a standard method for expressing doses, substitution of the apothecary system may contribute to an error. For example, a nurse needing 1/200 grain (0.3 mg) nitroglycerin tablets used 2 x 1/100 grain (0.6 mg each, or 1.2 mg total dose) instead.

Abbreviations

Medication errors often occur because of a failure to standardize abbreviations. If an abbreviation is idiosyncratic, it would not be found even if the reader consulted a medical dictionary. Problems also exist with the use of computer mnemonics and acronyms used to designate cancer chemotherapy regimens.

The abbreviation with the greatest potential to cause harm may be the use of "U" for the word "units." Patients have suffered permanent central nervous system impairment and death because of insulin overdoses caused by misreading the "U" as a zero or the number 4 or 6.

Many abbreviations have multiple meanings or are easily misread. "D/C" is commonly used to indicate both "discharge" and "discontinue." It is not always possible to ascertain the intended meaning from the context. For example, a physician wrote the following order: "D/C meds: digoxin, propranolol, regular insulin." His intent was that the three drugs be continued after the patient's discharge from the hospital. The clinical personnel assumed that the physician's intent was that the orders for the three drugs be discontinued. The patient went without these medications for 3 days. The error was discovered when a nurse noticed the discharge prescriptions clipped to the patient's chart.

Pharmaceutical companies inadvertently contribute to problems stemming from confusing abbreviations. One company used "HS" as part of the name for an estrogen product to designate that it was half the strength of the manufacturer's full-strength product. When some nurses and pharmacists saw prescriptions, they thought that "HS" meant *hora somni* (at bedtime). Patients erroneously received the full-strength product at bedtime. Table 5–3 in Chapter 5 lists some commonly used and frequently misunderstood abbreviations.

Ambiguous or Incomplete Orders

In 1995, the public was shocked to learn about a fatal medication error at the Dana Farber Cancer Institute in Boston, Mass. A 39-year-old woman being treated for metastatic breast cancer died of cardiotoxicity after a drug overdose. The medication in question, cyclophosphamide, was ordered in a dose of "4 g/m^2 days 1–4." The physician intended that a total of 4 g/m^2 be given over a 4-day period (1 g/m^2 daily for 4 days). A number of health professionals interpreted the order to mean that 4 g/m^2 be given each day for 4 days. Over the 4-day period, the woman received a total of 26.08 g of cyclophosphamide instead of 6.52 g—a massive overdose.

Incomplete orders may cause ambiguity. Examples include situations in which the route of administration, dose, or dosage form is not specified. For example, a prescriber wrote an order for a neonate for "digoxin 1.5 cc." She did not specify the concentration, even though two concentrations are available in the United States (0.5-mg/mL in 2-mL ampuls; and 0.1mg/mL in 1-mL ampul, which is designated for pediatric patients). A nurse administered the incorrect strength. Had either the concentration or the exact dose by metric weight been specified on the order, an overdose may have been averted.

Poor Drug Distribution Practices

A unit-dose drug distribution system has repeatedly been shown to reduce the incidence of medication errors. Such a system provides redundancies and fail-safes intended to identify errors or to increase the likelihood that they will be recognized. With the unit-dose system, medication orders are screened and transcribed by both nursing and pharmacy personnel. Doses are prepared, packaged, labeled, and checked by pharmacy personnel and dispensed to nurses, who perform additional checks for accuracy.

Many health systems implemented unit-dose programs during the 1970s and 1980s. More recently, many long-term care facilities and hospitals have eliminated certain aspects of the system as part of cost-containment efforts. In such institutions, for example, the pharmacy formerly provided unit-dose syringes for nurses to use to flush intravenous lines with sodium chloride or heparin. Today, multiple-dose vials kept as floor stock have replaced pharmacy-provided unit-dose syringes. If the wrong vial is about to be used or a syringe is unlabeled, there is no longer a system of redundant checks to detect these problems. The likelihood of an error is thus increased. The issue is not that one department is more accurate than another, but that fewer checks are being made throughout the system.

Computer-generated labels can also be a source of errors. If a pharmacist dispenses a medication on the basis of a computer-generated label instead of an original prescription, and the information entered into the computer was wrong, an error is inevitable. Automated dispensing equipment, used in the absence of proper checks and balances, has caused serious errors.

Even the way in which medications are stored can affect dispensing accuracy. For example, keeping a dangerous product next to another container that looks just like it has led to lethal drug mix-ups.

Granting access to medications by untrained, unsupervised personnel often presents serious problems. In some hospitals that do not have pharmacist services available around the clock, nurses have access to pharmacy after regular hours. In some instances, incorrect drugs are removed or drugs are used improperly, resulting in patient injury.

Dose Miscalculations

Dose miscalculations are particularly common with medications used for pediatric patients and with products administered intravenously. Several studies have shown that errors in dose calculations in pediatrics are not only common but also potentially grave: mistakes of 10-fold or more occur up to 15% of the time.[4]

Problems Related to Drugs and Drug Devices

Health professionals are taught to read labels three times: when obtaining an item, when using it, and when returning it to stock or discarding it. Poor packaging can hamper the health professional's best attempts to follow this advice.

Labeling and packaging problems are the second most frequent category of medication errors reported to the USP MERP. They account for over 20% of all reports.[2] Although extemporaneously prepared labeling and packaging are sometimes at fault, most reports find that commercial labeling and packaging were the cause. The problem often stems from the use of nearly identical packaging for two separate items. At the Veterans Administration Hospital in Omaha, Neb., three patients went into cardiorespiratory arrest after they received the neuromuscular blocking agent mivacurium instead of the antibiotic metronidazole. The manufacturer packaged each of the items in a foil moisture-protecting overwrap. The drug names were not apparent on the foil. They could be seen on the plastic intravenous bag through a window in the foil, but the bags had to be held in a certain way to make the label visible. Several pharmacists, technicians, and nurses mixed up the two drugs. After a detailed investigation, it was determined that the basic problem was the packaging. The packaging for these drugs has now been revised. The drug names are clearly visible on the outer foil wrap on both the front and back panels, as well as through the plastic window.

The design of certain drug devices facilitates, rather than precludes, medication errors. Automated intravenous compounders are a good example.

Several deaths have occurred because the wrong concentration of dextrose was placed into the compounder and adequate quality assurance checks were not made.

Infusion pumps, including those used for patient-controlled analgesia, also present safety challenges. Rates and drug concentrations have been misprogrammed. Intravenous lines have become crossed between two pumps or pump channels on dual-channel pumps, resulting in infusion of the wrong medication. The uncontrolled free flow of drug solutions, which happens when the gravity flow control clamp is not closed after the intravenous set is removed from the pump, has been a cause of death and injury. Although most pumps have a fail-safe clamp, others lack this feature.

Incorrect Drug Administration

Even when all previous steps of the medication ordering and dispensing process have been flawless, the possibility of failure related to drug administration remains. Getting the medication to the right patient by the right route and at the right time is essential. Patients are sometimes misidentified despite procedures for proper identification. Drugs may be given by the wrong route. For example, oral liquid medications such as Kaopectate® or an enteral feeding supplement meant for administration via a gastric tube have been given intravenously. Irrigations meant for the bladder have been injected intravenously. Ear drops have been instilled in the eye, and eye drops in the ear. Topical medications have been swallowed.

Lack of Patient Education

Health professionals who educate their patients take an important role in ensuring safe medication use. Patients who know what each of their medications is for, how it should be taken, what it looks like, and how it works are in an excellent position to help minimize the possibility of medication errors. It is essential for patients to be counseled and educated about their medications at all points of their care. Patients should be encouraged to ask questions, and they should expect to receive satisfactory answers.

••••
References

1. Leape LL, Bates DW, Cullen DJ, et al. Systems analysis of adverse drug events. *JAMA*. 1995; 274: 35–43.

2. Cousins DD. Preventing medication errors. *US Pharmacist*. August 1995: 70–75.

3. Davis NM, Cohen MR, Teplitsky B. Look-alike and sound-alike drug names: the problem and the solution. *Hosp Pharm*. 1992; 27:95–110.

4. Perlstein PH, White CC, Barnes B, et al. Errors in drug computations during newborn intensive care. *Am J Dis Child*. 1979; 133: 376–9.

Part II:

Medication Errors and Human Perspectives

A Systems Analysis Approach to Medical Error

Lucian L. Leape, MD

Adjunct Professor of Health Policy
Harvard School of Public Health
Boston, Mass.

An error may be defined as an unintended act (either of omission or commission) or as an act that does not achieve its intended outcome. Until recently, medical errors were seldom discussed. The reasons were not obscure. The public preferred to believe that errors in medical practice were rare. Health professionals, for a variety of reasons, sought to perpetuate that misconception. The adversarial climate produced by the threat of malpractice litigation exacerbated this "see nothing, do nothing" approach.

Wide publicity has been given to a series of apparently egregious errors that resulted in death or inappropriate surgery. This, combined with the recognition that more could be done in hospitals to prevent patient injuries resulting from errors, has led to a substantial increase both in investigations into the causes of medical errors and in the search for effective preventive mechanisms.

The toll of medical error is substantial. A significant number of patients suffer treatment-caused injuries while in the hospital.[1-5] The most comprehensive examination to date is the Harvard Medical Practice Study,[1,2] which reported the results of a population-based study of iatrogenic injuries in patients hospitalized in New York State in 1984. Nearly 4% of patients suffered an injury that prolonged their hospital stay or resulted in measurable disability. Approximately 14% of these injuries were fatal. If these rates are typical of the United States as a whole, one may estimate that 180,000 people die each year at least in part as a result of iatrogenic injury. An investigation of the causes of these injuries revealed that 69% were the result of recognizable errors and were therefore preventable.[6]

In 1991, Bedell et al.[5] reported the results of an analysis of cardiac arrests at a teaching hospital. They found that 64% of these events were caused by errors. Misuse of medications was the leading cause. Other studies[7-11] have shown that medication errors are common, accounting for 10% to 25% of errors. Most do not result in serious injury.[12]

Given the complex nature of medical practice and the multitude of interventions that each patient receives, a high error rate is perhaps not surprising. Delivery of a single dose of a medication is the end result of a complicated process involving 10 to 15 steps, each of which offers an opportunity for error. Using process steps instead of patient admissions as a denominator suggests that the medication error "rate" in hospitals may be as low as 1 in 1000 to 10,000.[13] Even a failure rate of 0.01%, however, is substantially higher than that tolerated in other industries, particularly hazardous fields such as aviation and nuclear power. Health care can, and must, do better.

Why do health professionals—doctors, nurses, and pharmacists in particular—have difficulty dealing with human error? One of the reasons, paradoxically, is the emphasis during training on error-free practice.[14] In everyday practice, the message is equally clear: Mistakes are unacceptable. Doctors, nurses, and pharmacists are expected to function without errors, which means that they feel ashamed and inadequate when errors inevitably do occur. This striving for perfection is laudable, of course, and is an important aspect of another goal of professional training: developing a sense of responsibility for the patient. If one is responsible for the patient, one also feels personally responsible for any errors that occur.

The high standards of practice that are taught to nurses, pharmacists, and doctors are often reinforced in hospital practice by an unforgiving system of censure and discipline. Attempts are made to eliminate errors by requiring perfection and responding to failure (error) by blaming individuals. Errors are usually someone else's fault, caused by a lack of sufficient attention or, worse, lack of caring. In severe cases, the person at fault may be fired or subjected to retraining.

Not surprisingly, this "blame and train" approach to medical error creates strong pressure on individuals to cover up mistakes rather than admit them.[15] Even if punishment is not overt, the realization that their colleagues will regard them as incompetent or careless makes many health professionals reluctant to admit or discuss their errors. The threat of malpractice litigation provides an additional incentive to keep silent.

Students of error and human performance reject the "blame and train" approach to error prevention. Although the nearest error leading to an accident is usually a human one, the causes of that error are often well beyond the individual's control. Systems that rely on perfect performance by individuals to prevent errors are doomed to fail, for the simple reason that all humans err, and frequently. If doctors, nurses, pharmacists, and administrators are to succeed in reducing errors in health care, they must change the way they think about errors and why they occur. Fortunately, a great deal has been learned about error prevention in other disciplines, yielding information that is relevant to the hospital practice of medicine.

Psychological and Human-Factors Research and Error Analysis

Cognitive psychologists and human-factors specialists have been concerned with the biology, psychology, and sociology of errors for several decades. By developing models of human cognition and studying complex environments such as airplane cockpits and nuclear power plant control rooms, they have learned a great deal about why people make errors and how to prevent them. The principles developed by experts in these fields are pertinent to an understanding of how to redesign health care systems to reduce errors. In simple terms, there are two modes of mental functioning: automatic and problem solving.

Most mental functioning is automatic—effortless and rapid. We don't have to "think" to eat or to drive a car to work, for example. This automatic mode is unconscious, rapid, and effortless; like the new microprocessors, it occurs in a parallel processing mode. While our minds are under "attentional control," we have to pay attention only when there is a change.

At other times, intense mental activity is required for problem solving, which can entail the application of a rule or the use of stored knowledge. In contrast to the automatic mode, problem-solving thought processes are conscious, slow, and sequential, and therefore difficult.

Errors That Occur in the Automatic Mode

Errors that occur when an individual is functioning in the automatic mode are called "slips." They usually result from distractions or failure to pay attention at critical moments. A familiar example is setting out in an automobile to go somewhere and finding that one has driven to work instead. Psychologists' term for this phenomenon is "capture." Another common error mechanism is loss of activation, in which attention is distracted and a thought process is lost. An example of loss of activation is entering a room and failing to remember what one came in for.

Both physiologic and psychological factors can divert attentional control and make slips more likely. Physiological factors include fatigue, sleep loss, alcohol, drugs, and illness. Psychological factors include other activity ("busyness") as well as emotional states, such as boredom, frustration, fear, anxiety, and anger. All lead to preoccupations that divert attention. Psychological factors, though considered internal or endogenous, may be triggered by external factors such as overwork, interpersonal relations, and other forms of stress. Environmental factors such as noise, heat, visual stimuli, and motion can also divert attention and lead to slips.

Errors That Occur in the Problem-Solving Mode

Errors of problem-solving thought ("mistakes" in human-factors jargon) are more complex. They include rule-based mistakes, which occur when a wrong rule is chosen—either because one misperceives the situation and applies the wrong rule or because one simply misapplies a rule. Knowledge-based mistakes occur when the problem solver confronts a situation for which he or she possesses no programmed solutions. Errors arise because of lack of knowledge or because of misinterpretation of the problem.

Familiar patterns are assumed to have universal applicability because they usually work. We see what we know. It is simpler to apply a pattern than to rethink each situation. Errors can arise from discrepancies in pattern matching; sometimes we unconsciously match the wrong patterns. One form of pattern mismatching is caused by biased memory. Decisions are based on what is in our memory, but memory is biased toward overgeneralization and overregularization of the commonplace.[16]

Another aberration of thought that leads to error is the availability heuristic. This is the human tendency to grab the first answer that comes to mind and to stick with it despite evidence to the contrary. This tendency may be compounded by another mechanism, confirmation bias, which is the natural inclination to accept evidence that confirms one's hypothesis and to reject evidence that negates it. Many other mechanisms have been described. The important point is that these things happen every day to all of us.

Rule- and knowledge-based functioning are affected by the same physiological, psychological, and environmental influences that produce slips. Stress is often cited as a cause of errors. Although it is often difficult to establish a causal link between stress and specific accidents, there is little question that both slips and mistakes are increased under stress.

Three clear lessons emerge from this research. First, errors are normal. Everyone errs every day. To err is indeed to be human. Second, errors result from well-known cognitive mechanisms—mechanisms that are complex, but understandable. Third, distractions are a common cause of errors. Errors truly result from a "normal" pathology.

Systems Causes of Errors

Although insights from cognitive psychology and human-factor research help us understand how and why people make mistakes, they offer limited help in devising methods to prevent errors. It may be possible to avoid distractions, for example, or at least to recognize when one is at risk of being distracted, but any individual is severely limited in his or her ability to "think straight" all the time. Successful methods of preventing errors require additional insight and understanding.

The major breakthrough in thinking about errors was the recognition that systems factors play a major role in increasing the likelihood that an individual will make an error. A watershed event in this understanding was the nuclear power plant accident at Three-Mile Island in 1979. Although initial investigations revealed the expected operator errors (i.e., "human error"), it became clear that preventing many of these errors was beyond the capabilities of the specific individuals operating the system at the moment the accident occurred. Many of the errors were caused by faulty interface design or breakdowns that were not discernible by the operators or their instruments. The errors were the result of major failures of design and organization that occurred long before the accident.

Investigations following the accident at Three-Mile Island revealed that faulty design provided gauges that gave a low pressure reading both when pressure was low and when the gauge was not working. Therefore, the operator thought the pressure was low—when actually the gauge was broken. Also, the system had a control panel on which 100 lights started flashing simultaneously: faulty maintenance had disabled a safety back-up system. Operators had been trained how to respond to each light individually, but not how to prioritize them should multiple lights go on at once. Thus, although an operator error may have been the proximal cause of the accident, the root causes had been present in the system for a long time.

Faulty systems design has two effects: it causes operator errors, and it makes them impossible to detect in time to prevent an accident. The operator at Three-Mile Island was "set up" to fail by poor design, faulty maintenance, inadequate training, and poor management decisions. Together, these factors created a situation in which a minor operator error could result in a serious injury.

Reason[17] terms errors resulting from these situations *latent errors*—errors whose effects are delayed. Latent errors may be described as accidents waiting to happen. The effects of active errors, by contrast, are felt immediately (see Chapter 20).

Psychological precursors, one type of latent error, are working conditions that predispose to errors.[17] Inappropriate work schedules, for example, can result in high workloads and undue time pressures, two conditions that induce errors. Poor training can lead to inadequate recognition of hazards or inappropriate procedures that may lead to accidents. A precursor can be the product of more than one management or training failure. For example, excessive time pressure can result from poor scheduling, but it can also result from inadequate training or faulty division of responsibilities. Because they can affect all cognitive processes, precursors can cause an immense variety of errors that result in unsafe acts.

The primary objective of systems design for safety is to make it difficult for individuals to err. Even with the best system, however, errors will inevitably occur. A mechanism is needed for recognizing and correcting errors before they cause accidents. Ideally, systems should be designed to automatically correct errors when they occur. If this is impossible, mechanisms should be in place to detect errors as soon as possible so that corrective action can be taken. Therefore, in addition to designing the work environment to minimize psychological precursors, designers should provide feedback mechanisms in the form of monitoring instruments. They must also build in buffers and make provisions for redundancy. Buffers are design features that automatically correct for human or mechanical error. Redundancy is duplication (or triplication or quadruplication) of critical mechanisms and instruments. If a system is redundant, a single failure does not result in loss of the function.

Accident prevention efforts must focus on root causes—errors in design and implementation of systems, not the errors themselves. Most errors result from the failure to use basic human-factors principles in the design of tasks and systems. Excessive reliance on memory, lack of standardization, inadequate availability of information, and poor work schedules all create situations in which individuals are more likely to make mistakes.

Industrial Models

Aviation, nuclear power generation, and space travel employ technology that is at least as complicated and risky as that used in health care.

Nonetheless, these industries have developed highly reliable systems for minimizing human error. For example, airline travel in the United States is indeed safe: more than 10 million departures and landings take place each year with an average of fewer than four crashes.

The difference between the approach used in the aviation industry and that used in medicine is that the aviation industry designs its systems for safety. Preventing accidents is a principal objective of aircraft design and flight procedures. First, aircraft designers assume that errors and failures are inevitable. They therefore design systems to absorb them by building in multiple buffers, automation, and redundancy. Second, procedures are standardized to the maximum extent possible. Specific protocols must be followed for trip planning, operations, and maintenance. Pilots go through a checklist before each takeoff. Third, the training, examination, and certification process is highly developed and strictly enforced. Airline pilots take proficiency examinations every 6 months. Much of the content of these examinations is directly concerned with safety procedures.

Finally, safety in aviation has been institutionalized. The Federal Aviation Administration regulates all aspects of flying and prescribes safety procedures, and the National Transportation Safety Board investigates every accident. The adherence of airlines and pilots to safety standards is closely monitored. A unique feature of the aviation industry is the Aviation Safety Reporting System, which provides immunity against disciplinary action for pilots, controllers, or others who report a dangerous situation, such as a near-miss midair collision. This program has been highly successful in ensuring the prompt reporting of unsafe conditions, communication problems, and traffic control inadequacies. The Aviation Safety Reporting System receives more than 5000 notifications each year.[18]

The Medical Model

By contrast, accident prevention has not been a primary focus of hospital medicine. Health care personnel typically react to a specific accident and focus on the error rather than attempt to understand the systemic cause. For example, a typical response to a dosing error is the institution of an additional checking stage. Human-factors experts recognize the futility of concentrating on solutions to the unsafe acts themselves. Other errors, unpredictable and infinitely varied, will soon occur if the underlying systems failure goes uncorrected. Correcting systems failures will not eliminate all errors, because individuals still bring various abilities and work habits to the workplace. Nonetheless, the correction of systems errors will substantially reduce the probability of error.

Most important, designers of medical systems rely largely on faultless performance by individuals to prevent errors rather than designing systems to prevent or absorb errors. They expect individuals not to make errors rather than assume that they will.

There are, of course, exceptions. For example, the advent of unit dosing, a major systems change in medication dispensing, has markedly reduced medication dosing errors. In intensive care units, monitoring is sophisticated and extensive (though perhaps not sufficiently redundant). In addition, equipment and procedures for anesthesia have been developed that make it difficult for personnel to commit errors. The success of these efforts has been dramatic. Whereas mortality from anesthesia was 1 in 10,000 to 20,000 a decade or so ago, it is now estimated at less than 1 in 200,000.[19] Anesthesiologists have led the medical profession in recognizing systems factors as causes of errors, in the design of fail-safe systems, and in training to avoid errors.[20-22]

Measuring Errors

Health care organizations that wish to reduce errors need to develop reliable methods for measuring them. Although it is systems that will ultimately need to be changed, the errors themselves provide clues as to which systems failures need to be targeted for redesign. Moreover, changes in the error rate are the measure of effectiveness of system changes. Unfortunately, accurate and reproducible measurement of errors is difficult. The purpose of measuring is to discover errors, quantify the extent and types of errors, and document trends.

Discovering Errors

Most health care organizations rely on spontaneous reporting to identify errors. This method is not only inadequate but also misleading, because the punitive nature of most hospitals' responses to error reporting effectively stifles such reporting. Typical incident reports identify only 2% to 5% of reportable adverse drug events.[23] It is unlikely that any meaningful insight into the nature or extent of errors will be obtained unless a more representative sample of errors is obtained. This will not occur unless personnel are provided with immunity from discipline and are convinced that they will not be punished. When immunity is provided, the yield is sometimes astonishing.[24]

Identification of errors, as well as investigation of all errors that cause injuries, should be a routine part of hospital practice. Only when errors are accepted as an inevitable, though manageable, part of everyday practice will it be possible for hospital personnel to shift from a punitive to a creative frame of mind that seeks out and identifies the underlying systems failures.

Quantifying Types of Errors

It is neither feasible nor necessary to measure all types of errors on a continuous basis. Periodic, focused data collection is sufficient. Once systems changes have been selected, specific indicator errors can be identified and measured intensively over a short period to determine the base error rate.

Documenting Trends

Once indicator errors have been identified and systems changes have been introduced, error rates should continue to be measured periodically to assess the effectiveness of the systems changes. It is helpful to present such data over time in the form of control charts that show the baseline rate, upper and lower control limits (usually three standard deviations), lowering of the error rate with the intervention, and maintenance of the improvement over time.

Measuring errors may be expensive, but the consequences of errors are more so. In industry, the savings from reduction of errors and accidents more than make up for the costs of data collection and investigation. In hospitals, the additional savings from reduced patient care and liability costs for hospitals and physicians are substantial. A recent study estimated the cost of each preventable adverse drug event to be $4685.[25]

A Framework for Systems Analysis

Once the extent of errors is known in a health care system (e.g., the medication system, the radiology department, or the emergency room), the next question is to determine where remedial efforts can be most profitably targeted. Systems failures can be grouped into two broad categories: design failures and organizational and environmental failures.

Design Failures

Many hospital systems were never "designed" in the true sense—they just grew. Errors occur because the processes used in these systems have not been well thought out. Basic human-factors principles have been disregarded in the design of these systems. Design failures can be classified into three categories: process design, task design, and equipment design.

Process design failures result from failure to analyze the purposes of the system and how best to achieve them. What are the objectives of the system? How can it best meet users' needs? What are its potential hazards? One must think through the system and determine the consequences of actions that can go wrong at each point.

A recent study[13] by my colleagues and me revealed that failures in just three systems accounted for more than half of the errors that either caused an adverse drug event or were "near misses" (intercepted errors). These three systems were drug knowledge dissemination, checking dose and identity of drugs, and making patient information available.

Drug knowledge dissemination is a major problem. Because of the number, variety, and complexity of drugs, it is impossible for any individual to recall all that he or she needs to know in order to use a drug appropriately and safely. Health professionals need to have drug information available at the time decisions are made and in a form they can easily use.

Methods for tracking and identifying drug, dose, and patient are often primitive when compared with those used in industry. Supermarkets keep better track of groceries than many hospitals do of medications.

Creative ways need to be developed for making patient information more readily available: displaying it where it is needed, when it is needed, and in an accessible form. Computerizing the medical record, for example, would facilitate bedside display of patient information, including tests and medications.

Task design failures result from the failure to incorporate human-factors principles into planning tasks. Norman[16] has pointed out the importance of designing tasks to minimize errors and has recommended a set of principles that have general applicability. Tasks should be *simplified* to minimize the load on the weakest aspects of cognition (i.e., short-term memory, planning, and problem solving). The power of *constraints* should be exploited. One way to do this is with *forcing functions*. These are design features that make it impossible to perform a specific erroneous act (for example, the lock that prohibits release of the parking gear of a car unless the brake pedal is depressed). *Standardization* of procedures, displays, and layouts reduces errors by reinforcing the pattern recognition that humans perform well. Finally, where possible, operations should be easily *reversible* or, when not reversible, difficult to carry out.

Checklists, protocols, and computerized decision aids could be used more widely. For example, physicians should not have to rely on their memories to retrieve a laboratory test result, nor should nurses have to remember the time a medication dose is due. Computers can do these tasks more reliably than humans.

Standardization is one of the most effective ways to prevent errors; examples in the airline industry include maintenance protocols and pilot checklists. The advantages of standardizing drug doses and times of administration, for example, are obvious. Is it acceptable to ask nurses to follow six different "K scales" (directions for how much potassium to give according to the patient's serum potassium levels) solely to satisfy idiosyncratic physician prescribing patterns? Other areas in which standardization would be beneficial include information displays, methods for common practices (such as surgical dressings), and the location of equipment and supplies in a patient care unit.

Forcing functions can be used to structure critical tasks so that errors cannot be made. For example, a computerized system for medication orders can be designed so that a physician cannot enter an order for a lethal overdose of a drug or prescribe a medication to which a patient is known to be allergic.

Equipment design failures result from the failure to apply basic human-factors principles to the design of equipment displays and controls. It is astonishing that most people using most of the equipment in hospitals do not understand how that equipment works. This is primarily a design problem; manufacturers have not seen to it that equipment offers the user information and controls that are readily understandable. In other words, the manufacturers, too, have failed to apply basic human-factors principles.

It is also remarkable that it is possible to connect an epidural catheter to a syringe with medication prepared only for intravenous use. A simple forcing function design, such as has long been used with oxygen and nitrous oxide connections in anesthesia, could prevent this error.

Organizational and Environmental Failures

Organizational and environmental failures, unlike design failures, can often be remedied by changes that can be implemented at the departmental or unit level (i.e., the pharmacy or nursing unit). Such changes do not require institution-wide changes. Three types of organizational failures may induce errors: psychological precursors, inadequate team building, and training failures.

Psychological precursors are conditions in the workplace, such as schedules, work assignments, and interpersonal relationships, that cause stress and lead to errors. These include environmental factors, such as excessive heat, inadequate light, crowded space, and high noise levels, as well as excessive workloads, long working hours, and poor managerial styles.

Although the influence of the stresses of everyday life on human behavior cannot be eliminated, stresses caused by a faulty work environment can be. Elimination of fear and the creation of a supportive working environment are powerful methods for preventing errors.

Team building requires a supportive environment and skilled leaders who can encourage individuals to work together effectively, help each other avoid mistakes, intercept errors, and reduce psychological precursors. Hospitals have historically been poor team builders because doctors and nurses have functioned semiautonomously and autocratically.

Training is essential. If personnel neither understand their responsibilities nor possess adequate skills, they will be more likely to make errors. Health professionals need more training in error prevention and identification. They need to learn to think of errors primarily as symptoms of systems failures. Many interns need more rigorous instruction and supervision than is currently provided. Young doctors need to be taught that safe practice is as important as effective practice.

Obstacles to Systems Redesign

The modern hospital presents many obstacles to those who seek to change its practices. Recognition is the first step in designing methods to overcome these obstacles. At the Institute for Healthcare Improvement Breakthrough Collaborative to Reduce Adverse Drug Events, I and my colleagues have identified five major obstacles that are found in most hospitals: (1) complexity of the system and lack of ownership, (2) lack of availability of information, (3) tolerance of stylistic practices, (4) infrequent occurrence of events, and (5) fear of punishment.

Complexity and Lack of Ownership

Hospital systems involve a wide variety of personnel and interlocking flows of materials and information. Many individuals have interests in multiple operations, and each system and subsystem have multiple stakeholders. No one has complete control of any of these systems. There are no owners. The system for ordering, dispensing, and administering medications is a good example of the challenges posed by complex systems. The medication system is characterized by multiple players (physicians, nurses, pharmacists, clerks, and technicians), multiple choices (drugs, names, routes, and doses), and multiple hand-offs that are frequent and fragile.

Unavailability of Information

Information transfer can pose a major challenge to knowledge-based problem solving. In our study[13] of systems analysis of adverse drug events, lack of knowledge about drugs and lack of information about the patient were two of the most common systems failures; they accounted for 40% of injury-producing errors. Health care providers need to have information available when it is needed, where it is needed, and in a form that they can readily use.

Tolerance of Individualistic Practices

Hospitals often cater to the idiosyncrasies and special demands of individual physicians. In drug prescribing, for example, tolerance of illegible and nonstandard orders and of differences in prescribing practices contributes to the likelihood of error. Similar tolerance is found of the authority of nursing unit managers to follow individual preferences, such as for times of administering medications, and the authority of the pharmacy to set its own schedule for delivery of drugs. Changing such long-standing practices can be a formidable challenge.

Infrequent Occurrence of Events

Despite alarming statistics, serious errors are uncommon in the experience of most hospital professionals. This low error rate leads to complacency. It also means that a change targeted at a low-frequency problem can result in a substantial increase in overall work for a low yield.

Fear of Punishment

Most hospitals impose strong overt or covert sanctions against those who make mistakes. As a result, most failures are not reported, making recognition, monitoring, and evaluation difficult.

Conclusion

Few American institutions are as ripe for systems redesign as hospitals. The current drive for efficiency will necessitate reexamination of the most serious form of inefficiency: injury-producing errors. Significant improvements will require major commitments to error reduction by each organization's leadership, as well as acceptance by all professionals and administrators that error is an inevitable aspect of the human condition. Unless errors are recognized as symptoms of systems flaws, not of character flaws, substantial progress in reducing medical errors is unlikely.

References

1. Leape LL, Brennan TA, Laird N, et al. The nature of adverse events in hospitalized patients. Results of the Harvard Medical Practice Study II. *N Engl J Med.* 1991; 324: 377–84.

2. Brennan TA, Leape LL, Laird N, et al. Incidence of adverse events and negligence in hospitalized patients. Results of the Harvard Medical Practice Study I. *N Engl J Med.* 1991; 324: 370–76.

3. Schimmel EM. The hazards of hospitalization. *Ann Intern Med.* 1964; 60: 100–10.

4. Steel K, Gertman PM, Crescenzi C, et al. Iatrogenic illness on a general medical service at a university hospital. *N Engl J Med.* 1981; 304: 638–42.

5. Bedell SE, Deitz DC, Leeman D, et al. Incidence and characteristics of preventable iatrogenic cardiac arrests. *JAMA.* 1991; 265: 2815–20.

6. Leape LL, Lawthers AG, Brennan TA, et al. Preventing medical injury. *Q Rev Biol.* 1993; 8: 144–49.

7. Barker KN, Allan EL. Research on drug-use system errors. *Am J Health Syst Pharm.* 1995; 52: 400–06.

8. Lesar TS, Briceland LL, Delcoure K, et al. Medication prescribing errors in a teaching hospital. *JAMA.* 1990; 263: 2329–34.

9. Raju TN, Thornton JP, Kecskes S, et al. Medication errors in neonatal and paediatric intensive-care units. *Lancet.* 1989; 374–79.

10. Classen DC, Pestonik SL, Evans RS, et al. Computerized surveillance of adverse drug events in hospital patients. *JAMA.* 1991; 266: 2847–51.

11. Folli HL, Poole RL, Benitz WE, et al. Medication error prevention by clinical pharmacists in two children's hospitals. *Pediatrics.* 1987; 79: 718–22.

12. Bates DW, Boyle D, Vander Vliet M, et al. Relationship between medication errors and adverse drug events. *J Gen Intern Med.* 1995; 10: 199–205.

13. Leape LL, Bates DW, Cullen DJ, et al. Systems analysis of adverse drug events. *JAMA.* 1995; 274: 35–43.

14. Hilfiker D. Facing our mistakes. *N Engl J Med.* 1984; 310: 118–22.

15. McIntyre N, Popper K. The critical attitude in medicine: Need for a new ethics. *Br Med J.* 1989; 287: 1919–23.

16. Norman DA. *To Err Is Human.* New York: Basic Books; 1984.

17. Reason J. *Human Error.* Cambridge, Mass: Cambridge University Press; 1990.

18. Perrow C. *Normal Accidents: Living with High-Risk Technologies.* New York: Basic Books; 1984.

19. Orkin FK. Patient monitoring during anesthesia as an exercise in technology assessment. In: Saidman LJ, Smith NT, eds. *Monitoring in Anesthesia.* 3rd ed. London: Butterworth; 1993.

20. Gaba DM. Human errors in anesthetic mishaps. *Int Anesthesiol Clin.* 1989; 27: 137–47.

21. Cooper JB, Newbower RS, Kitz RJ. An analysis of major errors and equipment failures in anesthesia management: Considerations for prevention and detection. *Anesthesiology.* 1984; 60: 34–42.

22. Cullen DJ, Nemeskal RA, Cooper JB, et al. Effect of pulse oximetry, age, and ASA physical status on the frequency of patients admitted unexpectedly to a postoperative intensive care unit and the severity of their anesthesia-related complications. *Anesth Analg.* 1992; 74: 181–88.

23. Cullen DJ, Bates DW, Small SD, et al. The incident reporting system does not detect adverse drug events: A problem in quality assurance. *Jt Comm J Qual Improv.* 1995; 21: 541–48.

24. Bates DW, Cullen DJ, Laird N, et al. Incidence of adverse drug events and potential adverse drug events: Implications for prevention. *JAMA.* 1995; 274: 29–34.

25. Bates DW, Spell N, Cullen DJ, et al. The cost of adverse drug events in hospitalized patients. *JAMA.* 1997; 277: 307–11.

3.

Failure Mode and Effects Analysis in Medicine

J. W. Senders, PhD

Professor Emeritus, University of Toronto
Toronto, Canada
Consulting Scientist, Institute for Safe Medication Practices
Huntingdon Valley, Pa.

S. J. Senders, PhD

Department of Anthropology—Peace Studies Fellow
Cornell University
Ithaca, N.Y.

We begin this chapter with a brief history of failure mode analysis and failure mode and effects analysis. We then discuss the inadequacy of the traditional linear-narrative approach to failure analysis. We conclude with a description of how these techniques, as well as a new concept called human error mode and effects analysis, can be applied to analyzing pharmaceutical naming, packaging, and labeling, as well as to purchasing, prescribing, dispensing, and using pharmaceuticals.

FMA Techniques

The purpose of failure mode analysis (FMA) is to discover the potential risks in a product or system. FMA involves examining a product or system to identify all the ways in which it might fail. FMA can be used to predict failures as well as to analyze why they occurred. The term *failure mode* may refer to specific types of failure (e.g., fractures, burns, or deviations from expected values) or to degrees of failure (e.g., catastrophic, partial, or minimal).

FMA was first used in engineering discourse in the early 1960s.[1] By the mid-1970s, it had become a standard term in electronics, structural and mechanical engineering, chemistry, and the aerospace industry.

Failure mode and effects analysis (FMEA), also introduced in the 1960s, is a risk assessment method based on the simultaneous analysis of failure modes, their consequences, and their associated risk factors. Like FMA, it can be used not only in the design stage (to prevent failures or mitigate their consequences) but also in post-hoc analysis. Because it is concerned with the effects of failure, FMEA has been used most extensively in areas characterized by high risk, such as nuclear power plant operations, or by high cost, such as the weapons and aerospace industries.

Both FMA and FMEA have been used to reduce the frequency and consequences of failures. The two forms of analysis, however, have different genealogies: FMA is an outgrowth of quality control concerns, whereas FMEA stems from risk assessment.

The human factor has long been recognized as an aspect of systems failures. Although no attempts to include human factors within the rubric of FMA or FMEA are known to us, work integrating the fields was done in the early 1960s[2–4] and has continued into the 1990s.[5]

Failure Analysis

Failure analysis is a central activity of human culture. The search for explanations of all events, especially of negative ones, is central to human understanding of order.

Historically, failure analyses were constructed from a linear perspective. In this approach, one needed only to retrace the chain of events until the fault was found. Such analyses were well suited to preindustrial mechanical and engineering failures. Because artisan production was sequential, most failures could be traced to particular events, techniques, or materials.

Industrial and mass production, by contrast, generally involves numerous subsystems in the production of a single product. Its development called for a new, systemic type of failure analysis. No longer could failures necessarily be traced to a single event; combined effects had to be considered. Moreover, the growing market for reliable industrial products, and the increasing complexity of the products themselves, demanded systemic analyses of both production and product failures. The rise of the military as the preeminent consumer of industrial products encouraged the rapid development of systemic analysis.

FMA and FMEA both use what could be called systemic, as opposed to linear-narrative, analysis. Systemic analysis does not demand that events take the form of a single story; instead, it requires a simultaneous imagining of all possible stories. Neither FMA nor FMEA refers to a specific methodology; instead, they define terms of inquiry. FMA asks, "What has failed, what could fail, and how?" FMEA asks, "Given the various possibilities for failure, what are the potential consequences of each?"

To apply FMA and FMEA, one must first define *failure*. In general, a failure is said to occur if a component or a collection of components of a system behaves in a way that is not included in its specified performance criteria. Fundamental to FMA and FMEA is an analysis of the system in question, including a detailed specification of all possible sites of failure—components, subsystems, processes, interactions, and functions. Each site must then be analyzed in terms of possible failure modes, and if they are available, the probabilities of those failures. Finally, for each identifiable site of failure, one must identify the consequences and calculate the associated cost.

Human Error Mode and Effects Analysis

Failures in mechanical, material, and production processes are amenable to systemic analysis. It seems clear that careful examination of a system can reveal the various kinds of failure that can occur. Further, there is general acceptance of the idea that if a failure occurs, one can calculate its consequences, provided that one is aware of the interaction between the elements involved.

Human failures, by contrast, are burdened by historical and cultural habit that equates human error with "blame," a term better suited to linear-narrative than to systemic analysis.[6] Most estimates of the fraction of accidents resulting from human error range between 70% and 90%.

It is astonishing that methods commonly applied to the nonhuman components of systems are not applied to humans, the major source of system failure. This lack stems from the view that human errors are unpredictable. Such is not the case. Human errors are not drawn from an infinite set of possibilities. Instead, they are drawn from the limited set of meaningful things that an individual can do in any defined situation. These actions may be termed the *affordances* of the work environment. Because the spectrum of errors is limited, they are theoretically capable of a priori discovery and analysis. To draw from a time-honored example, Murphy's law asserts: "If something can go wrong, it will." The task in the first instance is to discover what can be done wrong; in the second, to predict what would happen when it is done. These observations could serve, in short, as the basis of a human error mode and effects analysis (HEMEA).

Applying HEMEA to Medication Errors

The prevention of medication errors offers an excellent opportunity to explore the application of HEMEA. What would happen if we were to apply HEMEA to devices, prescriptions, packages, labels, and instructions—in short, to all aspects of medicine?

If we follow a medication or drug device from the point of its manufacture to its administration to a patient, it becomes evident that there are many opportunities to select an incorrect product and substitute it for the correct one. Each opportunity for incorrect selection is an opportunity to examine the consequences (the effects) of that selection and to estimate its associated risk. For example, the prediction of the outcome of administering an incorrect medication is a matter of pharmacology and physiology. Given the status of the patient, if the correct medication is withheld and a specified incorrect medication administered, it is possible, within limits, to predict the consequences.

Some medications are relatively benign. Their misuse does not lead to illness or death. Some patients are not in a physiological state in which the failure to use the correct medication will lead to illness or death. If both are true, the error will be of little consequence. In a recent case, for example, a patient was supposed to receive ear drops. The physician wrote "OD" (for once a day). The nurse read it as "OD" (right eye) and instilled the ear drops into the patient's right eye. It was only when the patient was about to leave the office and asked the nurse when he would receive his ear drops that the error was discovered.

In this instance, the substance given to the patient was pharmacologically benign and the delay in administering the ear drops led to no discernible effect. In another context, the same kind of error could have been lethal or permanently injurious. The error gives the HEMEA analyst a clue that either there should be a set of mandatory, standardized abbreviations or, perhaps better (though impractical), all abbreviations should be forbidden in prescription writing. The origin of the problem was in the use of a nonstandard abbreviation and in the use of abbreviations at all.

A second type of error involves packaging. For example, if a preloaded 5-mL syringe of 20% lidocaine 1000 mg is substituted for a similar syringe with a 2% concentration, the outcome may be fatal. The obvious remedy would be to design the 20% concentrate in a way that would make it impossible to inject as a bolus. This error has occurred many times, yet no effort has been made to redesign the syringe, simple as it would be to do so. Information on the high possibility of this error was not rapidly disseminated. The product was removed from the market after more than 12 years and about 100 deaths had occurred since the first reported error.

Mechanical design errors are also common. Improper assembly of infusion pumps has led to the free flow of medications into patients. This has happened so often that it should be possible to know virtually all the ways in which such devices can be misassembled. HEMEA would reveal that if the reservoir were improperly clamped, it would still appear to be properly seated and that if the pump were operated in that state, there would be free flow. The HEMEA approach would also emphasize that if one person has done something incorrectly, it is probable that another person will do the same thing. Yet manufacturers continue to resist the idea that redesign is necessary. Each reported misuse of these devices provides the evidence needed to identify a future potential error, not only in the particular medication or device reported but in all medications similarly packaged, labeled, or prescribed and in all similar devices.

Reported adverse outcomes are usually classified according to the medication or device involved rather than the underlying mechanism of error. For this reason, there is no opportunity to learn from one accident what needs to be done to prevent other accidents involving different kinds of medications or other devices in different situations.

"Read the label. Read the label. Read the label." —An Effective Error Deterrent?

Incorrect administration of medication frequently arises from a selection error. Although selection errors may occasionally be detected by rereading the label, this is not a dependable safeguard. In one case, a physician picked up a vial of concentrated saline and read the label three times. He noted that the product was "injectable" and that it was a "single-dose" vial. These phrases assured the physician that he had the correct medication in hand. The precise concentration designation (23.4%) appeared only once on the vial, and it happened to be beneath the physician's thumb at the time he read it. The first reading was inadequate, but the next two added nothing to the safety of the process.

The error occurred despite three readings because the manufacturer had made no effort to find out how people picked up vials of that sort and thus to learn that the essential information on concentration might be hidden by the user's hand. If a reasonable sample of people had been allowed to handle the vial under observation before it went to the market, the possibility that the concentration would be unreadable might have become apparent and the label could have been modified.

Medication errors continue to be made. The admonition to "read the label" has clearly been ineffective. What is needed is a carefully designed investigation of the underlying mechanisms of reading behavior and an equally careful test of alternative designs of labels and strategies of reading. Has there ever been an analysis showing a reduction in the probability of such accidents as a consequence of multiple readings? The command to read the label three times means nothing unless there is also a way of ensuring that the readings are statistically independent of one another.

All materials that come in two or more forms and that present a risk if the wrong form is used should be multiply labeled with the critical information. In that way, no matter how a container is picked up, even a casual examination would reveal the nature of the contents. In addition, all substances that present a risk of injury or death if injected should be tactually discriminable, as described on page 3.7. If the eye is not used, the hand inevitably will contact the relevant information.

Reporting Medication Errors

We have stated that the range of human error is not infinite; errors are limited to the affordances of the situation. It is difficult for even the most experienced analyst, however, to imagine everything that someone might do incorrectly. Therefore, it becomes critically important to develop a uniform and rational system of reporting errors, including those that have not resulted in patient injury. A database of error modes will assist those who have difficulty analyzing a design for the kinds of misuses that human ingenuity can devise.

A standard method for failure reduction in mechanical and electronic systems is the introduction of redundancy into critical subsystems. The same method should be applied to the reduction of human errors. Multiple sensory channels can be used for error prevention. The packaging for very dangerous products should feel different from that of other products. For example, the outside of a vial or preloaded syringe should be bumpy, rough, square, or even have a combination of these tactile characteristics. Before any such distinguishing characteristic is adopted, however, a complete statistical analysis should be performed of the accidents that the measure is designed to prevent. This will make it possible to assess the benefits and compare them with the costs.

Errors will continue to be made. Accidents, on the other hand, can largely be prevented by intelligent and imaginative use of additional cues that announce that an error has occurred and that make it possible for the error to be corrected before damage has been done. Where possible, physical design should be used to prevent error from being translated into injury.

History of Ergonomics in Design: Tactual Discriminability as a First Line of Defense

In 1857, a bill to regulate the sale of poisons was introduced into the British Parliament. One clause in the bill ordered that "all medicines containing any poison should be supplied in quadrangular blue glass bottles, labelled in conspicuous capitals, white on black ground, the word POISON being also embossed in raised letters on the four sides of the bottle."[7] The design was clearly the result of analysis and thought applied to the problem of reducing what we now call "medication errors." The proposal was well human-engineered:

- The black background of the printed word "POISON" serves by its blackness as a warning. It has been mandated in recent times in the United States that potassium chloride containers have a black cap.
- There is maximum contrast between the word POISON and the background. The modern use of various colors on labels often, on the other hand, reduces the contrast and readability of the label.
- The word "POISON" is embossed on all four sides of the bottle. This would markedly reduce the probability that the words would be overlooked because they were covered by the hand of the individual grasping the bottle. It also guards against the possibility of the loss of a printed "POISON" label.
- The bottle is rectangular in cross-section and made of blue glass. The former provides tactual, the latter visual, identifiability. This would be especially true if bottles of this shape and color were reserved for poisons.

Alas, the government fell before this bill became law. It was in the Pharmacy Act of 1868 that authority was given to the Pharmaceutical Society to make regulations (subject to the approval of the Privy Council) for the selling, keeping, and dispensing of poisons. A "bottle rendered distinguishable by touch for liniments, embrocations, and lotions, etc., containing poisons" was stipulated by the society.[1]

Stimulated by the bill and the society's specification, inventors designed and applied for patents on a host of methods aimed at ensuring that poisons were not inadvertently used. Many of their methods had quite modern flavors. Thus, we see the use of "spines" on the cap of a poison bottle in one application, and protrusions on the body of the bottle in at least two others. Such devices would provide instant tactual identification of poisons and materials that presented a hazard if injected via the wrong route.

Inventors of the 19th century, in other words, did what inventors might do today: They proposed shape, color, texture, upside-down labeling, luminous glass, sounding alarms, and puzzle locks. All they lacked was the sophistication of modern experimental design for assessment of their inventions. But then, many manufacturers do not use that tool today. Figure 3–1 shows a few of the many admirable solutions proposed more than a century ago.

The tactile feel of an object can assist in its identification by touch alone, much as color can do for sight. For unknown reasons, neither color nor feel has been used in North America, at least in recent times. The fact that 10% of men may be color-blind has been used as an argument against color-coding. The argument is specious; that the rate of adverse events might be reduced by as much as 90% through the use of color seems not to have been understood.

Another common objection has been that there are not enough identifiable shapes or colors to ensure that confusion does not occur. This is true if absolute identifiability were necessary, but it is not. If all medical personnel learned just one thing—that if something feels like a hedgehog, do not inject it—many deaths and permanent injuries could be avoided.

The moral of this tale is to be like a hedgehog and not like a fox. "The fox knows many things, but the hedgehog knows one great thing" (Archilocus, 680 BC).

Figure 3-1

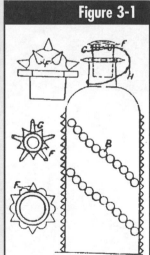

Textured bottles and caps were proposed a century ago for identifying poisons.

Conclusion

Methods of failure analysis such as FMA and FMEA provide models for the detection and reduction of accidents resulting from machine failures. For such models to be effective, however, the human factor must be taken into account. We therefore recommend the widespread adoption of HEMEA in the analysis of medical systems. The HEMEA approach will save lives.

••••
References

1. Kimball EW. *Failure Analysis*. National Symposium on Reliability and Quality Control; 1962: 117–28.

2. Meister D. *The Prediction and Measurement of Human Reliability*. Presented at the IAS Aerospace Systems Reliability Symposium, Salt Lake City, Utah, April 16–18, 1962.

3. Brady JS, Daily A. Evaluation of personnel performance in complex systems. Atlas Crew Procedures Laboratory Technical Memorandum. Space Laboratory Report GM 6300.5-1431; April 1961.

4. Shapero A. Human engineering testing and malfunction data collection in weapon systems test programs. Wright Air Development Division Technical Report 60-36. Dayton, Ohio; Wright Air Development Division; February 1960.

5. Hahn HA. Human factors issues in qualitative and quantitative safety analysis. Submitted to the Russian Institute, Los Alamos National Laboratory, NMex; 1993.

6. Denning PJ. Human error and the search for blame. RIACS Technical Report TR-89.46; 1989.

7. Bell J, Redwood T. *Historical Sketch of the Progress of Pharmacy in Great Britain*. London: Pharmaceutical Society; 1880.

One Hospital's Method of Applying Failure Mode and Effects Analysis

4.

Michael R. Cohen, MS, FASHP

Institute for Safe Medication Practices
Huntingdon Valley, Pa.

Chapter 3 introduced the concept of failure mode and effects analysis (FMEA) and described how it may be used in error prevention. This chapter discusses how FMEA may be applied in health care settings, through the example of one hospital.

Overview of the Use of FMEA in Preventing Medication Errors

FMEA is an ongoing quality improvement process that is best carried out by a multidisciplinary team.[1] FMEA acknowledges that errors are inevitable and predictable. It anticipates errors and designs a system that will minimize their impact. For each medication, FMEA asks what will happen if a health provider

- mistakes one medication for another because of packaging,
- administers the wrong amount of drug,
- gives a drug to the wrong patient,
- administers a drug by the wrong route or at the wrong rate,
- omits a dose,
- gives a drug at the wrong time, or
- takes any other action that may produce a medication misadventure.

In some cases, FMEA reveals that the patient can tolerate the error or that the error will be intercepted by the system of checks and balances that is part of a health system's quality improvement system. In other cases, FMEA reveals that specific steps must be put in place to address potential errors with significant impact—errors that are intolerable. Figure 4–1 illustrates how the FMEA system works.[1] The goal is to create "error traps" that will prevent accidents and ensure patient safety.

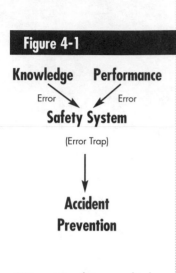
FMEA in Health Care

FMEA can often be easily integrated into a hospital's continuous quality improvement program.[2,3] For example, a committee at Memorial Mission Hospital of Asheville, N.C., used FMEA to identify significant failure modes in specific drug administration processes and to rank them in order of priority.[2] The following failure modes were identified:

- Storage of lethal drugs on floor stock,
- Errors in calculating doses,
- Errors in calculating flow rates,
- Failure to check patients' arm bands before administration of medication,
- Storage of excessive drugs in nursing unit floor stock.

Committee members assessed the identified failure modes on the basis of three factors:

A. Likelihood of their occurrence,
B. Severity of the failure should it occur, and
C. Probability that the error would be detected before a patient would be harmed.

Committee members ranked each factor on this list, and each member's score was combined for each factor. The products of these calculations (A x B x C) for all members were totaled to create a "criticality index." This index was used to rank the potential problems in order of priority. Priority items became the target of prevention efforts. On the basis of its analysis, the committee implemented solutions to four of the listed failure modes. Steps to be followed in implementing FMEA are summarized in Table 4–1.

Stomatis[4] has written an exhaustive review of the technique and application of failure mode and effects analysis.

Conclusion

When systems are in place to anticipate and prevent medication errors, the drug use process will be safer. Each system can be thought of as a layer of safety within the overall medication system. Other strategies that may enhance safe medication use include tactile clues, well-placed warning signs, and legible labels (see Chapter 3). Many systems under development, such as electronic alarms and bar code technology, as well as increased computerization, hold promise for improving safe medication use. Documentation and in-service education are essential.

Despite these welcome developments and advances, medication errors will continue to occur. Medication packages, devices, and drug delivery processes must therefore be continually subjected to FMEA.

Table 4-1

Steps in Implementing FMEA

1. Form a multidisciplinary group.

2. Help members gain an understanding of the process (e.g., create a flow diagram).

3. Brainstorm ways in which the process could fail (i.e., what could go wrong?).

4. List the effects of the failures on the process.

5. List the root causes that can generate the failure mode.

6. On a 10-point scale, estimate the following:

   — Likelihood of failure,

   — Severity of the failure, and

   — Probability that the failure will be detected.

7. Compute the criticality index.

8. Brainstorm actions that could reduce the criticality index, starting with failure modes that received the highest score.

9. Implement actions.

10. Follow up and assess action by recalculating the criticality index.

References

1. Cohen MR, Senders J, Davis NM. Failure mode and effects analysis: a novel approach to avoiding dangerous medication errors and accidents. *Hosp Pharm.* 1994; 29: 319–30.

2. Williams E, Talley R. The use of failure mode and criticality analysis in a medication error subcommittee. *Hosp Pharm.* 1994; 29: 331–37.

3. McNally KM, Page MA, Sunderland VB. Failure mode and effects analysis in improving a drug distribution system. *Am J Health Syst Pharm.* 1997; 54: 171–77.

4. Stomatis DH. *Failure Mode and Effects Analysis: From Theory to Execution.* Milwaukee: American Society for Quality Control; 1995.

High-Alert Medications: Safeguarding Against Errors

Michael R. Cohen, MS, FASHP

Institute for Safe Medication Practices
Huntingdon Valley, Pa.

Charles M. Kilo, MD, MPH

Institute for Healthcare Improvement
Boston, Mass.

Although most medications have a wide margin of safety, a few drugs have a high risk of causing injury when they are misused. These may be termed "high-alert medications." Although errors may not be more common with these drugs than with others, their consequences may be more devastating.

High-alert medications can be targeted for specific error reduction interventions. For example, they can be packaged, stored, prescribed, and administered differently than other medications. Forcing functions (i.e., methods that make it impossible for the drug to be given in a potentially lethal manner) can also be developed and instituted for these products.

This chapter consists of two major parts. In the first part, we present a general framework that may be applied to safeguard the use of high-alert drugs. This is followed by a discussion of several concepts for changes that may improve the safe use of these products. In the second part, we discuss several of the most commonly used high-alert drugs (Table 5–1) in detail. For each drug, we summarize the nature of the problems associated with its use, outline key areas for improvement, and present techniques for monitoring error reduction strategies. Recommendations are based on the experience of others who have used this methodology, the professional literature, and concepts drawn from human-factors knowledge of principles of error reduction.

Part I

High-Alert Drugs: A Framework for Improvement

Three principles may be used to safeguard the use of high-alert medications: (1) reducing or eliminating the possibility of errors, (2) making errors visible, and (3) minimizing the consequences of errors. These principles provide a framework for developing error reduction strategies. To safeguard high-alert drugs, each of these three primary principles should be employed whenever possible.

Principle 1: Reduce or Eliminate the Possibility of Error

The primary means of reducing adverse drug events and medical errors is to ensure that they do not occur in the first place—in other words, to prevent them. Ways of reducing the possibility of error include reducing the number of medications in the formulary, reducing the available concentrations and volumes, and removing high-alert drugs from clinical areas.

One example of the application of this principle is to remove all concentrated potassium chloride from floor stock. This measure will reduce errors associated with inadvertent intravenous administration of high-concentration potassium. Another example of this principle is to change the labeling for dobutamine and dopamine to reduce the chance of errors resulting from the fact that not only does the packaging of these two drugs look alike, but their names sound alike.

When errors do occur, their root causes should be explored. Organizations should ask why the error occurred and what system changes can be instituted to prevent its recurrence.

The Institute for Safe Medication Practices (ISMP) publishes informational features on medication errors and their root causes in professional journals and press reports. A biweekly facsimile or electronic mail alert system, *ISMP Medication Safety Alert!*, communicates error advisories based on reports submitted to the U.S. Pharmacopeia (USP) Medication Errors Reporting Program (MERP). USP's Practitioner Reporting Network publishes the *USP Quality Review*, which often discusses medication errors. The Food and Drug Administration (FDA) publishes medication safety information. Information provided by these sources should be monitored and used for error prevention. If an incident happens in one health care setting, there is a strong likelihood that it will recur elsewhere.

Principle 2: Make Errors Visible

It is unlikely that all errors will be prevented before they reach the patient. The second safeguard, therefore, is to make errors visible when they do occur. Having two individuals independently check infusion pump settings for high-alert drugs is one way to make errors visible. If an incorrect rate of infusion is programmed into a patient-controlled analgesia (PCA) device, a second, independent check prior to initiating the infusion should make the error visible.

Principle 3: Minimize the Consequences of Errors

It is also possible to make changes that will reduce the adverse effect of an error. For instance, fatal errors have occurred when the contents of 50-mL vials of lidocaine 2% were injected instead of mannitol, which was packaged in a vial of similar appearance. Had lidocaine been available only in 10-mL vials and had it been confused with another drug vial of the same size and erroneously administered, the overdose would not be fatal.

Key Change Concepts for Safeguarding High-Alert Drugs

The following suggestions show how the three principles just discussed may be incorporated into a system to safeguard high-alert drugs.

Build in System Redundancies

Although everyone makes mistakes, the probability that two individuals in the same institution will make the same error in association with the same medication for the same patient is quite small. For this reason, a system of redundancies, sometimes called check systems, whereby one person checks the work of another, is essential. Compare, for example, the following two systems of drug distribution:

1. In the floor stock system, a nearly complete pharmacy is maintained on every unit in a hospital or nursing home. Acting alone, the nurse interprets and transcribes a physician's order, chooses the proper container from hundreds available on the shelves, prepares the correct amount, places the dose in a syringe or cup, labels it, takes it to the patient, administers it, and verifies that the dose has been administered. The floor stock system includes certain automated point-of-use dispensing systems (see Chapter 10).

2. The unit-dose and intravenous admixture system intentionally incorporates many check systems or redundant steps.[1] Such redundancies have been shown to reduce accident rates.[2] The steps associated with administration of a medication under such a system are presented in Table 5–2.

In a unit-dose system, the work of pharmacy technicians must be checked by pharmacists. In critical procedures, the work of the pharmacist is checked by a second pharmacist. For example, independent checks should be made when setting pump rates and concentrations for PCA and infusion of high-alert drugs. All pediatric and geriatric dosages, as well as all dosages of high-alert medications, should be checked independently by at least two persons. Maximum doses should be established for high-alert medications. If an order exceeds these doses, a timely peer review process should be employed to determine the safety of the order before the drug is dispensed or administered.

Use Fail-Safes

Product design has a strong impact on error prevention. A prime example is intravenous infusion pumps. Hospitals commonly use pumps that require the operator to close a gravity flow control clamp to stop the flow of the solution. Many personnel are unaware of this important step; even those who do know how to operate the pumps sometimes forget to clamp the tubing. As a result, patients have been harmed by the free flow of intravenous solutions. If these solutions contain toxic medications, the risk is even greater.

Because these performance and knowledge deficiencies are predictable, measures can be taken to overcome them. For example, most electronic infusion devices now use intravenous sets with an automatic fail-safe clamping mechanism. Safe medication use dictates that all intravenous pump sets have built-in free-flow protection that cannot be overridden.

Reduce Options

The more options available for any medication (e.g., different concentrations and volumes), the more likely it is that an error will occur. Concentrations and volumes of all high-alert medications should be standardized to reduce options to a minimum. The result will be a decrease in the size of the formulary, a reduction in the floor stock, and a reduction in the possibility of errors.

For instance, instead of having the option of prescribing heparin in concentrations of 20,000 units per 250 mL, 20,000 units per 500 mL, 25,000 units per 500 mL, and so forth, only one option should be routinely available. Dosage charts should be made available that standardize dose adjustments of 50 units for each 1-mL change.

Use Forcing Functions

Forcing functions are techniques that reduce the possibility that a medication can be administered in a potentially lethal manner. A case in point is the use

Table 5-2

Steps in the Medication Use Process

1. A physician writes the order.

2. A unit secretary reads and transcribes the order.

3. A nurse checks the secretary's work.

4. A pharmacy technician reads the order and enters it into a computer.

5. The computer checks for drug interactions, proper dose, and allergies.

6. A pharmacist reviews the technician's work and performs a clinical screening.

7. The order and a computer-generated label move to the filling area, where a technician checks the order against the label.

8. A pharmacist checks the technician's work.

9. A nurse receives the drug and checks the nursing record against the medication that has been dispensed.

10. The nurse administers the drug, telling the patient the name of the drug, the dose, and its purpose, thereby allowing the patient to serve as a double-check.

11. Unused drugs are returned to the pharmacy, where a technician reviews them for mistakenly unadministered doses.

12. The technician follows up as needed.

of "lock-and-key" designs that ensure that parts from different systems are not interchangeable. For example, one should not be able to inject liquid added to a syringe meant for oral use into an intravenous line. If the parts from these two different systems fit, someone will inevitably try to inject an oral drug. Oral "syringes" for nonparenteral liquids have tips to which needles and intravenous tubing cannot be attached.

Preprinted order forms and computer order entry are other forcing function strategies. On preprinted order forms, clinicians can be "forced" to choose only from a limited number of printed medications of available dosages. Using preprinted order forms also helps to standardize the ordering process.

Externalize or Centralize Error-Prone Processes

Preparing intravenous solutions in patient care areas can be hazardous. Distractions, nonstandard concentrations, lack of nursing expertise, and erroneous calculations may all lead to errors.

Most high-alert drugs given by intravenous infusion are available in pre-mixed form. Using commercially prepared products reduces the risk of error because it relegates the error-prone process of solution preparation to the factory.

If commercial forms are not available, intravenous solutions should be prepared in the pharmacy. All institutions that delegate this responsibility to the pharmacy must provide competency-based training programs and ensure the development and use of quality assurance procedures to safeguard the preparation of these medications.

Outsourcing certain complicated parenteral solutions is another way to reduce error potential. Some hospitals have outside pharmacies prepare cardioplegic solutions, total parenteral nutritionals, and IV antibiotics. This can relieve congestion in the hospital pharmacy and assure that appropriate quality assurance steps exist in the drug preparation process. When outside facilities are used, they must certify that they meet the FDA's Good Manufacturing Practices.

Use Differentiation

All medications on a formulary should be examined for potential look-alike and sound-alike problems. Once these problems have been identified, safeguards should be introduced. They may include removing one of the products from the formulary, storing the products in separate locations, and using auxiliary labels.

For example, one might affix labels to Norvasc® containers because this product is frequently confused with Navane®. Auxiliary labels, such as "For oral use only," "For External Use Only," or "For the Ear Only," can be used to differentiate products and to call attention to a well-known problem. Additional auxiliary labels include "Caution—Read Label Carefully: Look-Alike or Sound-Alike Drug" and "Warning—Highly Concentrated Drug—Must Be Diluted Prior to Administration." Label manufacturers can custom-design other warnings.

Another option is to change labeling to emphasize different portions of a drug name. For instance, it is much easier to differentiate "DOBUTamine" and "DOPamine" than "dobutamine" and "dopamine."

It is best to label medications by their generic name rather than by brand name, because this limits the number of names that are likely to be used. However, if generic names are confusing, brand names may be safer to use.

Suppliers should be chosen wisely; not all manufacturers package and label high-alert drugs as safely as they could. Feedback concerning problems should be provided to group purchasing organizations, the manufacturer, USP, ISMP, and FDA.

Store Medications Appropriately

Many medication errors happen because a health care worker has chosen the wrong container. Look-alike packaging and poorly designed labeling contribute to such errors. Drug manufacturers should be urged to make their packaging more distinct.

Hospitals can reduce the possibility of this type of error by paying special attention to how products are arranged and shelved. Pharmacy staff should separate potentially dangerous drugs with similar names or similar packaging. If a drug is moved that would normally be stored next to one with which it could be confused, a reminder note should be left in its place indicating where it is now being stored.

On the patient's body, IV tubes and enteral connections and access ports should be as far apart from each other as possible. There have been reports of accidental intravenous injection of medications into epidural catheters whose ports resemble central intravenous access ports.

Screen New Products

The Pharmacy and Therapeutics Committee should inspect all new drugs and drug delivery devices. Medications should be examined for poor labeling and packaging (e.g., illegible print, name and strength not listed prominently or expressed properly). The committee should also be on the alert for see-through glass ampuls that are not easily read, as well as look-alike packaging and sound-alike names.

When selecting new pumps or delivery devices, decision makers should use failure mode and effects analysis, which provides a means for the systematic analysis of the potential for error and its consequences (see Chapters 3 and 4).

Standardize and Simplify Order Communication

Guidelines for ordering should be created, disseminated, and enforced. Preprinted order forms and computer order entry work best, provided that they have undergone rigorous multidisciplinary review.[3]

Recommendations from the National Coordinating Council for Medication Error Reporting and Prevention (NCC MERP) should be incorporated into the development of these guidelines. (A copy of "Recommendations to

Correct Error-Prone Aspects of Prescription Writing," published in 1996, is available by calling NCC MERP at 301-881-0666.)

Use of abbreviations is an especially problematic aspect of order communication. The health care facility should maintain a list of abbreviations, terms, and symbols that should not be used. Such a list is presented in Table 5–3.

Verbal (i.e., spoken) orders are particularly susceptible to errors and should be avoided when possible. All verbal orders should be repeated to the person who placed them. Some experts believe that all verbal orders should be confirmed by two persons.

Note that computerized order entry by physicians would eliminate steps 2 through 4 in Table 5-2, and thus would make the process errors associated with these steps impossible.

Limit Access

Ideally, a hospital pharmacy should be open and staffed by pharmacists 24 hours a day, 7 days a week. Restricting access to the pharmacy during times when it is closed reduces the possibility for medication error.

Many hospitals have devised systems that limit access to certain dangerous substances yet continue to make them available in a safe manner when necessary during hours when the pharmacy is closed. For example, if magnesium sulfate must be stored in a patient care area to prepare intravenous fluids, it could be locked up with narcotics in order to reduce access and possible misuse. Auxiliary labeling could be affixed to each vial to warn staff about the nature of the drug. Maintaining a limited after-hours formulary and stocking only limited amounts in the smallest drug containers are additional ways of restricting access.

Use Constraints

Constraints provide an effective means of limiting use of high-alert medications. Examples include requirements for approval prior to use, pharmacy screening of all orders for high-alert medications, automatic stop orders, and dose or duration limits.

Use Reminders

Labels can be placed on drug containers or in drug storage locations to remind staff of potential problems with high-alert medications. Computer fields in drug inventory databases can be programmed to flash warnings during order entry.

Table 5-3

Medication errors associated with abbreviations and symbols

Abbreviation ᵃ	Intended Meaning	Error	Recommendation
Apothecary Symbols	One Dram ℥ʲ Minim ♏	Not understood or misread; symbol for dram mistaken for the number three and symbol for the number one mistaken for a capital letter t, symbol for tablespoon; minim misread as mL	**DO NOT USE**
Drug Names *Abbreviations:*			
ARA-A	Vidarabine	Cytarabine (ARA-C)	
AZT	Zidovudine (Retrovir®)	Azathioprine (Imuran®)	
CPZ	Compazine® (prochlorperazine)	Thorazine® (chlorpromazine)	
DPT	Demerol® – Phenergan®–Thorazine®	Diphtheria–pertussis–tetanus (vaccine)	
HCl	Hydrochloric acid	Potassium chloride (KCl)	
HCT	Hydrocortisone	Hematocrit (Hct) or hydrochlorothiazide (HCTZ)	
HCTZ	Hydrochlorothiazide	Hydrocortisone (HCT)	
$MgSO_4$	Magnesium sulfate	Morphine sulfate (MS)	
MS	Morphine sulfate	Magnesium sulfate ($MgSO_4$)	
MTX	Methotrexate	Mitoxantrone	
Stemmed names:			
NITRO drip	Nitroprusside	Nitroglycerin	
NORFLOX	Norfloxacin (Noroxin®)	Norflex® (orphenadrine)	
PIT	Pitocin® (oxytocin)	Pitressin® (vasopressin)	
Symbols			
/(slash mark)	Separates two doses or indicates "per"	1 (numeral "one"); e.g., "25 units/10 units" read as "110 units"	Spell out "per."
+	Plus sign	Misread as 4 (numeral "four"); e.g., "+6 units" misread as "46 units"	Spell out "and."
⌀	Phenyl or pheno' (e.g., phenobarbital)	Misread as symbol for "stop" or "no"	Use full name of drug.
>,<	Greater than, less than	Mistakenly used opposite of intended	DO NOT USE.
()	Parentheses	Misread as letter "l"	Avoid use in orders.
µg*	Microgram	Misread as milligram (mg)	Use "mcg."
Decimal Points			
Zero after decimal point (e.g., 1.0 mg)	1 mg	Misread as 10 mg	Terminal zeroes are dangerous; DO NOT USE.
No zero before decimal when less than whole unit (e.g.,.1 mg)	.1 mg	Misread as 1 mg	Always use zero before decimal.

ᵃ Items marked with an asterisk (*) appear on NCC MERP's list of abbreviations that should not be used.

USE FULL NAMES OF DRUGS

Table 5-3 (continued)

Medication errors associated with abbreviations and symbols

Abbreviation [a]	Intended Meaning	Error	Recommendation
Other Abbreviations			
AU, AS, AD*	Both ears, left ear, right ear	Misread as Latin OU (both eyes), OS (left eye), or OD (right eye)	Write out full intended meaning.
BT	Bedtime	BID (twice daily)	Use "hs."
cc*	Cubic centimeters	Misread as "U" (units)	Use "mL."
D/C*	Discharge or discontinue	Medications have been prematurely discontinued when D/C (intended as "discharge") was misinterpreted as "discontinue" when followed by a list of drugs	Write out "discontinue" and "discharge."
HS*	Half strength	Misread as Latin "HS" (hour of sleep)	Write out strength of medication.
i/d	One per day	TID (three times daily)	Write out "daily."
IVP	Intravenous pyelogram	Intravenous push	Write "IV pyelogram"
IVR	Intravenous rider ("piggyback")	Intravenous push	Write "IV rider" or "IV piggyback."
PT	Physical therapy	Prothrombin time	Write out intended meaning.
q hs, q 6PM, etc	Nightly at bedtime, every evening at 6:00, etc.	Every hour, every 6 hours, etc.	Use "hs" or write out "6 PM nightly."
Q.D., q.d.*	Latin for "every day"	Period after "Q" mistaken for "I" and has led to medications being administered four times daily (qid) rather than once daily	Write out "daily."
Q.O.D., q.o.d.*	Latin for "every other day"	Mistaken for "QD" or "qd" or for "QID" or "qid"; if "o" is poorly written, it may look like a period or "I."	Use "q other day."
SC* or SQ	Subcutaneous	Mistaken for "SL" (sublingual)	Write out "subcutaneous."
ss	Sliding scale (insulin) or $\frac{1}{2}$ (apothecary)	Mistaken for "55"	Write out "one half" or use "$\frac{1}{2}$."
TIW*	Three times a week	Misinterpreted as "three times a day" or "twice a week"	Write out "three times a week."
U*	Units	Misread as zero (0), four (4), or cc	Write out "units."
x3d	For three days	Mistaken for "three doses"	Write out "for 3 days."

[a] Items marked with an asterisk (*) appear on NCC MERP's list of abbreviations that should not be used.

Standardize Dosing Procedures

Calculating doses on the basis of weight or other factors such as renal function is often an error-prone process, particularly for vasoactive intravenous medications. To simplify dosing and avoid the need to make calculations, standardized dosage charts or tables (e.g., expressed in micrograms per kilogram per minute) should be employed. These charts must take multiple factors into consideration, including solution concentration, patient weight, and rate of infusion. They can be produced in the form of a label and affixed to infusion containers.

Standardization of drug preparations is also necessary. For example, in the pharmacy it is important to standardize preparation and checking of chemotherapy orders, total parenteral nutrition (TPN) solutions, cardioplegic solutions, and similar preparations.

Part II

Part I of this chapter presents general principles that apply to the safe use of all high-alert medications. Part II provides an approach to improving the use of specific high-alert medications. Table 5–4 can be referred to in order to quickly ascertain the key steps for improving the safety of high-alert drugs.

High-Alert Drugs[1,4–6]

Adrenergic Agonists

Epinephrine, Isoproterenol, and Norepinephrine

Problems:

- In operating rooms, adrenergic agonists are often drawn up into unlabeled syringes or put into unlabeled or incorrectly labeled cups or pans. A recent example was the death of a child in Florida who was given intravenous epinephrine that had been poured into a pan labeled "lidocaine with epinephrine."

- In addition, these agents are provided in varying concentrations. For instance, epinephrine comes in concentrations of 1:1000 and 1:10,000. This is confusing to many health care personnel and inconsistent with most concentrations, which are referred to in terms of milligrams per milliliter (mg/mL).

- Isoproterenol is available in 1- and 0.2-mg ampuls. If the dose ordered is "1 amp," the wrong amount may be administered.

Aim: Reduce errors in administration of adrenergic agonists resulting from poor labeling or confusion about concentrations and dosages.

Key Improvements:

- Safeguard preparations:

  — Communicate orders in a standard fashion. Refer to intravenous doses in terms of metric weight (i.e., milligrams) rather than concentration, amps, or volume. (Note: The concentration may be important for drugs used topically or injected locally.)

  — Label all containers, including syringes and cups, into which drugs are placed. Label both sides of containers of drugs for intravenous infusion.

- Reduce options:

  — Remove phenylephrine (Neo-Synephrine®) and other adrenergic agonists from the formulary if there is no need for them. Use pre-filled syringes whenever possible.

  — Simplify preparation of solutions by using premixed solutions, preparation instructions, and dosing charts.

  — Perform independent double-checks. Before administering intravenous drugs, have a second nurse independently check pump settings, drug concentration, and line attachments.

  — Use heart monitors on patients with a central intravenous line.

Measures:

- Inspect operating room and intensive care unit (ICU) procedures to ensure compliance with proper labeling practices.

- Follow up on all orders for intravenous beta-blockers.

Dopamine and Dobutamine

Problems:

- These medications are subject to mix-ups because of similarities in their names, the settings in which they are used (e.g., ICUs), and the types of patients for whom they are used (e.g., patients with cardiac problems). Problems also occur because the two products are administered in similar doses, are provided in similar concentrations, and, if they are from the same manufacturer, have similar packaging.

- Intravenous flow rates are often confusing because they are based on calculations of micrograms per kilogram per minute.

- Extravasation is a problem when dopamine is given via peripheral veins.

Aim: Distinguish between two sound-alike names. Standardize dosing and display it in a manner that reduces the potential for dosing errors.

Key Improvements:

- Differentiate labeling:

  — Consider providing labels that differentiate critical parts of the names (e.g., "DOBUTamine" and "DOPamine").

  — Purchase premixed solutions from different manufacturers to ensure that they look different.

  — Differentiate packaging; for example, purchase dobutamine in 250-mL bags and dopamine in 500-mL bags.

  — Use preprinted order forms to standardize ordering and dosage.

  — Standardize concentrations to facilitate the use of dosing charts and eliminate the possibility of calculation errors. Base dosing on titration against clinical factors (e.g., blood pressure or heart rate).

  — Label intravenous bags and delivery pumps with dosage charts and equivalent delivery rates for these dosages.

Measures: Conduct rounds to confirm that the agents being delivered and their rates and concentrations match current orders.

Intravenous Esmolol and Propranolol

Problems:

- Esmolol ampuls have been confused with vials, resulting in administration of a concentrated product by direct injection. The contents of a vial of esmolol are much more dilute (100 mg/10 mL) than the contents of an ampul (2.5 g/10 mL). Patients who inadvertently receive the stronger concentration may develop bradycardia, electromechanical dissociation, or asystole that may be irreversible.

- With propranolol, the most common error is the accidental administration of an intravenous dose equal to the standard oral dose when switching a patient from the oral to the intravenous route. The intravenous dose is much smaller than the oral dose.

Table 5-4

Safety measures for high-alert drugs

Key Changes	Adrenergic Agonists	Intravenous Adrenergic Agonists	Amiodarone /Aminone	Benzodiazepines (Midazolam)	Calcium	Chemotherapy	Chloral Hydrate, Oral Midazolam	Digoxin	Dopamine/ Dobutamine
I. Standardize ordering, preparation, and administration									
Eliminate use of specific abbreviations						all			
Use standardized drug/dose expressions	x				x	x		dig	
Use preprinted order forms or ordering protocols						x			x
Order by metric weight, not by volume or ampul	x	x	x	x	x	x		x	x
Include dose formula with calculated dose				x		x	x (peds)	x (peds)	
Use drug preparation guidelines	x				x	x			
Use dosing charts	x					x			x
Standardize and limit drug concentrations/formulations	x	x		x	x	x	x	x	x
Use drug administration protocols			x	x		x	x		x
Use flow control pumps for continuous iv infusions	x	x			x	x			x
Use oral syringes for administration of oral products			x	x			x	x	
II. Externalize or centralize drug preparation									
Move drug preparation off units	x [IV]	x	x		x	x		x	x
Use commercially available premixed iv solutions	x								x
III. Distinguish or warn with labels, container size, or computer alerts									
Apply warning labels and/or distinguish drug names clearly		x (amps)	x			x	x		x
Establish dose limits and screen orders		x	x			x	x	x	
Use different-size containers/manufacturer (look-alike drugs)		x	x						x
IV. Limit or restrict drug access									
Remove drug from floor stock and dispensing cabinets		x (amps)	x			x	x		x
Sequester and lock drugs if stored on units			x				x		
Separate like products when using or storing		x	x						
Dispense the drug from pharmacy only		x (amps)	x			x	x		x
Use smallest size package, concentration, and dose for floor stock		x (vials)	x	x	x		x	x	
V. Limit or restrict drug use									
Formulary drug restrictions or criteria for use		x	x	x		x			
Eliminate or use acceptable alternatives	x							x	
Switch from iv to oral (or subcutaneous) use as soon as possible								x	
Certify/privilege staff to order, prepare, or administer drug	x	x	x	x		x		x	
VI. Perform independent double-checks									
Recalculate the dose				x	x	x	x	x (peds)	
Verify drug preparation		x	x			x	x	x	
Use peer review process for unusual drug, dose, regimen		x	x			x	x	x	
Double-check pump rate, drug, concentration, and line attachments	x	x			x	x	x	x	x
Involve the patient (family) through education	x	x			x	x	x	x	x
VII. Monitor the patient and respond to drug effects									
Obtain and communicate laboratory values via guidelines	cm (IV)			x	x	x	x	x	
Require CM and/or PO				cm, po			cm, po		
Require close observation/vital sign monitoring				x		x	x	x	x
Have antidotes and/or resuscitation equipment close at hand	x	x				x	x	x	x

Key Changes	Heparin IV and Warfarin	Insulin	Lidocaine	Magnesium Sulfate	Opiate Narcotics	Neuro-muscular Blockers	Potassium Chloride or Phosphate	Sodium Chloride Concentrate	Theophylline
I. Standardize ordering, preparation, and administration									
Eliminate use of specific abbreviations	u for units	u for units		MGSC4 MSO4					
Use standardized drug/dose expressions	x	x		x	x		x		x
Use preprinted order forms or ordering protocols	x		x	x	x		x		
Order by metric weight, not by volume or cmpl	x		x	x			x		x
Include dose formula with calculated dose	x				x (peds)		x (Kphos)		x
Use drug preparation guidelines					x				
Use dosing charts	x	x			x				x
Standardize and limit drug concentrations/formulations	x	x	x	x	x		x	x	x
Use drug administration protocols	x		x (IV)	x	x	x	x	x	x
Use flow control pumps for continuous iv infusions	x	x	x	x	x	x	x	x	x
Use oral syringes for administration of oral products					x				
II. Externalize or centralize drug preparation									
Move drug preparation off units	x	x (IV)	x	x	x (IV)	x	x (KCl)	x	x
Use commercially available premixed iv solutions	x		x	x				x	x
III. Distinguish or warn with labels, container size, or computer alerts									
Apply warning labels and/or distinguish drug names clearly	x	x	x		x	x	x	x	
Establish dose limits and screen orders	x	x	x	x	x		x	x	x
Use different-size containers/manufacturer (look-alike drugs)	x	x	x		x				
IV. Limit or restrict drug access									
Remove drug from floor stock and dispensing cabinets						x	x (KCl)	x (dialysis)	
Sequester and lock drugs if stored on units	x	x	x		x	x	x (KCl)	x	
Separate like products when using or storing		x (IV)				x	x	x	
Dispense the drug from pharmacy only	x					x			
Use smallest size package, concentration, and dose for floor stock	x				x				
V. Limit or restrict drug use									
Formulary drug restrictions or criteria for use	x	x		x		x	x		x
Eliminate or use acceptable alternatives									x
Switch from iv to oral (or subcutaneous) use as soon as possible	x	x			x		x		x
Certify/privilege staff to order, prepare, or administer drug	x				x	x			
VI. Perform independent double-checks									
Recalculate the dose	x	x	x	x	x (peds)		x (Kphos)		x
Verify drug preparation	x	x					x (Kphos)		
VII. Monitor the patient and respond to drug effects									
Use peer review process for unusual drug, dose, regimen	x				x		x		
Double-check pump rate, drug, concentration, and line attachments	x	x	x	x	x	x	x	x	x
Involve the patient (family) through education	x	x	x	x	x	x	x	x	x
Obtain and communicate laboratory values via guidelines	x	x		x	x		x	x	x
Require CM and/or PO			cm (IV)			cm, po	cm (Kphos)		
Require close observation/vital sign monitoring		x		x	x	x			x
Have antidotes and/or resuscitation equipment close at hand					x	x			

Abbreviations: cm = cardiac monitoring; IV = intravenous; Kphos = potassium phosphate; peds = pediatric patients; po = pulse oximetry.

Aim: Eliminate the possibility of errors in administration of intravenous esmolol and errors in dosing intravenous propranolol.

Key Improvements:

- Minimize the need for esmolol by selecting alternative agents.

- Standardize order communication. Do not allow esmolol to be ordered by "amp."

- Limit access—remove esmolol from patient care areas, night cabinets, emergency kits, and automated dispensing modules. Store only in pharmacy.

- Prepare intravenous infusions and syringes only in the pharmacy.

- Standardize solution concentrations.

- Administer esmolol only where resuscitation equipment, including a suitable pacemaker, is available.

- Have routine orders for intravenous propranolol screened by a pharmacist or second nurse prior to administration.

Measures:

- Track error rates with both drugs.

- Perform checks to ensure that esmolol ampuls are not available in clinical areas, if this has been adopted as an institutional policy.

Theophylline

Problems:

- Theophylline has a narrow therapeutic range, and it may interact with several commonly used medications (e.g., cimetidine and macrolide antibiotics). Close monitoring of theophylline levels is necessary, and dosage adjustments may be required.

- Theophylline is widely used, despite the availability of safer and more effective medications, such as inhaled beta-agonists and steroids. When theophylline is used intravenously, confusion may exist in calculating dosages and determining which concentration should be used.

- Liquid theophylline is often used in pediatric patients. Some health care facilities mix their own liquid theophylline. Errors in preparation may occur when pediatricians express dosages in volume (milliliters) instead of weight (milligrams).

- Personnel may be confused between aminophylline in vials and premixed intravenous theophylline solutions. (Aminophylline is only 80% theophylline.) Infant aminophylline doses have been prepared using milliliter measurements instead of milligrams. In one case, 7.4 mL (185 mg of 250 mg/10 mL solution) was given to a newborn instead of 7.4 mg.

Aim: Reduce the opportunity for interactions between theophylline and macrolide antibiotics (primarily erythromycin) and cimetidine, replace theophylline with safer and more effective medications, and reduce the opportunity for dosing errors.

Key Improvements:

- Use oral theophylline or other, safer medications (e.g., inhaled steroids) instead of intravenous theophylline.

- Set criteria for the use of intravenous theophylline.

- Develop and enforce standards for monitoring.

- Use premixed intravenous theophylline and limit the number of available concentrations. Have aminophylline doses for infants prepared only by the pharmacy.

- Standardize prescribing—write orders for intravenous solutions in milligrams rather than milliliters.

- Eliminate aminophylline floor stock.

- Provide equivalency labeling to reduce confusion between theophylline and aminophylline.

- Affix preprinted dosing charts on intravenous bags. Label both front and back.

- Have two individuals check intravenous rates for all new infusions and rate changes.

- Provide free-flow protection for all pumps.

- Provide computerized screening for drug interactions.

- Screen patients for conditions that may affect drug metabolism (e.g., tobacco use, liver disease, congestive heart failure).

- Encourage physicians to keep logs of patients' medications to alert them to potential interactions.

Obstacles: Physicians are used to prescribing theophylline for patients with asthma, despite the existence of more effective and less toxic alternatives.

Measures:

- Determine number of patients with asthma who are taking theophylline but are not being treated with optimal doses of anti-inflammatory agents (e.g., inhaled steroids with cromolyn sodium, inhaled anticholinergics, beta-adrenergic agonists).

- Determine number of hospitalizations related to theophylline toxicity.

- Screen laboratory results to determine the number of patients with serum theophylline levels of greater than 20 mg/dL.

- Adhere to monitoring standards.

- Determine number of emergency department admissions of patients with asthma.

Benzodiazepines (Midazolam)

Problems:

- Misunderstanding about the time of onset of midazolam's sedative effect often leads to errors associated with this medication. Many believe that the onset of action is immediate; however, it generally takes 5 to 10 minutes to reach its peak effect. If additional doses are given in the meantime, respiratory arrest, or even death, may occur.

- Overdoses have been associated with confusing labels. The concentration is displayed on the front panel as "1 mg/mL" or "5 mg/mL." Many users may erroneously believe that these numbers refer to the total amount in the vial. Depending on package size, the amount actually varies from 2 mg (1 mg/mL in a 2-mL container) to 50 mg (5 mg/mL in a 10-mL container).

Aim: Reduce errors caused by misunderstanding of the rate of onset of midazolam and by its misleading package label.

Key Improvements:

- Provide appropriate monitoring during midazolam use (e.g., use pulse oximetry, have resuscitation equipment in area).

- Restrict access—do not use midazolam for preoperative sedation except in the operating room, since appropriate monitoring equipment may not be available.

- Limit packaging options—use only one concentration if possible. Use the smallest package available.

Measures:

- Determine number of ICU admissions resulting from benzodiazepine toxicity.

- Determine rate of use of flumazenil and reasons for its use.

- Compare volume of use of midazolam with that at other hospitals performing similar procedures and with similar numbers of patients.

Intravenous Calcium (Calcium Gluceptate, Gluconate, and Chloride)

Problems:

- When ordering intravenous calcium, some prescribers fail to specify which salt is desired. There is a threefold difference in the primary cation between calcium gluconate, which contains 4.5 mEq of Ca^{++} per gram, and calcium chloride, which contains 14 mEq of Ca^{++} per gram. Calcium chloride dissociates more quickly and is more rapidly bioavailable than calcium gluconate. If a prescriber simply orders an "amp" of calcium intravenously, this difference may have serious implications. In addition, calcium chloride is more irritating than calcium gluconate when given intravenously.

- Confusion may also occur in ordering intramuscular calcium. Because of its irritant effect, calcium chloride should never be given by the intramuscular route.

- Prescribers who order calcium replacement therapy may be unaware of several factors that affect serum calcium. Foremost among these are serum phosphorus and albumin levels. The relation between calcium and phosphorus is not understood. At times, calcium phosphate may precipitate in the vasculature, resulting in organ injury, including renal dysfunction or failure. If serum phosphorus is low, larger quantities of calcium may be needed for replacement.

- Adverse drug events reported with calcium include

  — interactions with digoxin (rapid injection of calcium may cause bradyarrhythmias, especially in patients taking digoxin),

  — antagonism to calcium-channel blockers and elevations in blood pressure,

  — hypocalcemia or hypercalcemia resulting from inefficient monitoring of calcium levels,

— incorrect calcium-to-phosphate ratios in TPN solutions that may lead to precipitation and end organ injury or death (the precipitate is not visible when the TPN solution is mixed with lipids), and

— tissue necrosis caused by extravasation of calcium chloride.

Aim: Reduce medication errors with calcium.

Key Improvements:

- Make sure that orders specify the calcium salt.

- Standardize medications—use calcium gluconate or calcium chloride. Even when this is done, specify the calcium salt.

- Standardize preparation—prepare TPN solutions containing calcium and phosphorus only in the pharmacy under standard protocols.

- Have protocols for administration and monitoring that are similar to those used for potassium and magnesium.

- Order calcium only in milligrams.

Measures: Periodically review a sample of patients to whom intravenous calcium was administered to ensure its use was clinically justified.

Chemotherapeutic Agents

Problems: Chemotherapeutic agents are toxic by design. Because of the complexity and wide variety of dosing regimens, they are frequently associated with errors. (For a detailed treatment of this subject, see Chapter 15.)

Aim: Reduce errors associated with inappropriate dose calculations and administration of chemotherapeutic agents.

Key Improvements:

- Consider requiring certification before allowing practitioners to prescribe, dispense, or administer chemotherapy.

- Use carefully designed, preprinted order forms or computer order sets for all chemotherapeutic agents.

- Make sure all orders include patient's height and weight, so that body surface area can be calculated.

- Standardize dosing and delivery protocols.

- Establish dose limits:

  — ceiling for dose of a single drug,

  — daily dose ceiling,

— ceiling for total dose for a course of therapy, and

— ceiling for total lifetime dose.

- Require two independent calculations for all orders. Make sure orders include calculated dose and milligrams per meter squared (mg/m^2) or milligrams per kilogram (mg/kg) on which dose was based. Have two individuals independently check all chemotherapy pump settings before a drug is administered.

- Develop a standard administration procedure that includes the use of checklists.

- Avoid potentially confusing terminology (e.g., do not allow use of terms such as *platinum*, which may refer to cisplatin or carboplatin).

- Identify look-alike and sound-alike medication pairs and develop methods to distinguish between them. This can be done by using failure mode and effects analysis for each medication added to the formulary. Examples of potentially confusing names include cisplatin (Platinol®) and carboplatin (Paraplatin®), and vincristine, vinblastine, and vinorelbine.

- Develop protocols that require peer review in cases of disagreement between prescribers and clinical personnel.

- Do not use "U" for "units."

- Do not use an intravenous pump if only a bolus is needed.

- Use only premixed solutions.

- Make sure pumps are protected against free flow.

- Catheter flush should be only in inpatient care units. Do not allow therapeutic heparin or high concentrations in floor stock.

Obstacles:

- Staff members refuse to admit that a problem exists with chemotherapy administration.

- Poor packaging, labeling, and drug nomenclature contribute to problems.

- There may be difficulty in computerizing safety measures, such as establishing maximum doses and standardizing ordering methods.

Measures:

- Determine percentage of orders that exceed dosing standards (none should).

- Determine percentage of orders that need clarification and reason for clarification.

- Determine number of pharmacy interventions accepted.

- Match the medication administration record and intravenous flow chart to make sure the information agrees.

Chloral Hydrate (in Pediatric Patients)

Problems:

- Chloral hydrate is often used for sedation in the ambulatory setting, particularly in pediatric patients. Overdoses are sometimes caused by the fact that the drug is available in two concentrations (250 mg/5 mL and 500 mg/5 mL). A second cause of overdoses is that many physicians order chloral hydrate in terms of volume (e.g., teaspoons) rather than in milligrams.

- Chloral hydrate may be ordered as an as-needed sedative for agitated children. A child may receive multiple doses before the drug reaches its full effect, resulting in overdosage.

- Chloral hydrate is often administered by technicians or practitioners who are unfamiliar with proper dosing.

- Chloral hydrate is often used as a pediatric premedication; in such cases, responsibility for administration falls to the parent. If errors in dosing occur in the home, adequate treatment may be unavailable in case of overdose. Since nurses may not know whether the drug was given, or in what quantity, at home, excess doses may be administered.

Aim: Reduce the opportunity for medication errors associated with the use of chloral hydrate.

Key Improvements:

- Educate staff about the potential for errors.

- Allow only properly trained staff to administer chloral hydrate.

- Do not allow home use. If a child is to undergo a procedure, administer it after the child has arrived in the health care facility.

- Stock and prescribe only one concentration.

- Order in milligrams, not by volume or concentration.

- Dose children by weight, taking into consideration recommendations for doses in milligrams per kilogram.

- Do not order on an as-needed basis. If such orders are essential, limit the total allowable dosage (e.g., "up to 1 g").

- Monitor all children who have received chloral hydrate for preoperative sedation before and after the procedure. Have a resuscitation plan and equipment available.

Obstacles:

- The delayed onset of action may persuade many health professionals to favor administering the drug at home.

- The manufacturer offers the product in two strengths; one would be sufficient.

- Maximum pediatric doses in current compendia are unclear.

Measures:

- Review how often chloral hydrate is used in ambulatory settings.

- Review dosing for pediatric patients, as documented in medical records.

- Review number of orders for home use.

- Document the amount of the drug that is available in patient care areas (e.g., radiology, ambulatory settings).

- Test employee knowledge of dosing practices.

Digoxin

Problems:

- Most errors with digoxin occur in association with subacute or chronic use. They include problems associated with drug interactions and the drug's narrow therapeutic range. Individuals at particular risk include elderly patients receiving a high dose and patients on concomitant quinidine.

- Other problems include determining appropriate doses and conducting appropriate monitoring.

Aim: Reduce medication errors with digoxin.

Key Improvements:

- Provide patient education by certified staff in a well-structured setting.

- Increase patient monitoring through more frequent clinic visits or home testing of serum levels.

Measures:

- Measure digoxin levels.

- Monitor use of Digibind® (digoxin immune fab) with digoxin levels.

Heparin

Problems:

- Dose errors, concentration errors, and mix-ups of heparin with other drugs are common.

- Labeling of small-volume parenteral products from some manufacturers is a problem. The concentration (10,000 units per mL) may appear prominently, whereas the total volume (10 mL) does not. The practitioner may believe that the container holds 10,000 units when it actually holds 100,000.

- Both heparin and insulin are measured in units, and both are stored on the top of medication carts. As a result, the two products may be confused.

- Temporary increases in the heparin pump rate may cause errors if personnel do not later reset the pump.

- In settings where nonpharmacists have access to the pharmacy after hours, errors in mixing may occur.

- Heparin has been confused with vaccines because both are supplied as prefilled cartridge syringes that look alike and may be stored near one another.

- Heparin is associated with drug allergies and thrombocytopenia.

- If heparin units are abbreviated with a "U," the possibility of a 10-fold overdose exists.

- In newborns, heparin that is not preservative free may cause benzyl alcohol toxicity.

- Solutions of heparin may be extemporaneously prepared in various concentrations within the same facility. This may cause an error if a concentration is expressed in the order and it does not match the concentration supplied.

Aim: Reduce errors related to heparin delivery, reduce the variation in dosages used, and eliminate mix-ups with other medications.

Key Improvements:

- Standardize heparin solutions—use premixed solutions and reduce the number of concentrations available.

- Standardize administration procedures—place dose stickers on heparin bags and double-check all rate changes. If a bolus is ordered, give it from a syringe rather than temporarily modifying the rate of intravenous infusion.

- Differentiate products—use unit-dose syringes that look different from other parenteral products in routine use.

- Separate heparin, insulin, and other medications measured in units. Remove heparin from tops of medication carts and laminar flow hoods in the pharmacy.

- Standardize dosing using weight-based protocols:

  — Use the patient's actual weight as a basis for calculations.

  — Use standard dilutions; have the pharmacy place a label on each heparin bag that lists specific doses for each patient.

  — Double-check all dose calculations.

  — Draw blood for determination of activated partial thromboplastin time (aPTT) 6 hours after a rate change to determine the effects of the change.

  — Develop a standard format for making and communicating order changes to the pharmacy.

  — Double-check settings on infusion pumps after each rate change.

- Have infusion pump rate settings and line placement on dual-channel pumps independently checked by two persons.

- Develop and follow standard treatment guidelines.

- Use unit dose syringes that look different from those routinely used for other parenteral products.

- Purchase products that are well labeled. For optimal labeling, have the pharmacy place a label on both sides of the bag, taking care not to obscure the manufacturer's label. Have two people check the bag to ensure that labels are correct.

- If a bolus is needed, give it from a syringe rather than temporarily speeding up the pump rate.

- Do not use "U" for "units."
- Use only free-flow-protected pumps.

Measures:

- Determine percentage of aPTTs that are in the therapeutic range.
- Investigate reason for protamine use.
- Determine time until aPTT reaches therapeutic range in patients being initiated on heparin.
- Determine percentage of aPTTs over 100 for all patients on heparin.
- Determine rate of nonadherence to heparin protocols.
- Monitor patients to ensure correct infusion pump rate.
- Assure that heparin and insulin are not stored close to one another on drug carts, under the laminar flow hood, etc.

Hypertonic Saline

Problems:

- Rapid changes in serum sodium concentration caused by administration of nonisotonic saline are dangerous. This is particularly true when hypertonic saline is administered. Hypertonic sodium chloride injection is rarely necessary; nonetheless, this product is often kept on floor stocks in multiple concentrations. Five percent sodium chloride can be confused with 5% dextrose and sodium chloride. Three percent saline may be confused with 0.3% saline, which may be ordered as a nonstandard sodium chloride concentration. (Standard concentrations are dextrose with 0.2% sodium chloride injection and 0.45% and 0.9% sodium chloride injection, alone or in combination with dextrose.) Even the 3% product has 512 mEq/L, or 0.5 mEq/mL, of sodium.

- Pediatric ICUs may stock hypertonic sodium chloride in 23.4% or 14.6% concentrations for use in preparing enteral feedings. Dialysis units may use hypertonic solutions to increase blood volume and reduce cramping.

Aim: Reduce access to and use of hypertonic sodium chloride injection and restrict areas in which these products may be prepared.

Key Improvements:

- Allow only commercially available, standard concentrations of sodium chloride injection outside the pharmacy.
- Limit options—do not stock 5% sodium chloride injection.

- Set standards for administering concentrated sodium chloride solutions for use in treating hyponatremia. These standards should cover rate of administration and frequency of serum sodium monitoring.

- Limit titration of sodium for enteral feedings to the pharmacy. Remove from ICU stock.

- In dialysis units, stock a single concentration. Store in a locked area, limit access, and affix special hazard labeling.

Obstacles:

- Regulatory authorities have not established labeling standards to reduce medication errors associated with hypertonic forms.

- Nurses and others insist that concentrated forms be available.

Measures:

- Review the number of patients who receive hypertonic sodium chloride injection for hyponatremia.

- Monitor the availability of the product to ensure that it is available only in the pharmacy.

- Monitor use of the product in the pharmacy.

- Monitor to ensure proper storage and labeling in approved areas.

Insulin

Problems:

- Intravenous insulin is lethal if it is given in substantially excessive amounts or in place of other medications. Insulin and heparin are often mistaken for one another because both are administered in units and both may be stored in proximity to each other.

- Problems may arise when incorrect rates are programmed into an infusion pump.

- Overdoses have occurred when "U" is used as an abbreviation for "units" in orders: the "U" has been mistaken for an "O," resulting in a 10-fold overdose.

- Mix-ups may occur because of sound-alike names (e.g., Humalog® and Humulin®), multiple types of insulin (e.g., animal source and human source), and varying concentrations (e.g., U-500 and U-100).

- Insulin has been administered to the wrong patient.

Aim: Separate heparin and insulin, reduce the potential for errors associated with infusion pump administration, and eliminate incidents involving administration to the wrong patient and administration of the wrong form of the drug.

Key Improvements:

- Use "units" instead of "U."

- Store heparin and insulin separately, particularly in areas where they are used to prepare intravenous solutions (e.g., the pharmacy, intravenous admixture areas, and medication carts).

- Require two independent checks of all intravenous pump rate settings or rate changes involving insulin.

- Take precautions when writing and interpreting orders for insulin mixtures (e.g., Mixtard 70/30 premixed insulin).

- Standardize preparation and administration:

  — Never prepare U-100 insulin doses in tuberculin syringes. The metric scale may be confused with the apothecary scale (minims) on disposable syringes.

  — Use only a tuberculin syringe for U-500 insulin. If a U-100 syringe is used, doses may be incorrectly referred to on the basis of the U-100 scale. (A U-500 scale syringe is not available in the United States.)

- Since diabetic patients make errors with insulin because of poor eyesight, help them with tactile cues (e.g., place tape around regular insulin vials to differentiate them from NPH insulin). If necessary, diabetic patients may use their tongues rather than fingers to sense tactile differences.

- Caution patients that pharmacists may dispense the wrong type of insulin and that they should double-check their medication.

- Do not use slash marks to separate NPH and regular insulin doses. NPH 10/12 regular insulin has been confused with 10 NPH and 112 regular insulin because the slash mark was read as the numeral one (1).

- After dispensing insulin, do not place it back into the carton; this increases the risk that a vial will be returned to the wrong box (e.g., a vial of regular insulin placed into a box for NPH insulin), and the next person may automatically select the wrong product.

- Repeat all verbal (i.e., spoken) orders (e.g., say "one-six units" instead of "16 units"; otherwise, "sixteen" may sound like "sixty").

- Have nurses inform all alert patients that they are receiving insulin for diabetes. Patients not expecting this will immediately question the need.

- Use generic names to reduce confusion between brand names.

Obstacle: Following the procedures just described is time consuming.

Measures:

- Monitor and investigate all use of D50 injection or glucagon, which is likely to reflect hypoglycemia resulting from insulin overdose.

- Monitor and investigate all patients with serum glucose levels of less than 50 mg/dL by requiring automatic notification by the laboratory.

- Monitor adherence to protocols.

- Monitor drug storage methods in patient care areas.

- Monitor use of "U" in orders for insulin.

Oral Hypoglycemic Agents

Problems: Drug interactions are common with oral hypoglycemic agents. Warfarin, digoxin, thyroid medications, and beta-blockers are among the agents most frequently involved. This may worsen the hypoglycemia and alter the physiological response to it, thereby masking the symptoms. If physicians fail to adjust the dose with changes in diet or exercise, the patient may become hypoglycemic.

Aim: Reduce errors with hypoglycemics and improve patient compliance.

Key Improvements:

- Have pharmacy-managed diabetic clinics.

- Provide patient education by certified staff in a well-structured clinical setting.

- Increase patient monitoring through more frequent home visits or home testing.

Measures:

- Follow up on all uses of 50% dextrose and intravenous glucagon.

- Determine number of patients not taking medications as prescribed.

Potassium Chloride (KCl)

Problems:

- If potassium is injected too rapidly (i.e., at a rate exceeding 10 mEq of KCl infusion per hour) or in too high a dose, it may cause cardiac arrest. Potassium chloride should never be given as an intravenous push, and initiation of an infusion is never an emergency. Therefore, there is no need to store concentrated KCl outside of the pharmacy.

- Some doctors use the term "bolus" when ordering potassium at a rapid rate to treat acute hypokalemia. This term has been confused to mean that the dose should be given via intravenous push using a syringe.

Aim: Provide a method for administration that makes it nearly impossible for a patient to receive potassium chloride at a rate exceeding 10 mEq per hour.

Key Improvements:

- Remove all KCl vials from floor stock (including automated dispensing modules). Centralize intravenous KCl solution preparation in the pharmacy. Use premixed containers. Focus on timeliness of pharmacy preparation and delivery.

- If KCl must be left on floor stock, sequester it and treat it as a dangerous substance (see Note, page 5.32).

- Try to avoid mixing KCl extemporaneously. Purchase premixed solutions in 10-, 20-, and 40-mEq strengths in 50- to 100-mL minibags and large volume bags. Medical staff should work to standardize available solutions to ensure that premixed solutions maintained in the pharmacy or in patient care areas match the ordering preferences of prescribers.

- Standardize terminology. Do not use the term *bolus*.

- Use protocols for KCl delivery, including

    — when intravenous KCl is indicated (e.g., patient's serum potassium is <2.8, patient is on diuretics or other potassium-wasting medications),

    — maximum rate of intravenous delivery,

    — maximum allowable concentration,

    — guidelines for when continuous cardiac monitoring is necessary,

    — stipulation that KCl be given via a pump or other suitable infusion control device,

    — prohibition of delivery of multiple simultaneous KCl solutions (e.g., no intravenous KCl while KCl is being infused via TPN; Ringer's solution contains 4 mEq of potassium per liter),

— allowance for automatic substitution of oral KCl for intravenous KCl by pharmacy when appropriate, and

— use of preprinted potassium management order forms.

Obstacles:

• Nurses like the independence of having KCl available on the floor.

• Physicians desire KCl "riders."

• Access to product when pharmacy is not open 24 hours a day.

• Resource issues arise if the pharmacy cannot respond to intravenous KCl requests in a timely manner.

• ICU concern that intravenous KCl be given immediately.

• Perceived need for intravenous rather than oral potassium replacement.

Measures:

• Determine percentage of health care providers adhering to KCl guidelines.

• Determine rate of intravenous and oral KCl use and number of patients receiving intravenous KCl who could be treated with oral KCl.

• Monitor for adverse patient outcomes such as phlebitis and extravasation, increased length of stay, incidence of hyperkalemia (serum potassium >5.x after potassium replacement), incidence of hypokalemia after potassium delivery, use of Kayexalate®, use of intravenous insulin and glucose to treat hyperkalemia.

• These measures could be obtained by chart review on selected patients with hypokalemia, intermittent checks of patients receiving intravenous KCl, or review of laboratory data and pharmacy records.

• Track incidence of use of "bolus" in orders for rapid intravenous potassium replacement.

Lidocaine

Problems:

• Lidocaine mix-ups have occurred when lidocaine and heparin are obtained from a single manufacturer because their labeling is similar. Errors have occurred when 50-mL vials of lidocaine were confused with other drugs available in 50-mL vials (e.g., sodium bicarbonate, mannitol, and 50% dextrose).

Preventing Deaths from Potassium Chloride Concentrate

Direct injection of potassium chloride concentrate has resulted in numerous accidental deaths over the years. Because the most effective way to prevent this unnecessary tragedy is to remove the concentrate from patient care areas, we surveyed U.S. hospitals in January and February 1998 to determine how the medication is stored in these institutions. We received 449 usable responses, which represents slightly over 10% of our sampling size of 4000 hospitals. To ensure that respondents were not a biased group, we surveyed an additional random sample of 50 nonresponders by telephone. Since their answers were remarkably similar to those of our initial responders, we combined the data for a total of 499 responses.

We are encouraged by the responses. Whereas 10 years ago the opposite probably would have been true, most respondents now indicate that they have removed potassium concentrate from most patient care units. Areas where the concentrate is still stored include adult intensive care units and emergency departments. The exact percentages are listed in Table 5–5. Of the hospitals that volunteered information about additional storage sites, many reported that the concentrate is still stocked in the operating room and on dialysis units.

If the concentrate is stored in patient care areas, many respondents state that it is locked in a cabinet (sometimes a code cart) or automated dispensing unit. Some use special warning labels (for example, "must dilute"), place the concentrate in a zip-lock bag, or require nurses to sign it out. However, some still store the drug in nursing unit stock without special conditions for storage.

The reason that many respondents (331 of 382; 87%) removed the concentrate from most patient care areas was that they had read or heard about the potential for serious error. Others said that a "near miss" had occurred in their institution (19 of 382; 5%) or that an actual error had occurred that resulted in patient harm or death (11 of 382; 3%). Instead of the concentrate, most respondents supply patient care units with premixed mini bags and large-volume bags. The pharmacy prepares any unusual concentrations. Other pharmacies (54 of 381; 14%) send unit doses of the concentrate for specific patient orders.

The major reasons cited for not removing the concentrate from most patient care areas were opposition from nurses or physicians, no problems in the past, and lack of a 24-hour pharmacy. Cost concerns played a very minor role. It appears that most institutions have decided that storing potassium chloride concentrate injection in patient care areas is not a safe practice. However, there are still institutions that have decided to continue to store it outside the pharmacy and, even in some hospitals that have taken action, there are still areas of risk, such as adult intensive care units and emergency departments.

In addition, although absent from unit stock, vials of the concentrate are dispensed in unit dose fashion in individual patient bins, along with intravenous flush solutions. This practice is even more dangerous than providing potassium vials in unit stock because it makes it easier for a mix-up to occur. Although warning labels and special storage for potassium chloride concentrate injection are helpful, removing it from all nonessential areas is more effective. It is safest to stock premixed piggyback and large-volume bags in patient care areas, even in institutions without 24-hour pharmacy services. To minimize requests for unusual concentrations, pharmacists should work with the Pharmacy and Therapeutics Committee to develop a protocol that standardizes intravenous potassium concentrations and base solutions, favoring commercially available premixed solutions.

Table 5-5

Results of hospital survey on stocking of potassium chloride

Location[a]	Fax Results		Telephone Results		Combined	
	Present	Not present	Present	Not Present	Present	Not present
Adult medical/ surgical unit	25%	75%	24%	76%	25%	75%
Pediatrics	10%	90%	10%	90%	10%	90%
Neonatal	8%	92%	3%	97%	7%	93%
Adult ICU	41%	59%	50%	50%	41%	59%
Pediatric ICU	12%	88%	9%	91%	12%	88%
Neonatal ICU	13%	87%	7%	93%	13%	87%
Ambulatory units	8%	92%	7%	93%	8%	92%
Emergency department	44%	56%	30%	70%	43%	57%
Pharmacy	97%	3%	100%	0%	98%	2%

[a] ICU = Intensive Care Unit

Note ! (continued)

The February 27, 1998 edition of *Sentinel Event Alert*, published by the Joint Commission on Accreditation of Healthcare Organizations (JCAHO), suggests removal of potassium chloride injection concentrate from patient care areas. JCAHO has shared information about potassium errors with their surveyors, and the institution's approach to safe handling of potassium chloride injection concentrate may be among the probing questions during the survey. In addition, the U.S. Department of Veterans Affairs notified all Veterans Administration hospitals that the drug is to be removed immediately from all wards, intensive care units, surgical suites, and similar sites, encouraging the use of pre-mixed solutions instead.

- Multidose vials of lidocaine used as a local anesthetic may be contaminated as a result of poor aseptic technique.[7]

- Problems may arise because of misunderstanding how topical lidocaine is absorbed.

- The use of topical (viscous) lidocaine in the oral cavity for painful mouth lesions has caused aspiration due to oropharyngeal anesthesia and loss of sensation of food bolus that may be present in the oral cavity.

Aim: Reduce the potential for mix-ups, increase recognition of the risk of topical lidocaine absorption, and decrease the possibility of vial contamination.

Key Improvements:

- Use lidocaine only in single-dose vials. Do not place vials that hold more than 500 mg in patient care areas. Single-dose vials reduce the risk of overdose and eliminate the risk of contamination.

- Use premixed, adequately labeled solutions for all cardiology patients.

Obstacles:

- Economic constraints may force hospitals to use multiple-dose containers in patient care areas.

- Not all manufacturers use safe labeling practices for premixed intravenous lidocaine.

- There is a lack of education about the possibility of absorption after topical application.

Measures:

- Monitor compliance with protocols.

- Monitor compliance with restricted storage of multiple-dose vials, if applicable.

Intravenous Magnesium

Problems:

- Errors have resulted from mix-ups between the abbreviations "MS" or "MSO$_4$" for morphine sulfate and "MgSO$_4$" for magnesium sulfate.

- Other terminology problems have also led to errors; for example, "mg" (milligrams) and "mL" (milliliters) are confused, as are "mg" and "mEq" (milliequivalents).

• Infusion pump settings errors have led to fatal overdoses with free-flow intravenous solutions.

• Health professionals are often unaware that an excessive dose has been ordered and administer an overdose.

Aim: Prevent the use of erroneous terminology and reduce the possibility of overdose.

Key Improvements:

• Require protocols for the use of magnesium.

• Educate staff about proper dosing during orientation and in-service training.

• Establish and publicize maximum doses (e.g., post wall charts in pharmacy, enter dose maximums in computer).

• Do not permit the use of abbreviations for morphine and magnesium.

• Store containers holding more than 2 mL only in the pharmacy.

• Use only premixed containers for patients on intravenous magnesium replacement therapy and for women with preeclampsia.

• Standardize ordering methods (i.e., either in grams or milliequivalents).

• Require independent, redundant checks of all calculations, dose preparations, and infusion pump settings.

• Recognize the need for addressing problems relating to infusion pumps.

Measures:

• Test employee knowledge of proper magnesium dosing.

• Establish and monitor adherence to guidelines for magnesium administration.

• Monitor the inappropriate use of abbreviations in records of patients for whom magnesium sulfate has been prescribed.

Narcotics and Opiates

Problems:

• Narcotic accidents are among the most frequent of all serious incidents reported. One reason for errors with these drugs is that parenteral narcotics are usually stored in nursing areas as floor stock items. Doses are often identified, prepared, and administered by a single nurse; no redundant safety checks are performed.

- Mix-ups between hydromorphone and morphine are common. Hydromorphone is five times more potent than morphine.

- Oral liquid morphine may be consumed with the less concentrated forms, leading to overdoses.

- PCA accidents may involve errors in concentration, rate, drug, and route. PCA use by patients and their families may be problematic when, believing that the patient is in pain, families may activate the PCA.

- PCA and epidural lines are sometimes confused, leading to errors in route of administration.

- Allergic reactions are common.

- Pump-related errors have occurred.

Aim: Reduce errors associated with overdose of opiates, incorrect routes of administration, pump-related accidents, and opiate-related allergies.

Key Improvements:

- Educate staff about the possibility of mix-ups between hydromorphone and concentrated morphine.

- Standardize concentrations of intravenous solutions.

- Minimize the amount of drug in a single container.

- Ensure that naloxone or an equivalent is available in areas where narcotics are administered.

- Limit oral liquid items available in floor stock to conventional concentrations. Stock concentrated oral morphine and hydromorphone only in areas where patients with chronic pain are treated.

- Do not use potentially confusing abbreviations such as "$MgSO_4$" (magnesium sulfate) and "MSO_4" (morphine sulfate).

- Address concerns about unsafe parenteral infusion of these drugs.

- Implement protocols for the use of PCA and epidural medications that ensure independent double-checks of the appropriateness of drug, dose, pump setting, and line placement.

- Label the distal ends of epidural lines and intravenous lines to differentiate them.

- Question all patients receiving opiates about allergies.

- Use only generic names.

Obstacles:

- Untrained staff may be administering these products.

- Infusion control devices may be unsafe.

Measures:

- Determine number of patients admitted to the ICU as a result of narcotic-related problems.

- Monitor administration (pharmacy should monitor preparations, overall use, degree of analgesia or somnolence).

- Follow up on all uses of naloxone to determine if a narcotic error has occurred.

- Determine percentage of adherence to administration protocols, including the use of PCA.

Neuromuscular Blocking Agents

Problems:

- Outside of the operating room (e.g., in the emergency department, radiology department, or ICU), neuromuscular blocking agents have been inadvertently used in patients who are not receiving proper ventilatory assistance. Because their respiratory muscles are paralyzed, these patients may experience respiratory arrest. Some patients have died or have been permanently harmed.

- Patients have been extubated while an order for one of these agents still exists.

- Vials of neuromuscular blockers have been mixed up with other agents, such as vaccines.

Aim: Eliminate the potential for administration errors.

Key Improvements:

- Educate staff about past problems.

- Standardize ordering; do not allow "use as needed for agitation" orders. Never refer to neuromuscular blockers as "relaxants."

- Develop protocols to ensure proper storage and administration. These protocols should stipulate that neuromuscular blockers must be automatically discontinued when the patient is extubated and removed from a ventilator.

- Implement warnings to staff of potential adverse effects. For example, some hospitals place signs near where products are stored. Some place labels reading "WARNING: PARALYZING AGENT" on drug vials. Some manufacturers place these warnings prominently on package labels. Use these brands wherever possible.

- Limit access; neuromuscular blockers are best handled by anesthesia personnel.

- Do not store these agents outside of critical care areas.

- If they must be stored elsewhere, take precautions to reduce the possibility of mix-up with other agents (e.g., do not store neuromuscular blockers and vaccine products near one another in a refrigerator).

Measures:

- Test employee knowledge of proper use of these drugs.

- Check supplies to ensure proper auxiliary labeling (i.e., "WARNING: PARALYZING AGENT").

- Monitor to ensure drug is stored properly.

Phosphate Salts (Sodium and Potassium)

Problems:

- Phosphate is often given intravenously as potassium phosphate. The person ordering the phosphate may fail to consider the amount of potassium in the product.

- Commercially available vials may be labeled as "single dose." This may be misleading because the vials come in various sizes and some of them may contain several doses.

- Some prescribers order phosphate in terms of "amps" or "vials" rather than amount (expressed in millimoles [mmol]).

Aim: Reduce the potential for a potassium overdose associated with the administration of potassium phosphate.

Key Improvements:

- Educate staff about past problems.

- Administer phosphate replacement therapy via the oral route whenever possible.

- Use sodium phosphate instead of potassium phosphate when possible.

- Store intravenous potassium solution only in the pharmacy.

- Monitor patients' electrolytes; perform electrocardiography.

- Use guidelines for potassium phosphate administration based on patient's level of inorganic phosphate and other clinical factors (e.g., weight or age). The normal dose should not exceed 0.32 mmol/kg over 12 hours, repeated until serum phosphate is greater than 2 mg/dL.

- Use strict criteria for delivery rates when administering intravenous phosphate. Deliver via a pump.

Obstacles:

- Poor labeling of commercial products.

- Confusion among milliliters (mL), moles (mol), milliequivalents (mEq), and milligrams (mg) amounts listed on labeling.

Measures:

- Establish protocols.

- Intermittently monitor intravenous phosphate administration to ensure compliance with protocols.

- Review number of orders not using standard terminology, based on documentation of past and present patient records.

- Test employee knowledge of proper dosing and administration.

Warfarin

Problems:

- Improper dose adjustments.

- Failure to appreciate drug and food interactions.

- Improper monitoring of prothrombin time/international normalization ratio (PT/INR).

Aim: Decrease medication errors with oral agents. Increase percentage of patients whose INR falls within therapeutic range.

Key Improvements:

- Use pharmacy-run anticoagulation clinics.

- Provide patient education by certified staff in a structured setting.

- Increase monitoring (e.g., more frequent clinic visits or home testing).

Measures:

- Screen patients receiving warfarin whose PT/INRs are unduly high or low.

- Monitor the use of vitamin K.

- Examine all warfarin-associated admissions by screening for admission PTs/INRs that are out of the normal range.

• • • •
References

1. Cohen MR, Senders J, Davis NM. Failure mode and effects analysis: a novel approach to avoiding dangerous medication errors and accidents. *Hosp Pharm.* 1994; 29: 319–24, 326–28, 330.

2. Leape LL. Error in medicine. *JAMA.* 1994; 272: 1851–57.

3. Cohen MR, Davis NM. Developing safe and effective preprinted physician's order forms. *Hosp Pharm.* 1992; 27: 508, 513, 528.

4. Lacy C, Armstrong LL, Ingrim N, et al. *Drug Information Handbook.* 4th ed. Hudson, Ohio: Lexi-Comp; 1996.

5. Olin B, ed. *Drug Facts and Comparisons.* St. Louis, Mo: Facts and Comparisons; 1997.

6. McEvoy GK, ed. *AHFS Drug Information.* Bethesda, Md: American Society of Health-System Pharmacists; 1996.

7. Prott RT, Wagner RF, Trying SK. Iatrogenic contamination of multidose vials in simulated use. *Arch Dermatol.* 1990; 126: 1441–44.

Medication Errors Research

Elizabeth Allan Flynn, PhD
Kenneth N. Barker, PhD

Auburn University
Auburn, Ala.

Progress in improving medication distribution systems has now been traced for more than four decades. The goals of this research have been to measure medication error rates, compare the accuracy of different drug distribution systems, identify the causes of errors, and evaluate the effectiveness of error detection techniques. Research has revealed how often errors occur, what changes in the medication distribution system can decrease errors, and what factors affect error rates. Preliminary work has been done on the effect of automated drug dispensing devices on error rates.

The objectives of this chapter are to (1) describe the significance and frequency of medication errors, (2) summarize the nomenclature used in the medication error literature and the methods used to study medication errors, (3) critique medication error studies published in the past four decades, (4) review factors associated with medication errors that have been identified through research, and (5) demonstrate how error detection techniques have been applied in various settings. The chapter concludes with some research-based recommendations for error prevention.

Significance of Medication Errors

Clinical Significance

Several investigators have rated the severity of medication errors according to the potential for harm, based on their association with drugs of particular pharmacological categories. Barker and colleagues[1] classified 66.1% of 653 errors (excluding wrong-time errors) detected as "serious." ("Wrong-time" errors occur when a patient receives a dose outside of an acceptable time frame, such as within 30 minutes of the time the dose is due. Wrong-time errors are typically reported separately from other errors because some do not consider them significant.) Other investigators have reported similar results.[2–4]

Schnell[5] rated the clinical severity of individual errors on a scale of 0 to 100 according to the error category to which they were assigned. For example, wrong-dose errors received a rating of 80, whereas wrong-time errors received a score of 20. The clinical significance indices ranged from 28.0 to 47.1 when wrong-time errors were included and from 63.0 to 73.5 when wrong-time errors were excluded. These data were based on information from four hospitals and include both traditional and unit-dose drug distribution systems. There were no differences in the clinical significance ratings between the two types of systems.

Economic Significance

The economic consequences of medication errors include extended hospital stays, additional treatment, and malpractice litigation. Schneider and colleagues[6] reported that the mean cost of medication errors and adverse drug reactions at a university hospital ranged from $95 (for extra laboratory tests) to $2640 (for intensive care). The total cost of medication-related problems at that hospital in 1994 was estimated to be $1.5 million.[6] The cost of a single error as seemingly insignificant as administering glyburide 5 mg instead of diazepam 5 mg was measured at $13,941.72.[7]

Hynniman and coworkers[8] calculated the cost benefits of various drug distribution systems. They proposed that the ultimate criterion for evaluating the expense of a medication system should be the cost per dose delivered correctly. Results showed that a hospital with a unit-dose drug distribution system had a per-dose cost of $0.33 and an error rate of 3.5%. In a hospital with a floor stock system, the per-dose cost was similar ($0.32); however, the error rate was 11.5%. Three hospitals had a prescription order system; the cost per dose ranged from $0.38 to $0.54, and the error rates ranged from 8.3% to 20.6%. Other cost comparisons between drug distribution systems support the hypothesis that, when nursing and pharmacy costs are considered, the unit-dose system is the least expensive.[9,10]

The average indemnity payment for claims related to medication errors between 1985 and 1992 was $99,721.[11] Most medication error-related claims are settled out of court for much larger amounts.[12]

Frequency of Medication Errors

Table 6–1 presents a summary of error rates measured by observational studies of the medication administration process. (Observation is an error detection method that is described in detail later in this chapter.) On the basis of a number of studies, Barker and colleagues[13] estimated that errors (excluding wrong-time errors) occur at a rate of about one error per patient per day. However, error rates as low as two to three per patient per week have been achieved after the installation of unit-dose systems. Comparison of error rates reported by various studies should be made cautiously because of differences in error category definitions and methodologies. For example, some researchers define wrong-time errors as administration of a dose 30 minutes before or after it is due, whereas others use a range of 60 minutes.

Rates of pharmacy errors involving doses dispensed during the cart-filling process (termed *picking errors*) range from 0.04% to 2.9%.[14–20] Some state boards of pharmacy allow technicians to check other technicians after filling patient medication drawers instead of requiring that a pharmacist perform this task.[21] A comparison of the accuracy of checking unit-dose medication drawers by technicians and pharmacists found that the error rates by each group were similar. Both identified a cart-filling error rate of 1.2%; however, pharmacists overlooked more errors than did technicians.[22] The percentage of missed errors that could have resulted in patient harm was not significantly different in the two groups (25.2% for pharmacists and 32.0% for technicians); however, pharmacists overlooked 27 potentially serious errors, whereas technicians overlooked 16. A certification program for hospital pharmacy technicians to perform unit-dose cart checking has been described elsewhere.[23]

The source of information on medication profiles used in checking the carts has also been studied. A study of the rates of missing doses documented a decrease from 0.93% to 0.33% when nursing and pharmacy personnel checked the cart against the patient's medication administration record (MAR).[24]

Error rates in prescription-filling operations for ambulatory patients are summarized in Table 6–2. The rate of errors that could have had potentially harmful effects ranged from 1.5% to 4%.[25–27]

Table 6-1

Inpatient medication administration error rates in observation-based research

Year	Setting	TOE[b]	Error Rates (%)[a]		Drug Distribution Center		
			With wrong-time errors	Without wrong-time errors	Unit dose	Includes automation	Other
1962[33]			16.2	14.7			X
1964[34]	UAMC* pilot: before unit dose	1313	16.1	14.4			X
	UAMC* pilot: after unit dose	1124	7.2[c]	1.8[c]	X		
1966[1]	General hospital	9789	15.0	6.7			X
1967[85]	University of Iowa before DUDD*	6806	17.7[d,e]	0.4			X
	University of Iowa after DUDD*	11,001	8.8[d,e]	0.9	X		
1969[84]	UAMC* before unit dose	11,015	25.9	13.0			X
	UAMC* after unit dose	3043	12.0[c]	1.9[c]	X		
1970[2]	University of Kentucky	6061	f	3.5	X		X
	Kentucky Hospital A	1921	f	8.3			X
	Kentucky Hospital B	788	f	9.9			X
	Kentucky Hospital C	1432	f	11.5			X
	Kentucky Hospital D	1279	f	20.6			
1971[106]	North Carolina nursing home	235	59.1	24.7			X
	North Carolina nursing home	289	49.5	21.1			X
	North Carolina nursing home after unit dose	351	1.7	1.4	X		
1973[86]	Ohio State: Nurse administration	3678	f	5.3	X		
	Ohio State: Pharmacy technician administration	3447	f	0.6[c]	X[g]		
1975[88]	Johns Hopkins Hospital before unit dose	1428	f	7.3[h]			X
	Johns Hopkins Hospital after unit dose	1243	f	1.6[c,h]	X		
1976[5]	Canadian hospital A before unit dose	3123	37.2	8.9[c]			X
	Canadian hospital A after unit dose	3235	38.5	14.6	X		
	Canadian hospital B before unit dose	3443	42.9	14.5			X
	Canadian hospital B after unit dose	3069	23.3[c]	12.9[i]	X		
	Canadian hospital C before unit dose	3103	20.1	7.7			X
	Canadian hospital C after unit dose	2883	7.8[c]	2.0[c]	X		
	Canadian hospital D before unit dose	3134	38.5	9.6			X
	Canadian hospital D after unit dose	4445	23.1[c]	3.7[c]	X		
1976[40]	16 hospitals <100 beds	1197	24.6	17.5	i		
1982[109]	58 long-term care facilities	3051	f	12.2	i		
	10 hospitals with <150 beds	425	f	11.0	i		

Table 6-1 (continued)

1982[110]	Skilled nursing facility	415	34.2	4.8			X
	Skilled nursing facility	417	18	4.8			X
1984[12]	Sinai Hospital	2018	36.8	9.0	X		
1984[91]	Sinai Hospital: reevaluation	781	41.8	10.2	X		
	Sinai Hospital: reevaluation, after improvements	1003	40.3	12.3[i]	X		
1984[13]	Hospital with decentralized pharmacy system	873	15.9	6.7	X		
	Automated bedside device	902	10.6[c]	5.2[i]		X	
1986[4]	Intensive care nursery	389[k]	17.0	6.9			X
	Pediatric intensive care	231[k]	35.1	10.8			X
1987[35]	Ohio State: administration by technician	2028	4.4	1.6	X		
1991[111]	Pediatric hospital before unit dose (included left-at-bedside doses)	282	37.2[h]	10.3[h]			X
	Pediatric hospital after unit dose (included left-at-bedside doses)	241	21.2[h]	2.9[h]	X		
1994[95]	Long-term care facility, blister card	286[l]	2.1	1.4			X
	Long-term care facility, single unit-dose packaging	287	0	0		ATC Plus	
	Long-term care facility, multidose packaging	265	0	0		ATC Plus	
1995[57]	Teaching hospital	873	16.9	6.5		Medstation	
	Teaching hospital	929	10.4	2.0		Medstation Rx	
1995[112]	Long-term care facilities, before nurse education	Not reported	10.6	Not reported		Not reported	
	Long-term care facilities, after nurse education	Not reported	2.9	Not reported		Not reported	
1995[94]	British hospital, ward-based floor stock	2756	Not studied	3.0			X
	American hospital	919	Not studied	6.9		X	

*Abbreviations: DUDD = decentralized unit-dose dispensing; UAMC = University of Arkansas Medical Center.

[a] Percentage of total opportunities for error (TOE).

[b] Total opportunities for error.

[c] This value is significantly lower than the measurement for other drug distribution systems in the study at the $P \leq .05$ level of significance.

[d] In order to increase the comparability to other studies, these figures combine errors and discrepancies, but exclude "Left-at-bedside" discrepancies.

[e] Statistical analyses were not performed in this study.

[f] Wrong-time errors were not measured.

[g] Fifty percent of the packages used by nurses were in unit-dose form.

[h] Excludes omission errors.

[i] There was no significant difference between this value and its comparison value.

[j] Multiple drug distribution systems are included. The error rate is an average value.

[k] TOE Modified = number of omission errors added to doses administered and error rates recalculated from data in the study.

[l] Number of routine orders reported. The number of TOEs was calculated by dividing the number of errors by the error rate reported (6 errors divided by 0.021 = 286 opportunities for error).

Type of Pharmacy	No. of Errors	No. of Prescriptions	Dispensing Error Rate (%)
Community pharmacy: Patient follow-up[113]	29	223	13
Ambulatory pharmacy:[80]			
Pharmacists	48	929	5
Technicians	44	1055	4
Ambulatory pharmacy, teaching hospital[45]	1085	9394	12
High-volume military ambulatory pharmacy[81]	369	10,889	3
Ambulatory pharmacy[82]	37	3227	1
Ambulatory pharmacy[83]	195	5072	3
Ambulatory pharmacy[26]	552	9846	6
Community pharmacies[27,b]	24	100	24

[a] Studies were reviewed and error categories that were common to each study were included in the table to increase the comparability.

[b] Study was limited to having one of three different sample prescriptions filled a total of 100 times.

Nomenclature

Because various definitions have been used in medication error research, a common frame of reference is needed. The following definitions are used in this chapter:

- *Drug misadventure* is a broad label applied to adverse drug reactions, prescribing errors, and medication errors.[28,29]

- *Adverse drug events* are injuries from a drug-related intervention. They can include prescribing errors, dispensing errors, and medication administration errors.[30]

- A *medication error* is a deviation from the prescriber's handwritten or typed medication order or from the order that the prescriber has entered into the computer system.[1] Medication errors are typically viewed as related to administration of a medication, but they can also include errors in ordering or delivering medication.[31]

- *Dispensing errors* are deviations from the prescriber's order, made by staff in the pharmacy when distributing medications to nursing units or to patients in an ambulatory pharmacy setting.

- *Prescribing errors* are mistakes made by the prescriber when ordering a medication (e.g., miscalculating a chemotherapy dose).

Barker et al.[1] coined the phrase *opportunity for error* (OE) as the basic unit of data in error studies. An OE includes any dose given as well as any dose ordered but omitted. Because the dose in any given OE must be either correct or incorrect (i.e., either it is or is not an error), the error rate cannot exceed 100%. An OE includes only those doses of medication whose preparation and administration are both witnessed by an observer.

The following three situations are typically not counted as OEs:

1. A drug is left at the patient's bedside for self-administration, and its consumption is not observed.

2. A dose is associated with a written order uninterpretable by the observer.

3. A dose has been prepared and administered by a new nurse employee who is still learning the procedures, by a private duty nurse, or by a nursing student.

As defined by Barker et al.,[1] *total opportunities for error* (TOE) is the sum of all doses ordered and all unordered doses given. Studies may also define the TOE as all doses administered plus all doses omitted (i.e., ordered but not given), which leads to the same results.[32]

The *medication error rate* is the number of opportunities for error that are incorrect (in one or more ways), divided by the TOE. This figure is multiplied by 100 to arrive at a percentage.[1]

When reviewing studies, one must note the source of data on medication error rates. The Joint Commission on Accreditation of Healthcare Organizations (JCAHO) is testing an indicator that uses the number of reported medication errors divided by the total number of doses dispensed. This will result in a much different error rate than that which emerges when the number of observed errors is divided by the TOE.

Types of Medication Errors

Medication errors can be categorized by type. The categories are not always mutually exclusive; therefore, rates for different error types cannot always be simply added to obtain an overall error rate. The following terms must be borne in mind.

An *unordered* or *unauthorized drug error* (wrong-drug error) is the administration of a dose of medication that was never ordered for that patient.

An *extra-dose error* is a dose given in excess of the total number of times ordered by the physician, such as a dose given on the basis of an expired order, after a drug has been discontinued, or after a drug has been put on hold. For example, if a physician orders a drug to be given only in the morning and the patient receives a dose in the evening as well, an extra-dose error has occurred.

An *omission error* is noted if a patient fails to receive a dose of medication that was ordered by the time the next dose is due. If the patient refuses the medication, it is not generally counted as an OE. Doses withheld according to policy (e.g., "nothing by mouth before surgery") are not counted as errors or OEs. The observer detects omissions by comparing the medications administered at a given time with doses that should have been given at that time, based on the physician's written orders. If a dose was not given, an omission error is counted, barring another explanation.

A *wrong-dose* or *wrong-strength error* occurs when any administered dose contains the wrong number of preformed dosage units (such as tablets) or is, in the judgment of the observer, more than 17% greater or less than the correct dosage. (Seventeen percent is typical of the accuracy of measuring devices used in hospitals.) Some researchers use a narrower definition of wrong-dose errors for injectable doses that are measured by the nurse (e.g., any dose that is more than 5% or 10% different from the correct dosage would be in error).[1,5,33–35] In judging dosage, measuring devices provided for routine use by the institution (e.g., gradations on syringes and on medicine cups) are deemed acceptable. Wrong-dose errors are counted for ointments, topical solutions, and similar medications only when the dose was quantitatively specified by the physician (e.g., in inches of ointment).

Wrong-route errors occur when a medication is administered by a route that is different from the one ordered. Included in this category are doses given in the wrong site (e.g., the right ear instead of the left).

Wrong-time errors are defined as the administration of a dose more than 30 minutes before or after the scheduled time of administration in the absence of an acceptable reason. Acceptable reasons include situations in which a physician has ordered that a patient not consume anything by mouth, or when the patient is not in his or her room because of undergoing a procedure elsewhere in the hospital. As-needed (prn) doses should be administered no closer together than ordered. The time of administration of the previous prn dose is noted from the observer's notes, the MAR, or information in an automated drug dispensing device. The hospital's schedule is used to determine the time at which a dose should be given.

The schedule programmed into the pharmacy's computer system may be used to define correct administration times. If the physician did not record the time at which an order was written, wrong-time errors should not be recorded for doses given on that day until a second dose is given. The first dose given according to the standard administration schedule is considered to establish the schedule in effect, and subsequent doses on the same day may then be examined for wrong-time errors. Although each hospital may determine its own acceptable time range for administration of a dose, 30 minutes is commonly used because it has been shown that nurses can usually administer all their medications within 1 hour.[1]

A *wrong dosage-form error* is the administration of a dose in a form that is different from that ordered by the physician (e.g., giving a tablet when a suspension was ordered). Instances in which tablets are crushed are not considered wrong dosage-form errors because of the lack of information on the effects of crushing on the effectiveness of most tablets. Crushing an extended-release tablet is considered a wrong dosage-form error if it is likely that the timing of the release of the drug has been destroyed.

Deviations that do not fall into any of the above categories may be classified as "other." For example, the wrong rate of administration, wrong technique, or wrong preparation method may be placed in the "other" category if such errors are infrequent.[36]

The number of times in which each error category defined here was used has been reported for 14 observation-based studies.[36] The most commonly used error categories can be determined from this report and used in future studies.

Methods Used to Detect Medication Errors

Administration-based error rates detected by observation are one measure of the quality of drug distribution systems. Although JCAHO prefers such outcome-based measurements,[37] there are other ways to measure quality. For example, one may use structure criteria or process criteria.[38] Donabedian's model[39] theorizes a relationship between structure and outcome measures. There is evidence that compliance with certain structure standards is negatively correlated with observation-based error rates. Brown and coworkers[40] found high error rates in hospitals with low compliance scores, and vice versa. A correlation between structure and process criteria has been demonstrated in a community pharmacy.[41]

The next section of this chapter discusses the following six techniques for detecting medication administration errors:

1. anonymous self-reports,

2. incident reports,

3. the critical incident technique,

4. chart review,

5. direct observation,

6. a combination of self-report and observation.

Other techniques include urinalysis (which can detect the presence of unauthorized drugs[42] or the absence of ordered drugs), omission error detection (which is based on doses returned on the medication cart[43,44]), and examination of death certificates.[45]

Anonymous Self-Reports

Anonymous self-report methods provide a means by which the person committing or witnessing an error can report the mistake without being associated with it.[33] Advantages of this method are its low cost and the ability of staff to avoid the fear of disciplinary action. An important limitation of the self-report method is that the person witnessing the error cannot report it unless he or she is aware that a mistake was made. One study found that even if the nurse is aware of an error, he or she probably will not report it if:[33]

- a physician advises against reporting the error,

- the nurse believes that the error will not lead to patient harm, or

- the error is an omission or wrong-time error.

An ethnomethodological study by Baker[46] found that nurses would not report certain errors based on the following agreed-upon redefinitions of errors:

1. If it's not my fault, it's not an error.

2. If everyone knows, it is not an error.

3. If you can put it right, it is not an error.

4. If a patient has needs that are more urgent than the accurate administration of medication, it is not an error.

5. A clerical error is not a medication error.

6. If an irregularity is carried out to prevent something worse, it is not an error.

Barker and McConnell[33] discovered that only six anonymous reports of medication errors were filed over a 7-month period in a university hospital. Forty percent of the nurses in this study opposed this reporting method.

Incident Reports

An incident report is a written legal report of a medication error that has been documented by hospital staff. Hospital personnel who detect a medication error typically complete a form (required by the hospital) to report the incident. Guidelines, recommendations, and forms for reporting incidents are available.[47–53]

Medication error reports are collected and analyzed on national and international levels by the U.S. Pharmacopeia and the Institute for Safe Medication Practices. (More information can be obtained by calling 1-800-23-ERROR or at <www.usp.org> or <www.ismp.org> on the World Wide Web.)

One advantage of incident reports is that they provide an ongoing reporting mechanism for an entire hospital.[51] Observation, by contrast, typically samples only selected time periods in certain patient care areas. Some believe that the incident report method incurs lower costs than the observation method.[54] However, Shannon and DeMuth[55] found that the time per patient required for the observation of 20 patients was significantly less than that for incident report review. Brown[56] calculated that completing and analyzing one incident report in 1979 cost $6.71.

To submit an incident report, staff must be aware that an error has occurred. Research has shown that nurses are rarely aware of errors. It is possible that errors may be considerably underreported, resulting in a false sense of security. Barker and McConnell[33] demonstrated the inadequacy of incident reports as an error detection method. They found that incident reports documented 36 errors over a 1-year period. By comparison, 2 weeks' worth of data collected by direct observation on day, evening, and night shifts, when extrapolated over the same period, indicated that 51,200 errors may have occurred. In brief, the observation technique is capable of detecting far more errors than the incident report method.

Shannon and DeMuth[55] compared a combination of reviews of charts and incident reports with the observation method. Each method was performed simultaneously in a long-term care facility. Their results confirmed the earlier work of Barker and McConnell.[33] The observation method detected a mean error rate of 9.6%, whereas the paper review method yielded a mean error rate of 0.2%.

Other investigators have compared the number of incident reports filed with the number of errors detected by observation and have produced similar results.[1,12,31,57] In one study,[58] investigators considered the value of using error rates based on incident reports to evaluate the quality of drug distribution in hospitals and concluded that such analyses would not be meaningful.

Fear of disciplinary action is a deterrent to incident reporting.[51,59,60] Examples of punishments for administration errors vary widely and include remedial education,[51] counseling,[52,61,62] temporarily giving up one's nursing cap,[63] suspension without pay,[61] and termination of employment.[61,64,65] Some authors advise against associating any type of discipline with incident reporting.[51,60,66] Disciplinary action for dispensing errors is also controversial, especially when one considers that the error could be caused by poor system design. Recommendations for administering discipline have been published elsewhere.[67–69]

Critical Incident Technique

The critical incident technique is an event sampling method that involves in-depth analyses of a high number of individual errors with the goal of identifying common causes.[70–72] This method can involve direct observation of subjects or interviews of people who have committed an error. The sample size required for this type of research ranges from one hundred to several thousand critical incidents and is based on the complexity of the behavior being evaluated. The minimum sample size is reached when no new causes are observed and there are at least three examples in each error cause category.[73] Categories are formed by identifying common characteristics among the circumstances surrounding each error. Solutions are then developed for each category of problems.

One limitation of the critical incident technique is that it entails interviewing subjects and is strongly dependent on their subjective memories. An advantage of the critical incident technique over observation is the consideration of subjective information obtained from the participants relative to the causes of the errors detected. Disadvantages of this method include the difficulty of interpreting the data and of developing appropriate solutions.[73]

Chart Review

Chart review has been used in combination with stimulated self-report and review of medication records to detect errors and to compare them with the number of adverse drug events experienced by patients during the same time period.[74,75] This technique entails looking in the patient's chart for clues that an error has occurred. (One such clue, for example, might be the administration of an antidote for a drug overdose.) Chart review is most useful when the clinical significance of medication errors is the focus of the research. It could be more powerful if used in combination with observation.

Observation

The direct observation technique was developed by Barker and McConnell.[33] In this technique, an observer accompanies the person giving medications and witnesses the preparation and administration of each dose. The observer writes down in detail what the subject does when preparing the drug and witnesses its administration.[1] The notes are then compared with the physician's order. An error is counted if the subject did not carry out the order accurately. The error rate is then calculated as described earlier. The observation is termed *disguised* if the subject is unaware of the precise goal of the study. For example, subjects may be told only that problems with the drug distribution system are being studied. Barker[76] has described the factors that should be taken into account in planning and conducting a successful study using observation. An observer training program is being developed at Auburn University.

One advantage of the observation method is that it detects many more errors than other methods. This is partly due to the independence from the subject's knowledge of the occurrence of an error. Comments made by the nurse during observation can help identify correlations between errors and possible causes.[77] Another advantage of this method is objectivity. A trained observer provides an objective perspective. The observer provides a mechanism with which to avoid problems associated with the subject's willingness to report. The burdens of remembering to report and of reporting accurately are transferred from the subject to the observer. This is ideal for sensitive issues such as medication error reporting.[76]

One potential disadvantage of the disguised observation technique is fatigue. Observation is physically and mentally demanding.[76] This method can also be expensive because it requires a trained health professional with knowledge of medication names and appearances and the ability to read physician orders.[76] A third disadvantage is the influence of the observer. Care must be taken to minimize the effects of observation on the subjects by striving to remain unobtrusive and nonjudgmental.[76] Finally, the observer may process what he or she sees and hears incorrectly.[76] Careful training and proper category definitions can minimize this problem.

Barker and colleagues[1] checked for the possible effect of the observer on the observed by monitoring individual nurse error rates for five consecutive days. The consistency of each subject's medication error rate indicated that the observation did not affect the rate over time. Concern that observers would make a subject more nervous (leading to more mistakes) or more careful (preventing errors) seems unfounded. It has long been known that if observation is unobtrusive and nonjudgmental, the subject will resume normal behavior within 1 to 3 hours of the initial observation.[77]

In the participant observer approach, an employee collects data while performing the normal tasks of the job, but his or her coworkers are unaware that the study is taking place.[1,76] Mayo et al.[17] studied medication cart distribution errors using this technique. A pharmacy resident checked the contents of a medication cart against the MAR with a nurse and noted differences for investigation. Medication cart distribution errors were defined as any difference between what was found in the cart and what was on the MAR.

Self-Report and Observation

A combination of self-report and observation of discussions of the health care team during rounds and meetings has been used to detect adverse events.[78] Ethnographers attended rounds and noted how adverse events were identified by hospital staff. Adverse events were defined as "situations in which an inappropriate decision was made when, at the time, an appropriate alternative could have been chosen." The ethnographer observers did not ask any questions, nor did they appear to review patient medical charts for additional data. The method resulted in the identification of 204 adverse events in one of 20 drug-related categories; this represented 9.3% of all adverse events detected on three nursing units over a 9-month period. Twenty-seven of the adverse events were classified as serious. This method could be refined to focus on drug-related meetings, such as nurse change-of-shift reports, where adverse drug events may be discussed.

Other Error Detection Methods

A number of approaches have been used to study errors that occur before medication is prepared for administration to the patient (e.g., pharmacy dispensing errors). Although 100% dispensing accuracy does not guarantee error-free medication administration, it should increase the probability of success. Pang and Grant[24] studied the possible causes of missing doses using the critical incident method. An identified communication problem was resolved by implementing a new system under which the medication carts were double-checked against the MAR. This change led to a significant decrease (from 0.93% to 0.33%) in missing doses.

Observers have been used to double-check the accuracy of three processes: medication cart filling,[16,18,79] filling new orders,[17] and filling prescriptions.[25,26,80–83] The advantages and disadvantages of the observation method may apply to double-checking. Consideration should be given to whether the data collection should be disguised and to whether reliability checks of the error detection process should be performed. For example, will the investigator perform the double-check in the same location as the subjects? This could make the investigator vulnerable to the same stresses and environmental conditions as the subject and can result in missed errors. As long as the investigator does not have to fulfill any other duties and can concentrate on the task of inspection, it can be argued that error detection is accurate.

The objective of a research study should dictate the most appropriate error detection technique. The observation technique is superior in terms of validity and cost effectiveness. If the clinical significance of errors is under study, a chart review or patient follow-up component may be added to observation.

Review of Medication Error Research

The following critiques of observation-based studies provide an overview of major findings in medication error research performed over the past four decades. The studies discussed illustrate key methodological issues and provide examples of sound research methods. Following an extensive discussion of errors in the inpatient setting, separate sections are provided on the impact of automated medication dispensing devices, intravenous admixture errors, and errors in outpatient and community settings.

The 1960s

In 1962, Barker and McConnell[33] became the first to show that medication errors occur much more frequently than anyone had suspected—at a rate of 16 errors per 100 doses. Two years later, Barker and colleagues[34] performed a pilot study at the University of Arkansas Medical Center in which they compared the center's existing drug distribution system with an experimental centralized unit-dose dispensing system. When wrong-time errors were excluded, a significant decrease in the error rate (from 16.1% to 7.2%) was seen after implementation of the unit-dose system. The pilot study was later expanded to eight nursing units.[84] A significant difference was found between the two systems across shifts (day and evening) and services (medical, surgical, and pediatric). The unit-dose system offered features that would prove important for the accuracy of future medication systems, such as on-line, real-time data processing of medication orders; medication cart exchanges every 2 hours; and unit-dose packaging for 100% of medications administered.

In 1966, Barker and colleagues[1] conducted a comprehensive study of medication errors in a large general hospital. The work included analyses of the effect of the observer on the subjects, the role of situational factors, the personal psychological characteristics of nurses involved in errors, and observer comments about what may have caused the errors. Twenty-eight nurses were observed for five consecutive days. The combined error rate was 15.0% (6.7% excluding wrong-time errors) for 9789 OEs.

A study directed by Tester (1967)[85] at the University of Iowa Hospitals involved the detection of medication administration errors and discrepancies before and after implementation of a decentralized unit-dose dispensing system. The results require close examination because of unique error and discrepancy categories and the methods employed. They are, however, striking: excluding doses left at the patient's bedside ("discrepancies") and wrong-time errors, the error rates for each system were less than 1%. The nurse observers reviewed each patient's MAR before observation and may have been in a position to prevent errors. This is not only an ethical dilemma from a research perspective but also a potential liability problem. The denominator used in the calculation of the error rate was unclear, making it difficult to compare these results with those of other studies.

The 1970s

In 1970, Hynniman et al.[2] compared the error rate of the unit-dose system at the University of Kentucky Hospital with the error rates at four hospitals that used traditional methods of drug distribution (three used the prescription order system and one used floor stock). A critical departure from the recommended method for performing observation—namely, observers did not witness administration of the drug—limits the comparison of the study's results to those of other investigations. The implications of this change in method include the inability of the observer to detect wrong route, wrong administration technique, omission, and wrong rate of administration errors. While noting this limitation, the authors felt they could still use the error rates to compare drug distribution systems. On the basis of the definitions provided, it is not clear whether the error categories that could not be detected by the observer were included.

In 1973, Shultz and coworkers[86] compared the medication administration accuracy of registered nurses using a traditional system with that of an experimental, pharmacy-coordinated technician drug administration program that used the unit-dose system. The error rate of the traditional system was substantially lower than that of the experimental system. However, the study's design, which featured a static group comparison,[90] does not rule out other reasons for the decreased error rate. Although it is unclear how the error rate was calculated, the statistical results would have been the same because of the small number of omission errors. This study was repeated 10 years later to determine whether the low technician error rates were maintained.[32,35] The error rate remained less than 5%, despite changing from cart exchanges four times a day to once daily.

A 1975 study at the Johns Hopkins Hospital[88] explored the hypothesis that the medication error rate of a computer-based unit-dose drug distribution system would be lower than that of a multidose system. The former had a significantly lower error rate than the latter, but the experimental design did not entail measurement of the error rate on the nursing unit under study before the computer was installed. This study compared average error rates per patient instead of per drug distribution system. The results suggest that, on the average, patients on the unit-dose floor experienced fewer errors.

In 1976, Schnell[5] measured error rates in four Canadian hospitals before and after implementation of a unit-dose drug distribution system. The results should be analyzed cautiously because the presence or absence of a nurse's initials on the MAR was used to establish whether a dose was omitted. An unexpected increase in error rate (from 9% to 15%, excluding wrong-time errors) in Hospital A after implementation of the unit-dose system may have resulted from a rise in extra-dose errors. (There was less rigorous enforcement of the automatic "stop order" procedure by the pharmacy department, resulting in administration of extra doses.) The error rate difference would have been 8.5% before implementation of the unit-dose system and 5.8% after implementation if extra-dose and wrong-time errors were excluded. The decrease is statistically significant ($p < .05$).

The 1980s

In 1983, Rosati and Nahata[89] conducted a study of drug administration technique errors involving pediatric patients. These authors hypothesized that the manipulations sometimes required by pediatric doses may increase the risk of error. They found 28 technique errors during 217 administrations (12.9% error rate); the rate was 5.5% when wrong-time errors were excluded. Two problems can be identified in this study. The observer told the subject that he or she had committed an error immediately after administration of the drug to the patient. The effect of the observer on the subject due to this feedback may have altered the error rate. Moreover, the results of this study cannot be readily compared with those of other studies because it focused on a limited number of error categories. The situation also posed an ethical dilemma: if the observer is going to say that an error has been committed, why not prevent the error and note a potential error?

An interdisciplinary group headed by Barker performed an in-depth analysis of a unit-dose drug distribution system at a large hospital.[12] The initial error rate was 9.0% (183 errors, excluding wrong-time errors, per 2018 OEs). The rate was three to five times higher than that reported for some other unit-dose systems. Fourteen recommendations for improvement were made,[87] of which the hospital fully implemented two: the use of an MAR created in the pharmacy and an increase of pharmacy staff during peak workload periods. Four recommendations were partially implemented. These included an increase in the percentage of doses dispensed in unit-dose packages; the use of dispensing envelopes; more frequent deliveries; and dispensing prn drugs from the pharmacy upon request. Suggestions that were not implemented included computerized control of doses, computerized labeling of doses, and redesign of the pharmacy's facilities.

Two years after the recommendations were implemented as described, another study[90] found that the error rate had not changed significantly. This finding illustrates the importance of fully implementing all facets of the unit-dose system in order to achieve the lowest possible error rates.[91] It may also be an indication of other factors causing errors that are not affected by a change in the drug distribution system. For example, characteristics of the people involved in the system (e.g., visual impairment) and the lighting level on the unit may have contributed to the high error rates.[92]

In 1986, Tisdale[4] studied errors in an intensive care nursery and a pediatric intensive care unit in an effort to justify an upgrade of pharmacy services in these settings. The error rates reported were higher than the actual rates because the number of omission errors was not included in the denominator of the equation used to calculate the error rates.[32,36] The overall error rates were 23.7% (147 errors for 620 TOEs) and 8.4%, excluding wrong-time errors (52 errors for 620 TOEs), when the TOEs were adjusted to include errors of omission.[36] If wrong-time errors are excluded and the corrected ratios of errors to no errors are used, the chi^2 analysis with McNemar's test for correlated proportions is not significant for either location. Methodological problems included the use of the American Society of Hospital Pharmacists error category definitions[93] without adequate operationalization and the fact that the observer was aware of each patient's drug regimen prior to observation. The observer was allowed to intervene in the event of an impending error but did not have the occasion to do so.

The 1990s

In 1995, Dean and colleagues[94] compared medication error rates in a British hospital with those in a U.S. hospital. The British facility used a ward stock system in which a medication nurse obtained and prepared medications from a drug trolley that was moved to each patient's bedside during each pass. The physician wrote the medication order on the MAR. No transcriptions were required until a new MAR was needed. Instead of sending a copy of the medication order to the pharmacy, a ward pharmacist went to each patient's bedside to review orders on the MAR and wrote additional instructions to the nurse regarding administration. (For example, dose calculations for oral liquid medications and instructions such as "Take with food" were written by the pharmacist.) The U.S. hospital used a partially automated unit-dose drug distribution system with a MedStation device (Pyxis Corp., San Diego, Calif.) for controlled substances and some first doses, and for as-needed medications.

There was an important methodological difference in the way the observations were performed at the two hospitals. In the British hospital, the observers double-checked what the nurse was preparing against the MAR (which also represented the physician's original order). If the dose was wrong, the observer intervened in a way that prompted the nurse to identify the error and correct it. The observer recorded the error. The authors examined the data to determine whether the feedback given to correct the errors affected the frequency with which errors were made after the intervention. They found no effect. The error rate at the British hospital was 3.0%, whereas that at the U.S. hospital was 6.9%. Using the physician's original orders for a dual purpose (i.e., as MAR), eliminating transcription, and having the pharmacist clarify orders on the MAR were believed to contribute to the difference.

Studies of Medication Errors in Specific Areas or Operations

Automated Medication Dispensing Devices

Using the direct observation technique, Barker and colleagues[13] studied the effect of an automated bedside medication dispensing machine on medication errors. The system sounded an alert to notify nurses when medications were due to be administered and allowed access to only those medications that were to be given at that time. The bedside device system resulted in a significantly lower medication error rate than did the unit-dose system (10.6% and 15.9%, respectively). Although errors in all categories were committed during use of the automated system, rates for the majority of categories were lower for the automated system.

Cooper and colleagues[95] compared medication administration error rates for a blister card drug distribution system with those for an ATC-212 single unit-dose packaging system and the ATC Plus multidose packaging system

(Baxter Healthcare Corp., Chicago, Ill.) in a long-term care facility. The ATC Plus system packages all oral solid doses that are to be given at the same time in the same package. The nurse selects one package containing all oral solid doses due at that time from the patient's medication drawer. Packaging takes place in a central location, typically the pharmacy, and a pharmacist inspects each package for accuracy before it is delivered to the nursing unit. The blister card system produced a medication error rate of 8.0%, and the single unit-dose package system produced an error rate of 2.5%. No errors were detected with the multidose ATC Plus system.

The medication administration error rate for two nursing units using the MedStation system was determined by observation.[94,96] The MedStation system allowed nurses to obtain any medication stored in the device for any patient; there was no link to the patient's list of approved medications in the hospital's computer system. The medication error rate was 6.9%. Errors associated with the MedStation system are shown in Table 6–3. The error rate for all doses retrieved from the MedStation system was 17% (21 errors, 123 opportunities), whereas the error rate for doses retrieved from the traditional patient medication drawer on a unit-dose cart was 5% (43 errors, 796 opportunities).

Borel and Rascati[57] studied the effect of the Pyxis MedStation Rx system on medication errors. This system allows nurses access only to those medications in the MedStation Rx system that had been prescribed by a physician and approved by a pharmacist. This is made possible by a link to the patient's medication profile, which is maintained in the hospital computer system. It is possible, however, to override the system and obtain certain medications under certain circumstances (e.g., in emergencies) without prior approval by a pharmacist. The error rate for the unit-dose system was 16.9% (148 errors, 873 opportunities), and the error rate after implementation of the MedStation Rx system was 10.4% (97 errors, 929 opportunities). This difference is statistically significant. The new system decreased the relative frequency of omission errors but did not affect unauthorized drug errors and wrong-dose errors. The rate of wrong-time errors increased. The authors did not observe any instances in which a MedStation was refilled incorrectly. The authors reported that overrides did occur during the study but did not state whether any were associated with medication administration errors.

Intravenous Admixture Compounding

An observation study of intravenous admixture compounding error rates in sterile compounding centers in five hospital pharmacies measured a 9%

error rate (147 errors, 1679 doses). Of these errors, 1.5% were judged to be clinically significant. Wrong-dose errors (defined as a deviation of 5% or more from the dose listed on the pharmacy label) were the most common error category. Parenteral nutrition solutions prepared manually or with automation had higher error rates than any other type of product. These rates were 37% (manually prepared solutions) and 22% (prepared using automation).[97]

Dispensing Errors in Prescription-Filling Operations

When analyzing prescription-filling operations, it is necessary to be aware of differences in how the authors define a dispensing error as well as of differences in the error categories themselves. The results of the studies listed in Table 6–2 have been modified to include similar error categories. Other methodological techniques and pharmacy procedures that must be considered include noting who filled the prescription, the type of error detection system used (e.g., disguised observation, incident report, retrospective analysis[98]), whether errors were corrected before the medications were given to the patient, and who made the correction.

Effect of Work Environment and Workload on Medication Errors

Pharmacists and technicians can be affected by their work environment in a way that can increase or decrease the dispensing error rate. Research on associations between various factors and medication errors is summarized here. Kelly[99] has written an overview of pharmacy's contributions to adverse medication events and discussed procedural and systems problems and other sources of error in pharmacies.

Lighting

Buchanan and colleagues[81] studied the effect of lighting level on dispensing errors in a high-volume outpatient pharmacy. A total of 10,889 prescriptions were evaluated. Three different lighting levels were compared: 45, 102, and 146 footcandles (fc). There was a significant decrease in the dispensing error rate, from 3.9% to 2.6%, when the lighting level was increased from 102 to 146 fc.

Interruptions and Distractions

The relationship between interruptions and/or distractions and errors was the subject of a study in an ambulatory pharmacy.[83] The researchers inspected 5072 prescriptions over 23 days. The average dispensing

Type of Error	No. of Errors[a]
Unordered drug	
Ketorolac	1
Percocet®	4
Unipen®	1
Furosemide	1
Wrong dose	
Lorazepam (1 mg ordered, 2 mg given)	1
Promethazine i.v. (12.5 mg ordered, 25 mg given)	12
Meperidine i.v. (100 mg ordered, 50 mg given)	1
Total	21

[a] Based on 123 OEs.

Figure 6-1

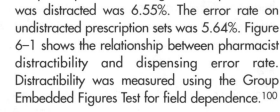

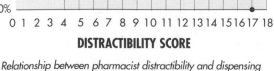

Relationship between pharmacist distractibility and dispensing error rates. Note: A high score indicates lower distractibility.[83]

Flynn & Barker, unpublished data, November 1996

error rate was 3.23%. Two video cameras recorded the work environment. Interruptions and distractions were detected and counted by reviewing the tapes.

Interruptions were defined as the cessation of productive activity because of an external stimulus prior to completion of a prescription-filling task. A total of 2022 interruptions were detected. Pharmacists were interrupted an average of three times per half-hour, and a peak of 17 interruptions in a half-hour period was observed. The error rate for uninterrupted prescription sets was 5.67%, and that for interrupted prescriptions was 6.65%. Interruptions per half-hour were associated with errors when controlling for prescription workload or pharmacist distractibility.

Distractions were counted if a pharmacist continued to work on a prescription-filling task while responding to an external stimulus. In the study, 2547 distractions were detected. Pharmacists were distracted approximately four times per half-hour; a peak of 16 distractions per half-hour was found. The error rate on prescription sets during which a pharmacist was distracted was 6.55%. The error rate on undistracted prescription sets was 5.64%. Figure 6–1 shows the relationship between pharmacist distractibility and dispensing error rate. Distractibility was measured using the Group Embedded Figures Test for field dependence.[100]

Noise

Certain noises and sounds have been found to decrease the rate of dispensing errors.[101] Unpredictable sounds, controllable sounds, and noise had a significant effect on pharmacists that resulted in a lower dispensing error rate. The effect of noise levels on errors was also assessed in this study. The error rate increased as loudness levels increased, but only to a point, after which it began to decrease.

Workload

State boards of pharmacy are considering imposing prescription quotas on pharmacists because of the potentially harmful effects of excessive workload on dispensing errors. Four studies have assessed this relationship. Three found that errors increased as prescription workload increased;[25,81,83] the remaining study[26] found no relationship. One study found that the risk of error increases when a pharmacist fills more than 10 to 12 prescriptions per half-hour (Figure 6–2).[83] Another study found that the percentage of hours during which one or more errors occurred increased as the workload increased.[25]

In the hospital setting, significant associations between medication workload and omissions, extra-dose, and wrong-time errors have been measured. There was not a significant correlation between medication workload and overall error rate or error rate (excluding wrong-time errors).[1]

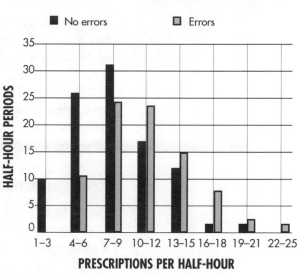

Figure 6-2

Relationship between prescription workload and risk of dispensing error.[83]

Flynn & Barker, unpublished data, November 1996

Other Factors

Significantly more wrong-time errors per OE occurred on the day shift. The dosage form most often involved in errors was oral liquids. Most errors occurred on routine orders (primarily wrong-time errors), as opposed to stat or prn orders.[1]

Applications of Error-Monitoring Techniques

Medication error detection by means of monthly observation[102] has been used as part of a quality improvement effort in an inpatient setting. Routine observation permits one to assess the impact of changes in a drug distribution system on the quality of service, using medication errors as an indicator. One use of this approach is to verify the accuracy of medication administration for drug distribution systems that have been outsourced.

The Health Care Financing Administration (HCFA) has used observation-based medication error rates to assess long-term care facilities since 1984.[103] HCFA's upper limit for medication errors in long-term care facilities is 5%, but they have proposed lowering it to 2%.[104] Any facility whose rate is higher will not receive Medicare reimbursement. In addition, if the observer detects any "significant" error, a deficiency report is filed.[103] A survey[105] found that 4000 of 15,000 nursing homes participating in

Medicare or Medicaid programs did not accurately carry out physicians' orders when administering medications.

A quality assurance program in a prescription-filling operation has been described.[98] A retrospective prescription checking program involved review of 16,000 prescriptions by comparing the original prescription with data entered in a computer. The program decreased the total error rate from 4.2% to 2%, and the rate of "serious" errors decreased from 0.6% to 0.1%. Most errors were corrected by changing an entry in the computer so that refills would be correctly dispensed. Serious errors were corrected by follow-up contact with the patient.[98]

Recommendations for Error Prevention

On the basis of published research, desirable medication automation system features that help prevent medication errors have been described.[106] These system characteristics are as follows:

1. Comprehensiveness: Control of the medication distribution system should start with entry of the order into the computer and should end with administration to the patient.

2. Focus: The system should accommodate error-prone dosage forms (e.g., injections, oral liquids, pediatric dosages).

3. Dispensing of unit doses: Medications delivered should not require further manipulation by the nurse.

4. Signals: To minimize omission and wrong-time errors, the device should remind the nurse when a dose is due.

5. Labeling: A machine-printed label should be affixed to the medication container when it arrives in the unit.

6. Machine identification: It should be possible to identify the dose, patient, and person administering the dose before the dose is administered. This can be done through bar codes or radio frequency tags.

7. Controlled access: Medications should be accessible only to approved personnel, as verified by the machine.

8. Capturing of dose administration: The time and place should be documented at the time the drug is given to the patient.

9. Drug-use information: Information needed by the nurse in order to facilitate correct administration of a medication should be provided at the point of administration.

10. Controls: All compromises or overrides of the system should be associated with a visible or audible alarm. Overrides should be documented
automatically at the time they occur.

Increasing the light to 146 fc significantly decreases dispensing error
rates.[81] This is a practical and reasonably priced improvement. Changes in
facility design should be directed at preventing pharmacist interruptions and
distractions as well as minimizing the effects of workload. The Indian Health
Service has effectively used patient counseling to reduce the number of dispensing errors.[107] This technique verifies the patient's identity, dispenses
from the chart (the original prescription order is used during counseling for
a final check), and shows the medication to the patient.

Conclusion

Thirty-five years of medication error research have contributed to reducing
errors. More research is needed as automated drug distribution systems are
developed and systems are outsourced or cosourced.

••••
References

1. Barker KN, Kimbrough WW, Heller WM. *A Study of Medication Errors in a Hospital.* Fayetteville, Ark:
University of Arkansas; 1966.

2. Hynniman CE, Conrad WF, Urch WA, et al. A comparison of medication errors under the University
of Kentucky unit-dose system and traditional drug distribution systems in four hospitals. *Am J Hosp
Pharm.* 1970; 27: 802–14.

3. Hall KW, Ebbeling P, Brown B, et al. A retrospective-prospective study of medication errors: basis for
an ongoing monitoring program. *Can J Hosp Pharm.* October 1985; 38: 141–43, 46.

4. Tisdale JE. Justifying a pediatric critical care satellite pharmacy by medication error reporting. *Am J
Hosp Pharm.* 1986; 43: 368–71.

5. Schnell BR. A study of unit-dose drug distribution in four Canadian hospitals. *Can J Hosp Pharm.*
1976; 29: 85-90.

6. Schneider PJ, Gift MG, Lee YP, et al. Cost of medication-related problems at a university hospital. *Am
J Health Syst Pharm.* 1995; 52: 2415–18.

7. Wou K. Costs associated with recurrent hypoglycemia caused by dispensing error. *Ann Pharmacother.*
1994; 28: 965–66.

8. Hynniman CE, Hyde GC, Parker PF. How costly is medication safety? *Hospitals.* September 16, 1971;
45: 73–74, 76, 80, 82–85.

9. Summerfield MR. *Unit Dose Primer.* Bethesda, Md: American Society of Hospital Pharmacists; 1983:
28–36.

10. Barker KN, Pearson RE. Medication distribution systems. In: Brown TR, Smith MC, eds. *Handbook of
Institutional Pharmacy Practice.* 2nd ed. Baltimore, Md: Williams & Wilkins; 1986: 341–42.

11. Physician Insurers Association of America. *Medication Error Study.* State of Washington: June 1993: 3.

12. Barker KN, Harris JA, Webster DB, et al. Consultant evaluation of a hospital medication system: analysis of the existing system. *Am J Hosp Pharm.* 1984; 41: 2009–16.

13. Barker KN, Pearson RE, Hepler CD, et al. Effect of an automated bedside dispensing machine on medication errors. *Am J Hosp Pharm.* 1984; 41: 1352–58.

14. Douglas JB, Wheeler DS. *Evaluation of Trained Pharmacy Technicians in Identifying Dispensing Errors.* P-244(E). Presented at the American Society of Hospital Pharmacists Midyear Clinical Meeting, Miami, Fla, December 7, 1994.

15. Woller TW, Stuart J, Vrabel R, et al. Checking of unit dose cassettes by pharmacy technicians at three Minnesota hospitals. *Am J Hosp Pharm.* 1991; 48: 1952–56.

16. Becker MD, Johnson MH, Longe RL. Errors remaining in unit dose carts after checking by pharmacists versus pharmacy technicians. *Am J Hosp Pharm.* 1978; 35: 432–34.

17. Mayo CE, Kitchens RG, Reese RL, et al. Distribution accuracy of a decentralized unit dose system. *Am J Hosp Pharm.* 1975; 32: 1124–26.

18. Taylor J, Gaucher M. Medication selection errors made by pharmacy technicians in filling unit dose orders. *Can J Hosp Pharm.* February 1986; 39: 9–12.

19. Hassall TH, Daniels CE. Evaluation of three types of control chart methods in unit dose error monitoring. *Am J Hosp Pharm.* 1983; 40: 970–75.

20. Hoffman RP, Bartt KH, Berlin L, et al. Multidisciplinary quality assessment of a unit dose drug distribution system. *Hosp Pharm.* March 1984; 19: 167–69, 173–74.

21. Chi J. Tech-check-tech, as sanctioned practice, gaining in states. *Hospital Pharmacist Report.* August 1994; 8: 14, 17.

22. Ness JE, Sullivan SD, Stergachis A. Accuracy of technicians and pharmacists in identifying dispensing errors. *Am J Hosp Pharm.* 1994; 51: 354–57.

23. Gray SL, Parker PE. *Hospital Certification of Technician Checking Technician in Unit Dose Cart Fill.* P-151(D). Presented at the American Society of Hospital Pharmacists Midyear Clinical Meeting, Miami, Fla, December 6, 1994.

24. Pang F, Grant JA. Missing medications associated with centralized unit dose dispensing. *Am J Hosp Pharm.* 1975; 32: 1121–23.

25. Guernsey BG, Ingrim NB, Hokanson JA, et al. Pharmacists' dispensing accuracy in a high-volume outpatient pharmacy service: focus on risk management. *Drug Intell Clin Pharm.* 1983; 17: 742–46.

26. Kistner UA, Keith MR, Sergeant KA, et al. Accuracy of dispensing in a high-volume, hospital-based outpatient pharmacy. *Am J Hosp Pharm.* 1994; 51: 2793–97.

27. Allan EL, Barker KN, Malloy MJ, et al. Dispensing errors and counseling in community practice. *American Pharmacy.* 1995; NS35: 25–33.

28. Manasse HR Jr. Medication use in an imperfect world: drug misadventuring as an issue of public policy, part 1. *Am J Hosp Pharm.* 1989; 46: 929–44.

29. Manasse HR Jr. Medication use in an imperfect world: drug misadventuring as an issue of public policy, part 2. *Am J Hosp Pharm.* 1989; 46: 1141–52.

30. Bates DW, Cullen DJ, Laird N, et al. Incidence of adverse drug events and potential adverse drug events: implications for prevention. *JAMA.* 1995; 274: 29–34.

31. Cullen DJ, Bates DW, Small SD, et al. The incident-reporting system does not detect adverse drug events: a problem for quality improvement. *Jt Comm J Qual Improv.* 1995; 21: 541–48.

32. Allan BL. Calculating medication error rates (letter). *Am J Hosp Pharm.* 1987; 44: 1044, 46.

33. Barker KN, McConnell WE. The problems of detecting medication errors in hospitals. *Am J Hosp Pharm.* 1962; 19: 360–69.

34. Barker KN, Heller WM, Brennan JJ, et al. The development of a centralized unit-dose dispensing system, VI: the pilot study—medication errors and drug losses. *Am J Hosp Pharm.* 1964; 21: 609–25.

35. Jozefczyk KG, Schneider PJ, Pathak DS. Medication errors in a pharmacy-coordinated drug administration program. *Am J Hosp Pharm.* 1986; 43: 2464–67.

36. Allan EL, Barker KN. Fundamentals of medication error research. *Am J Hosp Pharm.* 1990; 47: 555–71.

37. O'Leary D. Joint Commission charts new course for quality assurance (editorial). *Am J Hosp Pharm.* 1986; 43: 2403.

38. Hynniman CE. Quality assurance and performance standards. In: Brown TR, Smith MC, eds. *Handbook of Institutional Pharmacy Practice.* 2nd ed. Baltimore, Md: Williams and Wilkins; 1986: 633–34.

39. Donabedian A. *Explorations in Quality Assessment and Monitoring. Vol I. The Definition of Quality and Approaches to Its Assessment.* Ann Arbor, Mich: Health Administration Press; 1980: 79–97.

40. Brown WM, Blount CW, Harley GD. *Quality of Pharmaceutical Care in Small Hospitals. Unpublished report to the Missouri Regional Medical Program.* Kansas City, Mo; March 1976.

41. Jackson RA, Smith MC, Mikeal RL. The quality of pharmaceutical services: structure, process, and state board requirements. *Drugs in Health Care.* Winter 1975; 2: 39–48.

42. Ballinger BR, Simpson E, Stewart MJ. An evaluation of a drug administration system in a psychiatric hospital. *Br J Psychiatry.* 1974; 125: 202–07.

43. Goldstein MS, Cohen MR, Black M. A method for monitoring medication omission error rates. *Hosp Pharm.* 1982; 17: 310–12.

44. Hoffman RP, Bartt KH, Berlin L, et al. Multidisciplinary quality assessment of a unit dose drug distribution system. *Hosp Pharm.* March 1984; 19: 167–69, 73, 74.

45. Phillips DP, Christenfeld N, Glynn LM. Increase in U.S. medication error deaths between 1983 and 1993. *Lancet.* 1998; 351: 643–44.

46. Baker HM. Rules outside the rules for administration of medication: a study in New South Wales, Australia. *Image: Journal of Nursing Scholarship.* 1997; 29(2): 155–58.

47. Canadian Society of Hospital Pharmacists. CSHP guidelines for medication incident and medication discrepancy reporting in Canadian hospitals. *Can J Hosp Pharm.* 1986: 39: 67–69.

48. Trudeau TR. Pharmacy Q's and A's: Effective programs for adverse drug reaction and medication error reporting. *Hospital Topics.* 1980; 58: 42–47.

49. Wasiuta V. Reporting incidents: how many is too many? *Dimensions in Health Services.* 1982; 59: 16–18.

50. Wellman GS, Johnson GT. How to handle and control medication errors in the hospital setting. *Pharmacy Times.* 1986; 52: 111–13.

51. Tribble DA, Lamnin M, Garich JL. Ideas for action: reporting medication error rate by microcomputer. *Topics in Hospital Pharmacy Management.* November 1985; 5: 77–88.

52. Myles LJ, Naeger LL. The pharmacy medication error peer-review committee. *Hosp Pharm.* January 1987; 22: 50–52.

53. Hartwig SC, Denger SD, Schneider PJ. Severity-indexed, incident report-based medication error-reporting program. *Am J Hosp Pharm.* 1991; 48: 2611–16.

54. Lunik M, Gaither M. Medication errors; New form aids in discovery, analysis, and prevention. *Hospital Formulary.* 1991; 26: 666–67, 71.

55. Shannon RC, DeMuth JE. Comparison of medication-error detection methods in the long-term care facility. *The Consultant Pharmacist.* March/April 1987; 2: 148–51.

56. Brown GC. Medication errors: a case study. *Hospitals.* October 16, 1979; 53: 61–62, 65.

57. Borel JM, Rascati KL. Effects of an automated, nursing unit-based drug-dispensing device on medication errors. *Am J Health Syst Pharm.* 1995; 52: 1875–79.

58. Van Leeuwen DH. Are medication error rates useful as comparative measures of organizational performance? *Jt Comm Qual Improv.* April 1994; 20: 192–99.

59. Cohen MR. To report or not to report: that is the question (editorial). *Hosp Pharm.* March 1982; 17: 114, 16.

60. Duran G. Positive use of incident reports. *Hospitals.* July 16, 1979; 53: 60, 64, 68.

61. Cobb MD. Evaluating medication errors. *J Nurs Adm.* April 1986; 16: 41–44.

62. Betz RP, Levy HB. An interdisciplinary method of classifying and monitoring medication errors. *Am J Hosp Pharm.* 1985; 42: 1724–32.

63. Landrie RM. A study of medication errors. *Washington State Journal of Nursing.* Summer/Fall 1977; 49: 9–12.

64. Regan WA. Legal case briefs for nurses. IL: RN's delayed medication: fatality; NY: kidney disease: orders ignored. *Regan Report on Nursing Law.* September 1980; 21: 3.

65. Regan WA. Medication mistakes: fire the nurse? Case in point: Edgewood Nursing Center v. NLRB. *Regan Report on Nursing Law.* May 1980; 20: 2.

66. Germaine A, Rinneard B. How effectively do you use your incident/accident report? *Hosp Adm Can.* August 1976; 18: 24–26.

67. Noel MW. Effective discipline. In: Noel MW, Bootman JL, eds. *Human Resources Management in Pharmacy Practice.* Rockville, Md: Aspen Systems Corp; 1986: 111–24.

68. Anderson ER Jr. Disciplinary action after a serious medication error. *Am J Hosp Pharm.* 1987; 44: 2690, 92.

69. Hayman JN. Microcomputer-assisted monitoring of medication-dispensing errors. *Am J Hosp Pharm.* 1989; 46: 1806–09.

70. Safren MA, Chapanis A. A critical incident study of hospital medication errors, I: *Hospitals. Journal of the American Hospital Association.* May 1, 1960; 34: 32–34, 57–58, 60, 62, 64, 66.

71. Safren MA, Chapanis A. A critical incident study of hospital medication errors, II: *Hospitals. Journal of the American Hospital Association.* May 16, 1960; 34: 53, 65–66, 68.

72. Cooper JB, Newbower RS, Kitz RJ. An analysis of major errors and equipment failures in anesthesia management: considerations for prevention and detection. *Anesthesiology.* 1984; 60: 34–42.

73. Flanagan JC. The critical incident technique. *Psychol Bull.* 1954; 51: 327–58.

74. Bates DW, Boyle DL, Vander Vliet MB, et al. Relationship between medication errors and adverse drug events. *J Gen Intern Med.* April 1995; 10: 199–205.

75. Cullen DJ, Sweitzer BJ, Bates DW, et al. Preventable adverse drug events in hospitalized patients: a comparative study of intensive care and general care units. *Crit Care Med.* 1997; 25: 1289–97.

76. Barker KN. Data collection techniques: observation. *Am J Hosp Pharm.* 1980; 37: 1235–43.

77. Kerlinger FN. *Foundations of Behavioral Research.* 2nd ed. New York: Holt, Rinehart and Winston; 1973.

78. Andrews LB, Stocking C, Krizek T, et al. An alternative strategy for studying adverse events in medical care. *Lancet.* 1997; 349: 309–13.

79. Grogan JE, Hanna JA, Haight RA. A study of accuracy of pharmacy technicians working in a unit-dose system. *Hosp Pharm.* April 1978; 13: 194–95, 99.

80. McGhan WF, Smith WE, Adams DW. A randomized trial comparing pharmacists and technicians as dispensers of prescriptions for ambulatory patients. *Med Care.* 1983; 21: 445–53.

81. Buchanan TL, Barker KN, Gibson JT, et al. Illumination and errors in dispensing. *Am J Hosp Pharm.* 1991; 48: 2137–45.

82. Spader TJ. *Dispensing Errors and Detection at an Outpatient Pharmacy.* Chapel Hill, NC: University of North Carolina; 1994. Thesis.

83. Allan EL. *Relationships Among Facility Design Variables and Medication Errors in a Pharmacy.* Auburn, Ala: Auburn University; 1994. Dissertation.

84. Barker KN. The effects of an experimental medication system on medication errors and costs, I: introduction and errors study. *Am J Hosp Pharm.* 1969; 26: 324–33.

85. Tester WW. *A Study of Patient Care Involving a Unit Dose System: Final Report.* Prepared under US Public Health Service grant HM-00328-01. Iowa City, Iowa: University of Iowa; 1967.

86. Shultz SM, White SJ, Latiolais CJ. Medication errors reduced by unit-dose. *Hospitals.* March 16, 1973; 47: 106–12.

87. Campbell DT, Stanley JC. *Experimental and Quasi-Experimental Designs for Research.* Boston, Mass: Houghton Mifflin; 1963: 12–13.

88. Means BJ, Derewicz HJ, Lamy PP. Medication errors in a multidose and a computer-based unit dose drug distribution system. *Am J Hosp Pharm.* 1975; 32: 186–91.

89. Rosati JR Jr, Nahata MC. Drug administration errors in pediatric patients. *Quality Review Bulletin.* 1983; 9: 212–13.

90. Barker KN, Harris JA, Webster DB, et al. Consultant evaluation of a hospital medication system. Synthesis of a new system. *Am J Hosp Pharm.* 1984; 41: 2016–21.

91. Barker KN, Harris JA, Webster DB, et al. Consultant evaluation of a hospital medication system: implementation and evaluation of the new system. *Am J Hosp Pharm.* 1984; 41: 2022–29.

92. Buchanan TL. *On the Effect of Varying Levels of Illumination on the Prescription Dispensing Error Rate in an Army High-Volume Outpatient Pharmacy Service.* Auburn, Ala: Auburn University; 1989. Thesis.

93. American Society of Hospital Pharmacists. ASHP standard definition of a medication error. *Am J Hosp Pharm.* 1982; 39: 321.

94. Dean BS, Allan EL, Barber ND, et al. Comparison of medication errors in an American and a British hospital. *Am J Health Syst Pharm.* 1995; 52: 2543–49.

95. Cooper S, Zaske D, Hadsall R, et al. Automated medication packaging for long-term care facilities: evaluation. *The Consultant Pharmacist.* 1994; 9: 58–70.

96. Barker KN, Allan EL. Research on Drug-Use-System Errors. Presented at the Conference on Understanding and Preventing Drug Misadventures, Chantilly, Va, October 21–23, 1994. *Am J Health Syst Pharm.* 1995; 52: 400–03.

97. Flynn EA, Pearson RE, Barker KN. Observational study of accuracy in compounding i.v. admixtures at five hospitals. *Am J Health Syst Pharm.* 1997; 54: 904–12.

98. Boneberg RF, Kellick KA, Pudhorodsky TG, et al. *Results of a retrospective outpatient medication error prevention program at a Department of Veterans Affairs Medical Center.* Presented at the American Society of Hospital Pharmacists Midyear Clinical Meeting, New Orleans, La, December 1991.

99. Kelly WN. Pharmacy contributions to adverse medication events. Presented at the Conference on Understanding and Preventing Drug Misadventures, Chantilly, Va, October 21–23, 1994. *Am J Health Syst Pharm.* 1995; 52: 385–90.

100. Oltman PK, Raskin E, Witkin HA. *Group Embedded Figures Test.* Palo Alto, Calif: Consulting Psychologists; 1971.

101. Flynn EA, Barker KN, Gibson JT, et al. Relationships between ambient sounds and accuracy of pharmacists' prescription-filling performance. *Hum Factors: Special Section on Human Factors in Health Care.* 1996; 38: 614–22.

102. Flynn EA, *An affordable observation-based method for monitoring error rate and reducing errors.* Presented at the American Society of Health-System Pharmacists Midyear Clinical Meeting, Las Vegas, Nev; December 9, 1998.

103. Feinberg JL, ed. *Med Pass Survey: A Continuous Quality Improvement Approach.* Alexandria, Va: American Society of Consultant Pharmacists; 1993.

104. Gannon K. HCFA may tie its funding to med error rate. *Hospital Pharmacist Report.* October 1997; 11: 44.

105. Anonymous. Thousands of nursing homes do not follow drug orders, U.S. survey reveals. *Am J Hosp Pharm.* 1989; 46: 426, 434.

106. Barker KN. Ensuring safety in the use of automated medication dispensing systems. *Am J Health Syst Pharm.* 1995; 52: 2445–47.

107. Kuyper AR. Patient counseling detects prescription errors. *Hosp Pharm.* 1993; 28: 1180–81, 1184–89.

108. Crawley HK, Eckel FM, McLeod DC. Comparison of a traditional and unit dose drug distribution system in a nursing home. *Drug Intell Clin Pharm.* 1971; 5: 166–71.

109. Barker KN, Mikeal RL, Pearson RE, et al. Medication errors in nursing homes and small hospitals. *Am J Hosp Pharm.* 1982; 39: 987–91.

110. Reitberg KN, Miller RJ, Bennes JF. Evaluation of two concurrent drug-delivery systems in a skilled-nursing facility. *Am J Hosp Pharm.* 1982; 39: 1316–20.

111. O'Brodovich M, Rappaport P. A study pre- and post-unit dose conversion in a pediatric hospital. *Can J Hosp Pharm.* 1991; 44: 5–15, 20.

112. Ruffin DM, Hodge FJ. Pharmacists' impact on medication administration errors in long-term care facilities. *The Consultant Pharmacist.* 1995; 10: 1025–32.

113. Wertheimer AI, Ritchko C, Dougherty DW. Prescription accuracy: room for improvement. *Med Care.* 1973; 11: 68–71.

Caregivers' Reactions to Making Medication Errors

Zane Robinson Wolf, PhD, RN, FAAN

La Salle University School of Nursing
Philadelphia, Pa.

Michael R. Cohen, MS, FASHP

Institute for Safe Medication Practices
Huntingdon Valley, Pa.

Primum non nocere. First, do no harm.

This time-honored standard directs nurses, pharmacists, and physicians to the primary goal of health care: to act with and on the behalf of patients to improve their health and well-being. Health care providers' fundamental priority is the welfare of the people they serve. As caregivers and healers, they are most fearful of causing harm, however inadvertent or unintentional, rather than doing good.

The public has implicitly placed its trust in health care professionals. Society expects that nurses, pharmacists, and physicians will devise systems to provide safe, competent care and that the professionals within the system will police themselves. The minimum standard for all actions taken on behalf of the public seeking health care services is patient safety. Consequently, when nurses, physicians, and pharmacists make medication errors and cause harm to patients, both the providers and patients are violated.

When an error occurs, formal punishment by the individual's profession, in the form of license suspension or withdrawal, is sometimes administered in response to very serious situations resulting from professional impairment, negligence, or misconduct. Much more frequently, the individual may be inappropriately punished via the lost respect of his or her fellow health care professionals.[1] This loss of self-respect can be even more devastating than professional reprimand.

The human suffering experienced by caregivers following such events is the focus of this chapter. Specifically, the reactions of caregivers after making a medication error are explored. Support for the content of this chapter comes from themes identified in a content analysis of literature dealing with human error in general and medication errors in particular (see "Suggested Reading" at the end of this chapter).

The Drive for Perfection Confronts Human Fallibility

When clinicians provide care to patients, they use their intellectual abilities to design, implement, and evaluate the outcomes of daily "experiments." How patients will respond to medication and other regimens is not always predictable. Although clinicians do not think of patient care as experimentation, their clinical practice nonetheless includes some experimental elements, albeit on a case-by-case basis. The term *therapeutic trial*, often used to describe the practice of charting a patient's response to a given medication or procedure, gives credence to this concept. The uncertainties of the outcomes of clinical practice and patient management are often accompanied by the knowledge that clinicians sometimes make mistakes. Still, health care providers are often puzzled when procedure fails them.

During training and practice, health care professionals are immersed in an environment where there is no place for error. Precision and perfection predominate. The logic has been as follows: If clinicians are well educated and follow policies, procedures, and other guidelines, medication errors will not happen. Apart from conferences on morbidity and mortality, physicians are afforded few forums in which to report or discuss the errors they have made, and they are not encouraged to do so by their profession or their peers.[1-5] Nurses and pharmacists likewise have no formal opportunities for such discussions.

Despite this drive for perfection, the realities of a modern health care delivery system dictate that drug-related errors are going to occur. Increased patient acuity and decreased numbers of professional staff provide all the evidence some caregivers need to advance this argument.

Medication errors are unavoidable. Humans are fallible beings who are going to make mistakes. More disturbing to seasoned clinicians is the probability that they will make more medication errors than they would otherwise, since they are involved with more patients. The possibility of making a mistake directly correlates with the frequency of prescribing, dispensing, or administering medications. Ironically, the tension that accompanies this fatalism could place the caregiver at even greater risk of making errors.

It is sobering to realize that every time a health professional provides care to a patient, a serious mistake is possible. This is as true for a pharmacist screening a new prescription order as it is for a nurse at the bedside or a physician entering prescription orders at a computer terminal. The ever-lurking likelihood of a treatment error is only one worry of concerned professionals; more upsetting is the thought that they may make a mistake that seriously harms or even kills a patient.

Although they intellectually understand the ever-present reality of error, some clinicians still have great difficulty admitting that they personally have made a mistake. To admit this would be the same as confessing that they are "bad" caregivers. They feel they have soiled their image as perfect clinicians.

Reason[6] notes the willingness of professionals to accept responsibility for their actions as part of a professional package that contains (after a long and expensive period of training) considerable power, high status, and financial rewards. In truth, some of the worst medication errors involve some of the best, most experienced practitioners. For example, there have been numerous incidents in which potassium chloride injection concentrate was given accidentally as a direct intravenous injection rather than as a constant infusion. Some of these cases have involved nurses with more than 20 years of experience, who had never previously been involved in any serious medication error.[7] We are all fallible.

To Report or Not To Report

Once an error has occurred, the question becomes whether to report it and, if so, to whom. One thing is certain: many events go unreported. Many health care providers, in fact, describe reported medication errors as the tip of the iceberg. Nurses, pharmacists, and physicians are uncertain about what to do when medication errors are made. Being able to deliberate about the clinical consequences of the error for the patient, as well as the professional consequences for the provider, is a luxury that few providers have. There may be little time for reflection. The clinician is left alone with his or her decision.

In some cases, the error may be easy to forget because the patient's condition does not change and the mistake is not likely to be discovered. Some nurses, pharmacists, and physicians do not report medication errors if there is no noticeable harm done to the patient, because to do so would be to admit to being less than perfect, making them vulnerable to being viewed as careless or incompetent.[1-5,8] Providers may cover the mistake by watching over patients, correcting the order, or taking action to dispel harm. They may deny that the event took place at all. Some physicians see themselves as the sole judges of their own mistakes, since no one else is the best judge of medical decisions.

Another approach is to rationalize errors—to choose not to recognize mistakes by describing clinical practice as an inexact discipline that combines art and science.[5] Alternatively, a provider may report the incident to a manager or to house staff; however, those individuals, too, may keep certain business insular. Being defensive about clinical actions and judgments maintains such isolation. Another approach is to admit the error only to a select few confidants.

Silence is dangerous: to oneself, to one's patients, and to one's colleagues. Warnings are missed that could help prevent injury. If the mistake is not disclosed to colleagues, no support can be offered. As a result, the emotional impact of the error persists.

Ultimately, it is concern about the patient that forces the clinician to admit the mistake. The professional does this with the foreknowledge that actions can be taken to reduce the harm incurred by errors. The health professional has the assurance that others may learn from the mistake and thus avoid making the same or similar mistakes.[1–5,8–10]

Disclosing Errors to Patients

If reporting a mistake to risk management or disclosing an error to other health care professionals is difficult, revealing an error to a patient or family is a truly arduous task. Among the consequences feared are not only the anger and rejection of the patient and family but also the threat of litigation.[2,5] In a study by Wu et al.,[4] house officers reported discussing a mistake with the patient or the patient's family in only 24% of cases.

Expecting the patient or his or her family to understand and forgive a human error that may have contributed to the patient's failure to improve, a worsening condition of the patient's, or even death may be somewhat optimistic. A survey administered to patients in an academic general internal medicine outpatient clinic by Witman et al.[11] demonstrated that 98% of respondents desire and/or expect their physician to acknowledge any error that has occurred in their care, regardless of the severity. This study also revealed a trend toward an increased likelihood to report the physician to a state medical board or to seek legal compensation for errors of greater severity. Respondents were also more apt to either report or sue the physician who failed to acknowledge the mistake.

Although this sample is small, the results underscore the importance of honesty in the physician–patient relationship and of patients' desire to be informed of all aspects of their care, including even minor errors.[11] The attention and concern demonstrated to the patient and family through the admission of the error and afterward may actually mitigate their response to the error.[2,11]

Dangers of Placing Blame

One common reason for failing to report errors is fear of punishment. It is often convenient for managers, patients, and families who are trying to come to terms with an incident to blame the practitioner. Although this reaction is universal, natural, emotionally satisfying, and legally and politically convenient, it has little or no remedial value. This is because it focuses on the last and probably the least remediable link in the accident chain, which in most cases is the direct care provider.[6]

Blaming leads to ineffective countermeasures such as disciplinary action, exhortations to "be more careful," retraining, and writing new procedures to proscribe those actions implicated in some recent accident or incident.[6] These are of little or no value and may even make matters worse, especially if they increase the fear of reporting. For this reason, the purpose of investigating errors should be to determine what system elements, such as poor labeling or packaging, short staffing, or long hours, were contributing factors.[1,10,12]

Because nurses are most often the ones at the medication–patient interface, it is understandable that they are involved in most medication errors. Inevitably, they are blamed for errors that are rooted in the system as well as in the work of other providers. Nurses have often been held responsible for the errors of physicians and pharmacists. Some are aware of a double standard: administrators often treat physicians' mistakes more lightly than those of nurses. In addition, physicians most often have separate (and often unequal) quality assurance programs. These separate peer review mechanisms prevent the open, honest interchange necessary to root out the causes and to implement system-related error prevention methods.

Emotional Impact of Disclosure

Once an individual does admit an error, he or she must face, on both a professional and a personal level, the resulting emotional impact. The emotional and spiritual distress that follow the error may be very overwhelming.

Confidence may be so shaken that some may consider leaving the profession. Some actually do.

Some individuals process the error intellectually. This may include determining how the error occurred, consulting with colleagues, validating their decision-making process, and providing extended follow-up patient care to prevent further complications. Other common reactions include embarrassment, humiliation, shame, anguish, self-disgust, self-doubt, fear, frustration, pain, guilt, sadness, anger, and depression.[1-5,13] Some health care providers have reported that they considered suicide after a patient's death that was linked to a medication error. These reactions may last for days to years. The individual's sense of devastation may never abate.[2]

Most health care professionals who have erred require reaffirmation of their professional competence and, in many cases, reassurance of their personal self-worth.[1-5,8,14] Professionals may be so troubled by the mistake that they doubt their continued ability to practice safely. They check and recheck medication orders. They may be especially vigilant when involved in a procedure similar to that in which they erred. This extreme caution regarding these procedures may work against the individual, making him or her more susceptible to future mistakes when carrying out other tasks on which he or she is less focused.[1-5,14]

Emotional support is crucial in the wake of reporting an event; however, the degree of such support, and the sources from which it is received, vary. Physicians are more likely to receive emotional support from a spouse or a close friend than from a professional colleague. Other health care professionals, such as nurses, may be more able to find supportive coworkers. Psychotherapy is an option for individuals seeking a safe forum in which to discuss their involvement in an error.

Accepting responsibility and being accountable for the error in a productive manner can be the start of the healing process that culminates in self-forgiveness.[2,5] Individuals should be held accountable for reporting potential and actual errors that are detected, analyzing root causes of the error, and recommending system-wide changes. The health care provider must then continue his or her career, more aware than before that every task and every decision has the potential for error. As a professional, one cannot allow this awareness to adversely affect performance.[1-5,13]

Role of Risk Management Programs

All institutions have risk management programs to which errors should be reported. An effective risk management program is based on honest, complete, accurate, and prompt reporting of errors.[1,15] This, however, is rarely achieved. In many cases, error reporting is viewed as a means for assigning blame and doling out punishment.[9,12,13,15–19] Such punishment may take the form of incident reports placed in the individual's personnel file, points assigned according to an arbitrary system, a written warning, probation, suspension, or even termination of employment. Serious medication errors may result in the filing of criminal negligence charges.[10,12,14,20]

Every error should be examined, not from the perspective of who is at fault but from the viewpoint of what elements in the system allowed it to happen. In this way, those who manage health systems can learn from the error and can determine what corrections are needed to prevent similar errors in the future.[1,9,10,12,13,15–17,19] Another way to prevent recurring errors is to review medication error reports in professional publications and include them in hospital newsletters.[9,16]

An institution's risk management program should stipulate that incident reports are to be used as tools to correct unfavorable elements within the system. Increased error reporting, facilitated by a nonpunitive system, will assist in identifying system problems that contribute to errors.

Need for Interprofessional Work

Clinicians can let the group know that they are "in this together" by relating stories of their own errors when a colleague makes a mistake. Nurses, for example, often share with one another the blame and the guilt for errors. With some medication errors, the blame is diffused among the nursing staff working on a certain unit.[21] However, the fact that nurses, physicians, and pharmacists often make a series of mistakes that end in drug errors has convinced them that more interprofessional work is needed. Calls for collaborative efforts targeted to prevent drug-related incidents are thus more frequent today than in the past.[1,15,17]

The interdisciplinary nature of the work required to reduce medication errors is obvious. Nurses are often held responsible for detecting the prescription and dispensing errors of physicians and pharmacists, respectively. If a nurse identifies a mistake made by a physician or pharmacist colleague, an error can be prevented. When a nurse fails to catch the mistake, however, he or she owns the medication error. Physicians or pharmacists may minimize their involvement in such an instance (by saying, e.g., "The nurse should have caught it").

In contrast, many clinicians appreciate providers who discover a potential error and who take steps to prevent it. Such appreciation should be turned toward working together and avoiding a "finger-pointing" mentality. Nurses, pharmacists, and physicians should put safety nets in place to prevent errors from happening. A formal discussion in a case conference attended by a multidisciplinary team could improve systems and prevent future errors.

Interdisciplinary acceptance of responsibility for medication errors is essential. Blame should be placed on systems rather than on nurses, pharmacists, or physicians.[1] System-wide innovations such as bar-code technology and on-line medication profiles may provide additional safety nets.

Conclusion

Medication errors are not sins or crimes, because they are unintentional. The language used to classify errors sometimes suggests otherwise; the literature speaks, for example, of errors of "commission" and "omission." The guilt and shame that health care providers feel when medication administration goes wrong point to the seriousness of the problem and perhaps explain the "sin" terminology.[2–5,22,23]

By accepting their human fallibility, nurses, pharmacists, and physicians can move away from guilt and blame and accept the fact that good people do make mistakes. Medication errors can be seen as unfortunate events and can be turned into opportunities to help prevent future errors. By collaborating through continuous quality improvement initiatives to identify system weaknesses, health professionals can begin to address the true cause of errors. Joining together will help caregivers identify solutions to the many problems that are inherent in medication administration.

●●●●
References

1. Leape LL. Error in medicine. *JAMA.* 1994; 272: 1851–57.

2. Christens JF, Livens W, Dun PM. The heart of darkness: the impact of perceived mistakes on physicians. *J Gen Intern Med.* 1992; 7: 424–31.

3. Newman MC. The emotional impact of mistakes on family physicians. *Arch Fam Med.* 1996; 5: 71–75.

4. Wu AW, Folkman S, McPhee SJ, et al. Do house officers learn from their mistakes? *JAMA.* 1991; 265: 2089–94.

5. Hilfiker D. Facing our mistakes. *N Engl J Med.* 1984; 310: 118–22.

6. Reason JT. *Human Error.* New York: Cambridge University Press; 1990.

7. Cohen MR. Ongoing potassium chloride concentrate errors kill patients: an issue of cost versus care? *Hosp Pharm.* 1996; 31: 187–88.

8. Kowalski K. From failures to major learning experiences. *Hosp Pharm.* October 1992; 27: 851–2, 4–5.

9. Cohen MR. Banish a system that blames. *Nursing 96.* January 1996: 15.

10. Anderson ER. Disciplinary action after a serious medication error. *Am J Hosp Pharm.* 1987; 44: 2690–92.

11 Witman AB, Park DM, Hardin SB. How do patients want physicians to handle mistakes? A survey of internal medicine patients in an academic setting. *Arch Intern Med.* 1996; 156: 2565–69.

12. Harnden L. Disciplinary responses to nurses' medication errors. *Dimensions.* May 1988: 26, 32.

13. Davis NM. Nonpunitive medication error reporting systems: tough to accept but safest for patients. *Hosp Pharm.* 1996; 31: 1.

14. Carley L. On probation. *Nursing 85.* September 1985: 88.

15. Honesty, incident reports and risk management (editorial). *Nursing Management.* 1981; 12: 7–8.

16. Cohen MR. Blaming employees for medication errors makes no sense. *Hosp Pharm.* 1996; 31: 322.

17. Davis NM. Is our medication error rate acceptable? *Hosp Pharm.* 1983; 18: 236.

18. Hancock MR. A pointless system? (letter). *Am J Nurs.* 1992; 92 (8): 18.

19. Green E. Quality Q&A (column). *Nursing Quality Connection.* September/October 1992: 7.

20. Nornhold P. Nursing on trial. *Nursing 97.* 1997; 27: 33.

21. Biordi DL. Nursing error and caring in the workplace. *Nursing Administration Quarterly.* 1993; 17(2): 28–45.

22. Wolf ZR. Medication errors and nursing responsibility. *Holistic Nursing Practice.* 1989; 4: 8–17.

23. Wolf ZR. *Medication Errors: The Nursing Experience.* Albany, NY: Delmar; 1994.

• • • •
Suggested Reading

Arndt M. Nurses' medication errors. *J Adv Nurs.* 1994; 19: 519–26.

Arndt M. Research in practice: how drug mistakes affect self-esteem. *Nursing Times.* 1994; 90: 27–30.

Baker H, Napthine R. Medication error: the big stick to beat you with. *Australian Nursing Journal.* 1994; 2: 28–30.

Baker H, Napthine R. Ritual + workloads = medication error. *Australian Nursing Journal.* 1994; 2: 34–36.

Booth B. Management of drug errors. *Nursing Times.* 1994; 90: 30–31.

Canavan K. ANA works to prevent medication errors. *American Nurse.* January/February 1996: 14.

Cassell J. Technical and moral error in medicine and in fieldwork. *Human Organization.* 1981; 40: 160–68.

Cohen MR. Cooperative approaches to medication error management. *Topics in Hospital Pharmacy Management.* 1991; 11: 53–65.

Cohen MR, Anderson RW, Attilio RM, et al. Preventing medication error in cancer chemotherapy. *Am J Health Syst Pharm.* 1996; 53: 737–46.

Collins SE. Nurse attorney notes. Professional nursing and unlicensed assistive personnel: a practice dilemma for the 90's. *Florida Nurse.* 1995; 43: 12–13.

Cullen DJ, Bates DW, Small SD, et al. The incident reporting system does not detect adverse drug events: a problem for quality improvement. *Jt Comm J Qual Improv.* 1995; 21: 541–42.

Elizabeth R. The mistake I'll never forget. *Nursing 90.* 1990; 20: 50–51.

Elnicki RA, Schmitt JP. Contribution of patient and hospital characteristics to adverse incidents. *Health Serv Res.* 1980; 15: 398–414.

Sin. In: *Encyclopedia Judaica.* New York: Macmillan; 1971: 1587–94.

Finkelstein P. Resign or be fired. *Minnesota Nursing Accent.* 1995; 67: 10.

Flynn ER, Wolf ZR, McGoldrick TB, et al. Effect of three teaching methods on a nursing staff's knowledge of medication error risk reduction strategies. *Journal of Nursing Staff Development*. 1996; 12: 19–26.

Foucault M. Georges Canguilhem: Philosopher of error. *I & C*. 1986; 7: 51–62.

Gladstone J. Drug administration errors: a study into the factors underlying the occurrence and reporting of drug errors in a district general hospital. *J Adv Nurs*. 1995; 22: 628–37.

Gorovitz S, MacIntyre A. Toward a theory of medical fallibility. *J Med Philos*. 1976; 1: 51–71.

Hackel R, Butt L, Banister G. How nurses perceive medication errors. *Nursing Management*. January 1996: 31–44.

Haggard HW. Error in medicine. In: Jastrow J, ed. *The Story of Human Error*. New York: Books for Libraries Press; 1967: 389–411.

Hilfiker D. *Healing the Wounds: A Physician Looks at His Work*. New York: Pantheon Books; 1985.

Hughes EC. Mistakes at work. *Journal of Economics and Political Science*. 1951; 17: 320–27.

Manthey M. Discipline without punishment, part I. *Nursing Management*. October 1989: 19.

Manthey M. Discipline without punishment, part II. *Nursing Management*. November 1989: 23.

McClure ML. Human error—a professional dilemma. *J Prof Nurs*. 1991; 7: 207.

McGuiness I. Sin (theology of). In: *New Catholic Encyclopedia*. New York: McGraw-Hill; 1967: 241–45.

Mizrahi T. Managing medical mistakes: ideology, insularity and accountability among internists-in-training. *Soc Sci Med*. 1984; 19: 135–46.

Napthine R. Pen power—doctors under scrutiny. *Australian Nursing Journal*. 1995; 3: 28–29.

National Coordinating Council for Medication Error Reporting and Prevention. *National Coordinating Council Defines Terms and Sets Goals for Medication Error Reporting and Prevention*. Rockville, Md: United States Pharmacopeia; 1996.

Norman JC. Nurses and malpractice. *Defense Law Journal*. 1991; 3: 103–08.

Paget MA. Your son is cured now; you may take him home. *Cult Med Psychiatry*. 1982; 6: 237–59.

Puckett F. Medication-management component of a point-of-care information system. *Am J Health Syst Pharm*. 1995; 52: 1305–09.

Redman BK. The ethics of leadership in pharmacy. *Am J Health Syst Pharm*. 1995; 52: 2099–104.

Rushton CH, Hogue EE. Confronting unsafe practice: ethical and legal issues. *Pediatric Nursing*. 1993; 19: 284–86.

Thigpen J. Minimizing medication errors. *Neonatal Network*. 1995; 14: 85–86.

Thompson MJ. Is there an attitude problem? *Minnesota Nursing Accent*. February 1991: 20–21.

Waters JA. Nurses' perceptions of reportable medication errors and factors that contribute to their occurrence. *Appl Nurs Res*. 1992; 5: 86–88.

Wolf ZR, McGoldrick TB, Flynn ER, et al. Factors associated with a perceived harmful outcome from medication errors: a pilot study. *Journal of Continuing Education Nursing*. 1996; 27: 65–74.

Part III:

Preventing Medication Errors: A Shared Responsibility

8.

Preventing Medication Errors Related to Prescribing

Michael R. Cohen, MS, FASHP

Institute for Safe Medication Practices
Huntingdon Valley, Pa.

Although the root causes of medication errors reside in systems, it is the responsibility of each health care professional to take every possible precaution to prevent them. The first individual who can take steps to prevent a medication error is the prescriber.

It is difficult to quantify the extent of errors related to medication prescribing, because many errors go undetected or unreported. Existing evidence suggests that the problem is substantial. Lesar and colleagues[1] reviewed medication prescribing errors in a hospital. They found an overall error rate of 3.99 clinically significant prescribing errors per 1000 orders over a 1-year period. The most common errors were associated with failure to alter drug therapy in patients with impaired renal or hepatic function (13.9%); failure to recognize a patient's allergy to the prescribed medication class (12.1%); use of an incorrect drug name, dosage form, or abbreviation (11.4%); dosage miscalculation (11.1%); and use of an unusual or atypical but critical dosage frequency (10.8%).[1]

In this chapter, the pitfalls associated with prescribing medications are discussed and suggestions are offered to help prescribers avoid them.

Written Orders

Need for Legibility

No matter how accurate or complete an order, it may be misinterpreted if it cannot be read. Illegible handwriting on medication orders and prescriptions is a widely recognized cause of medication errors.[2–6] Such errors have resulted in patient injury and death. Poor handwriting is also a source of legal concern: a 1997 report by the American Medical Association showed that medication errors secondary to misinterpreted physicians' prescriptions were the second most prevalent and expensive claim listed on 90,000 malpractice claims filed over a 7-year period.[7]

Poorly written orders may delay the administration of medications. They may increase the potential for a serious medication error stemming from an incorrect understanding of the intended drug, dosage, route of administration, or frequency. When personnel must be interrupted to clarify an order, work flow is interrupted. These interruptions can in turn affect someone's performance and further increase the chance of errors.

The prescriber's obligation to provide optimal patient care should in itself be adequate incentive to express all orders clearly. In addition, there are legal requirements that written orders be legible and that the prescriber's name be printed if the signature is not legible.[2] Prescribers with poor handwriting should take responsibility for clearly communicating the orders and prescriptions they write by taking time to write or print more carefully.[3] If the prescriber's handwriting is particularly poor, using a word processor or dictating orders, with appropriate review by the prescriber, may be necessary. Computers are playing a major role in solving the handwriting problem.[7]

Handwriting may be improved if the prescriber is seated while writing.[3] Many institutions, clinics, and physicians' offices set aside areas for order writing and dictation where the prescriber may be seated and isolated from distractions.[4]

An additional precaution that prescribers may take to ensure accurate interpretation of their orders or prescriptions is to speak to the nurse or pharmacist, as well as the patient, regarding the medication. This is especially helpful if the medication is new to the market or unfamiliar to other health care providers.

A physician, pharmacist, and pharmacy were sued as a result of a death caused by an illegible order. The physician intended to order Isordil® (isosorbide dinitrate), 20 mg every 6 hours (Figure 8–1). His handwriting was illegible, and the pharmacist misread the prescription as Plendil® (felodipine), a calcium channel blocker. The patient suffered a myocardial infarction and died. The plaintiffs maintained that the physician, pharmacist, and pharmacy failed to provide reasonable standards of medical and pharmaceutical care. They noted that the physician wrote poorly and that the purpose of the medication was not indicated on the prescription. The pharmacist was involved because he did not question the illegible prescription or

Figure 8-1

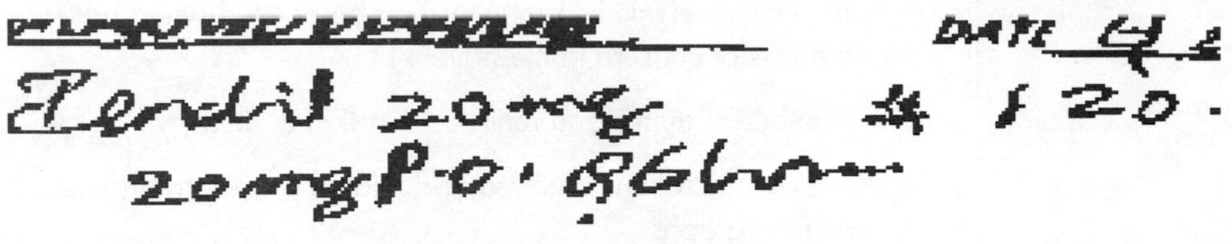

This prescription for Isordil was mis-read as "Plendil."

the high dose (the maximum dose of felodipine is 10 mg per day). The pharmacy was named because it failed to incorporate controls that could have prevented the error (for example, the pharmacy computer did not catch the excessive dose).

Need for Complete Information

It is the prescriber's responsibility to communicate complete information to all intended readers. A complete order should include the following:[8–10]

1. Patient name.

2. Patient-specific data.

3. Generic and brand names of the drug. Ideally, both should be expressed. If only one is used, the generic name is preferable, unless there is a possibility for confusion because another drug has a similar name or because a specific brand is desired. Research or chemical names, chemical symbols, abbreviations, and locally coined names should be avoided.

4. The drug strength should be expressed in metric units by weight (e.g., milligrams [mg], grams [g], milliequivalents [mEq], or millimoles [mmol]). The apothecary system should not be used.

5. Dosage form.

6. Amount to be dispensed, expressed in metric units. Package units (bottle, tube, ampul) should not be used.

7. Complete directions for use, including route of administration and frequency of dosing. Ambiguous orders, such as "take as directed," should be avoided unless they are accompanied by further directions. Specific instructions reinforce proper medication use by the patient, differentiate the intended medication from other medications, and allow the dispenser to check the appropriate dose for the individual patient and counsel the patient.

8. Purpose of the medication. This provides the pharmacist, the nurse, and the patient with an additional way to ensure that they have the correct medication. (This information may be omitted when patient confidentiality is of concern to the patient.)

9. Number of authorized refills or duration of therapy.

Specific considerations on these and related issues are discussed in the following paragraphs.

Specific Issues to Consider When Writing an Order

Patient-Specific Information. The prescriber must consider the individual patient when selecting a medication. A complete patient history, including age; weight; renal and hepatic function; concurrent disease states; results of laboratory tests; current medications (including over-the-counter medications, vitamin and mineral supplements, and herbal or homeopathic remedies); allergies; and medical, surgical, and family history is recommended. If the patient is a woman, the history should include pregnancy or lactation status.[1,9]

The history should be reviewed for potential contraindications to the medication being considered and possible interactions with other medications the patient is receiving. The prescriber should not rely on the checks and balances system within the health care system to verify the appropriateness of the drug, because this system is fallible. Moreover, the prescriber may have information in the patient history that is not readily available to other health care professionals. The prescriber should communicate pertinent patient information, along with the medication order, to other health care professionals so that they can be better prepared to assess the appropriateness of the order.[1,4]

Abbreviations. Abbreviations may appear to be great time savers. If not properly used, however, they consume the time of other health care professionals and increase the potential for medication errors.[11] Abbreviations may be misunderstood for a variety of reasons. An abbreviation may have more than one meaning; the reader may be unfamiliar with the meaning of the abbreviation; or, if poorly written, it may be mistaken for another abbreviation.[8,9,11–14]

Prescribers should avoid any nonstandard abbreviations, including Latin directions for use. Certain abbreviations are consistently misunderstood and should never be used. These include the following:[9,12,14]

- Drug names,
- Any abbreviation for the word *daily*,

- The letter "U" for the word *unit,*
- "µg" for *microgram* (use "mcg"),
- "QOD" for *every other day,*
- "sc" or "sq" for *subcutaneous,*
- "a/" or "&" for the word *and,*
- "cc" for *cubic centimeter,*
- "D/C" for *discontinue* or *discharge.*

A complete list of abbreviations that have been associated with medication errors and that should never be used appears in Chapter 5.

Expression of Weights, Volumes, and Units. Prescribers should express all weights, volumes, and units by using the metric system. The apothecary system can lead to errors because of many users' unfamiliarity with the units and their abbreviations, confusion between apothecary and metric system units, and errors in conversion from the apothecary system to the metric system.[9,14–16]

There are many examples of errors associated with the apothecary system. For example, the symbol for *minim* (M_x) has been confused with "mL," causing a 16-fold overdose. Nurses have thus given 10 mL of opium tincture instead of 10 minims. Syringes marked with a minim scale have been confused with insulin syringes, resulting in massive insulin overdoses. In one case the symbol for 1 dram (**ʒi**) was mistaken for 3 tablespoons (T), leading to a theophylline overdose in a child. The abbreviations for grain (gr) and gram (g) can easily be confused. There is also confusion about the interpretation of fractional doses, such as "gr 1/200." For example, a nurse gave 2 x 1/100-grain tablets of nitroglycerin when her supply of 1/200 grain tablets ran out. If the metric system had been used, it would have been obvious that 1/100 (0.6 mg) plus 1/100 (0.6 mg) does not equal 1/200 (0.3 mg).

Because of this confusion, the *United States Pharmacopeia XXIII/National Formulary XVIII* does not recognize the apothecary system as an official system for measurement of drug doses. All expressions of strength, including those on manufacturers' labels, medication orders and prescriptions, and dispensing labels, must be in metric units. The exception is cases in which it is appropriate to express the strength of the medication as a percentage of active ingredient.[15]

Expressing doses or quantities in terms of dosage form, volume, or packaging units is also unacceptable.[8,17,18] Some exceptions to this rule do exist; two examples are insulin and heparin, both of which are expressed in units. Volume may be used along with a strength or concentration or in cases in which the concentration or strength is not a factor (e.g., cola syrup). For example, it is acceptable (though redundant) to prescribe 5 mL of a solution of 100 mg/5 mL. It is also acceptable to prescribe by volume when there is no strength because of a combination of many ingredients or no active ingredient, as in cola syrup.

The importance of including strength of medications on prescription orders is illustrated by a case in which a physician prescribed intravenous digoxin for an infant (Figure 8–2). Because the order did not specify strength, the baby received 1.5 mL of the adult concentration, 0.25 mg/mL, instead of the pediatric concentration, 0.1 mg/mL. The child required digoxin immune Fab fragment (ovine) to bind and inactivate digoxin in her blood.

The following error illustrates the problems that may result from the use of apothecary symbols. A physician reduced the daily warfarin dosage for a patient in a long-term care facility from 3 mg to 2.5 mg. He wrote the order as "5 mg ss̄ [the apothecary symbol for one half] every day." The pharmacist dispensed the prescription with 5-mg tablets cut in half, and the nurse transcribed the order onto the patient's medication administration record exactly as it had been written.

A bottle of warfarin 5 mg remained in the patient's medication drawer, even though the patient had not taken 5 mg daily for some time. The other nurses overlooked the "ss̄" symbol in the medication book and administered 5 mg every day to the patient from the old bottle.

For 3 weeks, the patient, who had a history of stroke and congestive heart failure, received 5 mg instead of 2.5 mg of warfarin. He died, and the death certificate stated that gastrointestinal hemorrhage was a significant contributing factor.

A combination of factors led to these tragic consequences. First, the physician used a nonstandard abbreviation, "ss̄." Second, the discontinued pre-

Figure 8-2

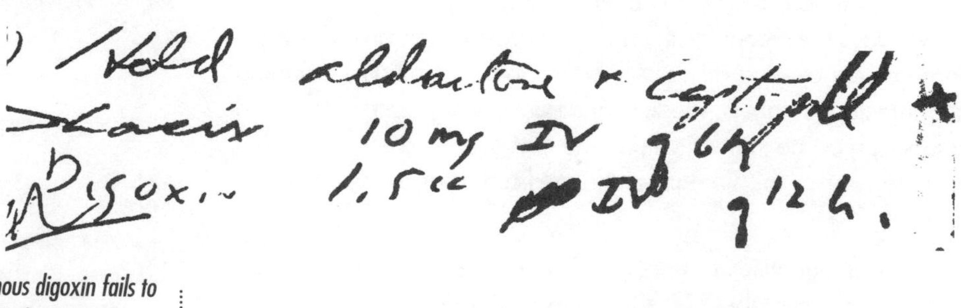

Order for intravenous digoxin fails to include strength. Medication orders must always include strength in metric weight.

scription was not removed from the medication drawer. Removing discontinued medications may seem wasteful for a health care institution, but errors like this are much more costly. Finally, because warfarin 2.5-mg tablets are available, these should have been prescribed. The pharmacist should have contacted the prescriber to have the prescription changed.

Decimals. Numbers containing decimal points are a major source of errors. They can easily be missed, especially on lined order sheets, carbon and no-carbon-required (NCR) forms, and faxes. If a decimal point is missed, an overdose may occur. Decimals should be written with great care and should be avoided whenever a satisfactory alternative exists.[8,13,14] For example, the prescriber should write "500 mg" in place of "0.5 g," or "125 mcg" instead of "0.125 mg."

A decimal point should never be left "naked." Decimal expressions of less than 1 should always be preceded by a zero (0) to enhance the visibility of the decimal.[8,9,12–14] "Trailing" zeroes (e.g., "1.0"), however, should not be used; that is, a whole number should never be followed with a decimal point and a zero.[8,9,12–14]

A space should appear between the name of the medication and the dose, as well as between the dose and the units.[13] For example, "Inderal40mg" may easily be misread as "Inderal 140 mg" instead of "Inderal 40 mg."

Drug Names. Names of drugs that look or sound alike increase the risk for medication errors. Overlapping dosage ranges within a look-alike or sound-alike pair compound the problem. Errors involving these medications may occur when the prescriber interchanges the two drugs while writing the order or prescription, when someone misinterprets a poorly written order or prescription and does not verify the correct drug with the prescriber, or when the person taking a verbal order or prescription does not hear the order correctly and fails to repeat the order to the prescriber.[4,19]

A common cause of name mix-ups is what human-factors experts call "confirmation bias." A practitioner confronted with a poorly written order may see the name with which he or she is most familiar and may overlook any evidence to the contrary. In many cases the practitioner never thinks of questioning the order.

Computer systems can reduce the risk of confirmation bias and drug name mix-ups. Many systems can be programmed to display on the monitor a clinical flag or a formulary note that contains important drug-related information. This feature can alert the person entering the order when a look-alike or sound-alike danger is present. When the drug name "Norvasc®" is entered into the computer at Erie County Medical Center in Buffalo, N.Y., for example, a formulary note appears on the screen and alerts the pharmacist that Norvasc® often looks like Navane®. The pharmacist can then take steps to confirm the order if necessary. The Erie County Medical Center uses such notes for more than 100 name pairs.

Prescribers must take extra care, by writing or speaking more clearly and taking steps to confirm that other health care providers understand what medication is intended, when they order medications for which there is a known look-alike or sound-alike. The error may be avoided by expressing the purpose for which the medication is prescribed, given that few look-alike or sound-alike drug pairs include two drugs with the same therapeutic indication.[8,9,19,20] An additional safety check is to educate the patient concerning his or her prescription medications. Including the purpose of the medication on the prescription and the label facilitates this safety check.[19]

A related type of error is caused by the addition of a suffix to an already-familiar drug name when a new dosage form is marketed. These suffixes can cause errors if they are omitted from the prescription; if they are misinterpreted as an abbreviation, dosage, or administration directions; or if they are ignored.[4,21] For example, when extended-release Procardia XL® was first marketed, many people thought they heard "Procardia® sl" (sublingual) when verbal orders were communicated. A list of problem suffixes has been published elsewhere.[22]

Purpose of Medication. Prescribers should indicate the purpose of the medication on the order or prescription. This provides pharmacists with an additional way to confirm that they have interpreted the order correctly. This is especially useful in preventing medication errors associated with look-alike drug names, because very few of these pairs have similar indications.[9,20,23] (A list of look-alike names is available from the U.S. Pharmacopeia at 1-800-272-8772. The "Safety Briefs" and drug name problem alerts published in *ISMP Medication Safety Alert!* help practitioners keep the information up to date.)

The pharmacist should place information concerning the purpose of the medication on the label. This provides patients with a way to confirm that they have the medication their physician has prescribed and gives them an additional means of distinguishing among the medications they are taking.[20,23] A prescription form designed to remind prescribers to include the medication's purpose is shown in Figure 8–3.

Many prescribers are concerned that placing information concerning the purpose of a medication order will violate patient confidentiality. Others resist it because of the time required or because of concern that insurers will deny payment of medications prescribed for off-label indications.[9,20,23] Use of the "Triple i" Safety Bar may allay some of these concerns (Figure 8–4). This vertical bar, displaying icons representing various therapeutic categories, appears on the right-hand side of some prescription blanks. The prescriber places a check in front of the appropriate icon.[23]

An error that underscores the importance of including the purpose on prescriptions occurred in association with an outpatient prescription for Florinef®. In this case, the physician neither wrote the strength on the prescription nor included directions for its use. The prescription was misread as Fiorinal®. Had the dose and directions been included, this error could have been avoided, because the recommended dose and directions for Fiorinal® differ from those for Florinef®. Including the purpose (the patient had Addison's disease and the drug was being prescribed to control electrolyte balance) would also have prevented the mix-up, since Fiorinal® is an analgesic.

Figure 8-3

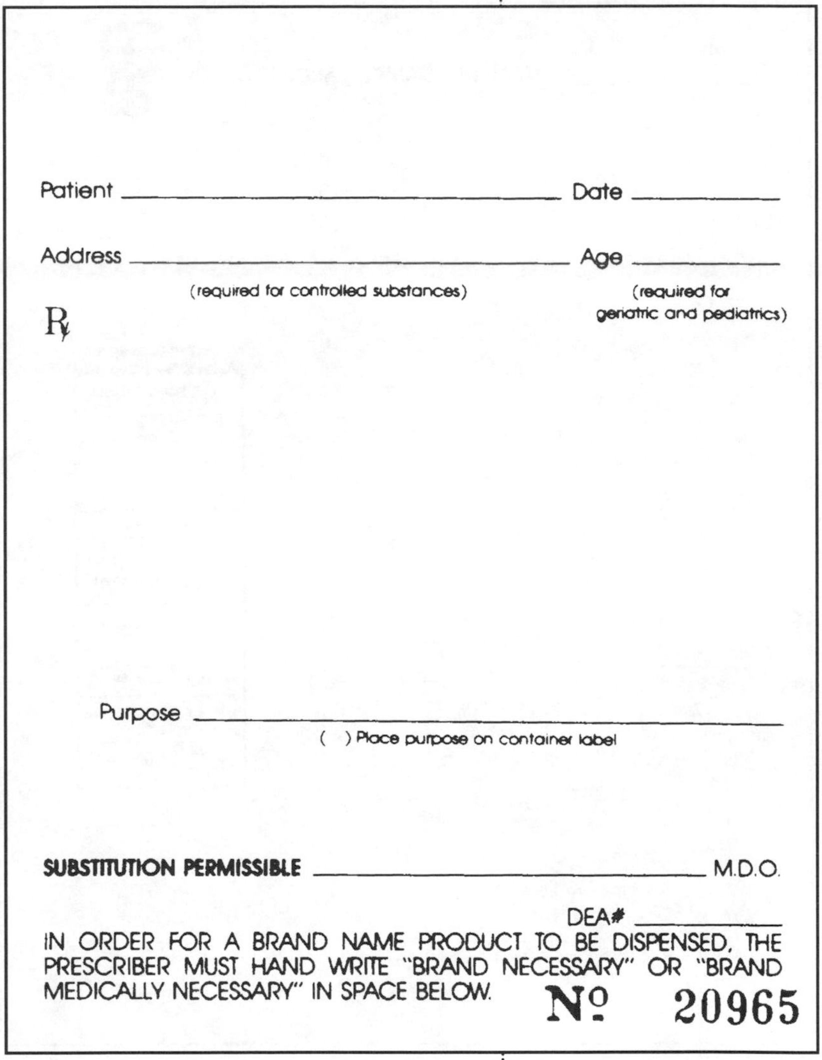

Patient _____ Date _____

Address _____ Age _____

(required for controlled substances) (required for geriatric and pediatrics)

℞

Purpose _____

( ) Place purpose on container label

SUBSTITUTION PERMISSIBLE _____ M.D.O.

DEA# _____

IN ORDER FOR A BRAND NAME PRODUCT TO BE DISPENSED, THE PRESCRIBER MUST HAND WRITE "BRAND NECESSARY" OR "BRAND MEDICALLY NECESSARY" IN SPACE BELOW.

№ 20965

Medication Order Systems and Error Prevention

Prescribers should be familiar with the medication ordering system of every institution at which they hold privileges.[8] They should make every effort to prescribe medications that are on the formulary, because other professionals within the institution are familiar with them and are less likely to make errors with these medications than with those that are not on the formulary.

Preprinted forms such as these, which specifically request the prescriber to indicate the purpose of the medication, are recommended.

Figure 8-4

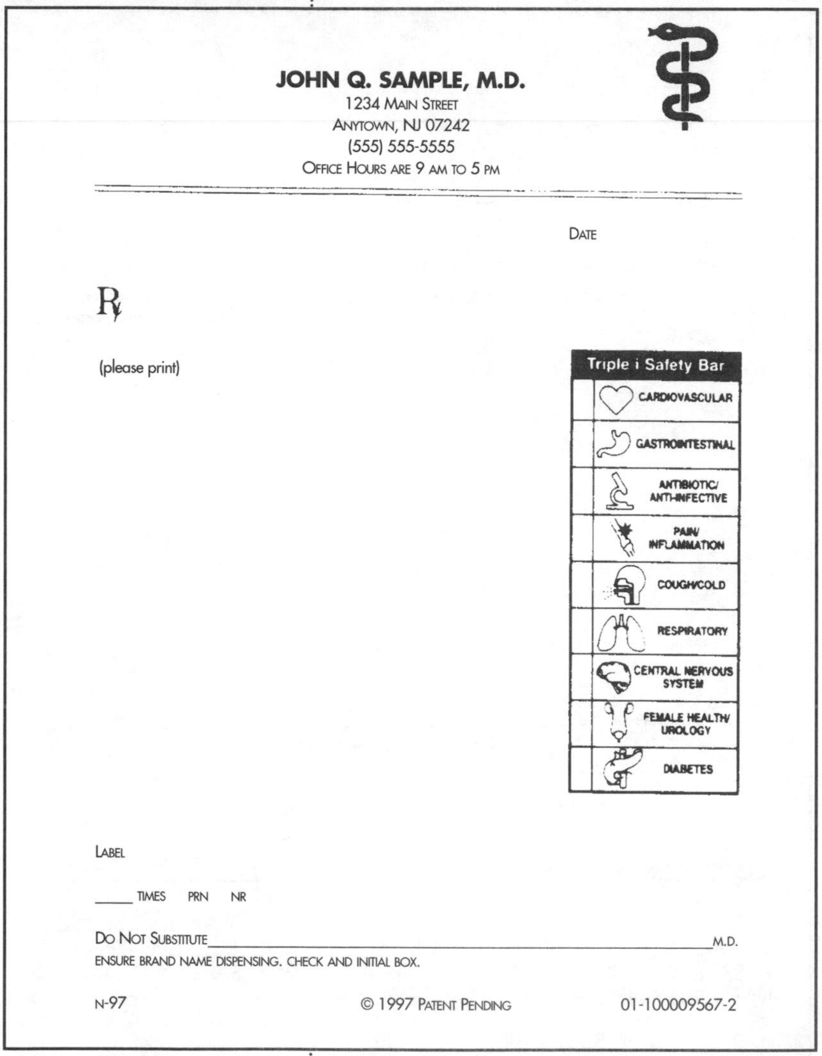

If a nonformulary medication must be ordered, prescribers should be familiar with ordering procedures in order to avoid delays in the initiation of therapy. They should write the medication order clearly and reinforce it in conversations with the nurse or pharmacist.

To avoid delays in initiation of therapy, the prescriber should understand how medication orders are processed. Orders are either taken from the chart and sent to the pharmacy as a carbon, NCR, or fax or are generated electronically through a computer system.

Prescribers should be familiar with standard medication administration times for institutional prescribing. Doses administered at odd intervals (e.g., every 11 hours), or those given at regular intervals but off the standard medication administration times, are more likely to be given at the wrong times or to be missed altogether than are those administered at standard times. It is usually preferable to adjust the dosage of a medication, rather than adjust the dosing interval, in order to maintain a standard interval. For example, if a patient with renal failure needs a dose adjustment for gentamicin, it is safer to order a smaller dose given on an even schedule (e.g., every 12 hours) than to order the medication in its normal dose to be administered every 16 hours.

JOHN Q. SAMPLE, M.D.
1234 MAIN STREET
ANYTOWN, NJ 07242
(555) 555-5555
OFFICE HOURS ARE 9 AM TO 5 PM

DATE

R⁄

(please print)

Triple i Safety Bar

CARDIOVASCULAR
GASTROINTESTINAL
ANTIBIOTIC/ ANTI-INFECTIVE
PAIN/ INFLAMMATION
COUGH/COLD
RESPIRATORY
CENTRAL NERVOUS SYSTEM
FEMALE HEALTH UROLOGY
DIABETES

LABEL

_____ TIMES   PRN   NR

DO NOT SUBSTITUTE_____M.D.
ENSURE BRAND NAME DISPENSING. CHECK AND INITIAL BOX.

N-97   © 1997 PATENT PENDING   01-100009567-2

The Triple i Safety Bar allows the prescriber to easily indicate the general purpose of the medication. Over 30 icons are available to satisfy the needs of individual specialties.

Finally, the procedure for modifying an order that has been written is important. Once a prescriber has written an order, he or she should not alter the original copy. If that copy has already been sent to the pharmacy, the change or correction will be missed, resulting in a medication error. To revise an order, the prescriber should write a new order and alert the nursing unit staff of it.[24]

If an error is made or an order change must be written, it should not be erased or otherwise obliterated. Instead, the prescriber should draw a single, thin line through all of the erroneous material, write the word *error* next to the lined-out area, and date and initial the error. Corrections should only be entered as new orders.

Preprinted Order Forms

To minimize communication system errors, one of the steps advocated by the Institute for Safe Medication Practices is to standardize communication by using preprinted orders. If preprinted orders are not carefully designed and checked, however, they may actually contribute to errors.

Many health care professionals feel a certain amount of comfort with preprinted orders, since such forms are usually approved by one or more committees within the institution before they are printed in mass quantities. All disciplines should be involved in the development, review, and approval of such forms.[25,26]

Recommendations for handwritten prescriptions and orders apply equally to preprinted forms. Generic drug names should be used. Reasons for drug administration should be specified whenever possible. The dose per meter squared (m^2) or per kilogram (kg) should be required on all chemotherapy and pediatric orders; a calculated dose must also be entered. The daily dose and the number of days it is to be taken should have to be entered on any multiple-day regimen.[25,26]

Use of the apothecary system, abbreviations, coined names, trailing zeroes, and printed order forms prepared by pharmaceutical companies should be avoided. Inclusion of commonly allergenic medications on a printed form may increase the risk of exposing allergic patients to such agents, because the prescriber can easily overlook the need to strike out the offending agent. Ambiguous statements such as "Unless allergic, give..." are not acceptable because they transfer clinical and legal responsibility to clinicians other than the prescriber and may fail to protect the allergic patient from receiving the medication. Rather, a uniform system should be developed and used to indicate orders that should or should not be followed. Providing a list of medications from which the prescriber may choose is not recommended because it is too easy to choose the wrong medication.[25,26] For instance, vincristine has been confused with vinblastine and carboplatin with cisplatin.

Because preprinted order forms have become the standard for many hospital-run protocols, algorithms, critical pathways, and guidelines, it is increasingly important for institutions to have in place some methods and rules to evaluate and use order forms. In addition to the recommendations just described, the following are recommended when institutions develop preprinted order forms:

- Do not use preprinted orders unless all disciplines are involved in the process for developing, reviewing, and giving final approval to the forms.

- Do not allow orders that do not coincide with hospital policy (e.g., many hospitals do not permit instructions to "renew all previous orders").

- Avoid using preprinted hospital order forms that are sponsored or prepared by pharmaceutical companies; such forms may promote a specific product or may list nonformulary items. Blank order forms for use in preparing preprinted orders should be accessible only through authorized personnel.

- Use generic drug names on forms and specify the reason for their administration whenever possible. The brand name should also be included for single-source items.

- No forbidden abbreviations or dangerous dose designations should appear on the forms. Each hospital should have a list of these forbidden terms and abbreviations.

- Require the dose per meter squared (m^2) or per kilogram (kg) for all chemotherapy and pediatric orders when a calculated dose must be entered.

- Express doses by metric weight (e.g., 5 mg) rather than by number of tablets, milliliters (mL), and so forth, unless the drug is not measured by weight (e.g., milk of magnesia).

- Avoid coined names and jargon such as *magic mouthwash* and *banana bag*, as they may be misunderstood by people who are unfamiliar with them.

- Enhance readability by using fonts and print styles that are of professional quality. Proper spelling and spacing are important (i.e., "propranolol20mg" is easily misread as "propranolol 120 mg").

- Lines on back copies of any carbonless order form are unnecessary and may hide decimal points or portions of a number or name. Instruct the printer to leave them off.

- Print a tracking number and revision date on the form to ease replacement.[25,26]

- Review all printed order forms every 2 to 3 years or when protocols change.[25,26]

Safe preprinted orders forms are no accident. A system must be in place to ensure the forms being used are safe. In one case there was a preprinted order sheet listing the protocol for managing acute pain on which the prescriber listed six different analgesics (three parenteral and three oral), all with dose ranges (e.g., "morphine 4–10 mg i.m. q 4 h," "Vicodin 1 tab p.o. q 4–5 h"), relying on the nurse to choose the drug, dose, dosage form, route, frequency, and parameters by which the drugs should be given. In addition, the long list of drugs was preceded by a statement to "use minimum drug amounts initially in patients less than 120 pounds or over age 65." Worse, the orders were followed with the statement, "May use any of the above medications as long as the patient is not allergic."

Simplification and standardization are two important methods for reducing errors. Orders such as that just described, which complicate clinical situations, are bound to increase the frequency of errors. Carrying out such orders entails separately transcribing each drug name. This increases the risk of transcription errors or errors in dose documentation. In most states, this type of order would be considered illegal, because it abrogates the physician's responsibility. Statements that transfer responsibility for checking allergies from the prescriber to others increase liability, including that of the hospital, if a patient receives a known allergen and has a reaction. An important checkpoint for allergy detection is eliminated, since the order implies that the person administering the medication, rather than the person who prescribed the drug, is solely responsible for performing the check. In the example just given, the statement about checking allergies followed, rather than preceded, the long list of drug alternatives, making it even more likely that this statement would be missed and that allergy screening would not be properly performed.

Printed forms should be edited for correct spelling; doses; spacing between drug name, dose, and unit of measurement; and compliance with hospital policy. Readability may be enhanced by using professional-quality font and print styles. It is advisable not to place lines on the back copies of duplicate order forms, because the lines may obscure decimal points or portions of words or numbers.[25,26]

Importance of Dosage Calculations

Patient-specific information (e.g., height, weight, age, and body system function) should be used to calculate the correct dose for an individual patient if the medication in question is influenced by these factors. For example, many renally eliminated drugs may be adjusted for renal function using creatinine clearance as a measure. Some drugs should be adjusted to reduce the risk of toxicity, whereas others may be adjusted to reduce expenses without sacrificing patient care.

Dosage calculations are a well-recognized cause of medication errors. Perlstein et al.[27] reported a study showing that 1 of every 12 dosages calculated by 95 registered nurses in an intensive care unit contained errors that would result in the administration of doses 10 times larger or smaller than those prescribed. Eleven pediatricians, given the same examination, scored higher than the nurses but still made errors at the rate of 1 of every 26 computations attempted.

Two solutions are most evident: performing routine, independent cross-checking, or avoiding calculations. Through standardization of drug concentrations and use of commercially prepared dosage forms, many calculations can be avoided, but the prescriber's cooperation is mandatory. Chapter 5 discusses the value of standardization of critical care drugs as a way to avoid calculation errors.

Cross-checking is especially useful when calculating doses for pediatric or geriatric patients, cancer patients, and patients in the critical care setting. In these and other situations that involve a potentially dangerous drug, an unfamiliar calculation, or an especially sensitive patient population, prescribers should include both the mg/kg and the mg/m^2 dose (or other dose expressed as unit per weight or unit per body surface area in metric units) used in their calculation, as well as the actual dose they have calculated.[28,29]

A 13-month study[30] at Albany Medical Center, N.Y., examined the nature of 200 consecutive prescribing errors arising from the use of dosage equations. Errors included those made with common calculations such as "mg/kg/day in four divided doses" and "mg/kg q6h." Most (69.5%) errors involved pediatric patients, which is hardly surprising when one considers that prescribing medications for children often requires the use of a dosage equation. Errors in the placement of decimal points, in mathematical calculations, and in expressions of dosage regimens accounted for 59.5% of the errors. The dosage equation itself, however, was misinterpreted in 29.5% of the errors. Examples include prescribing the entire day's dose as a single dose instead of properly dividing it into dosing intervals for that day, and using the entire day's dose each time for each dosing interval through-out the day. The "take-home" message is that medication errors are certain to occur when dosage equations are used. Some alternatives to using dosage equations include using preestablished dose ranges or tables, incor-porating a calculator into a computer order entry system, and requiring both the calculated dosage and the dosage equation to appear on orders to facilitate independent checks.[30]

The importance of cross-checking dosages is illustrated by an event that took place at a children's hospital in California. Because of an obscured decimal point, an order for "2.6 mg of hydralazine i.v. q 4–6 hours," which was prescribed for a 9-year-old patient with leukemia, was misread as "26 mg" (Figure 8–5). A nurse gave the incorrect dose, and the child became hypotensive and suffered cardiac arrest. He never regained consciousness and was removed from ventilatory support 4 days later.

When writing prescriptions for pediatric patients, physicians should include the dose in milligrams per kilogram (mg/kg) as well as the calculated dose.

Figure 8-5

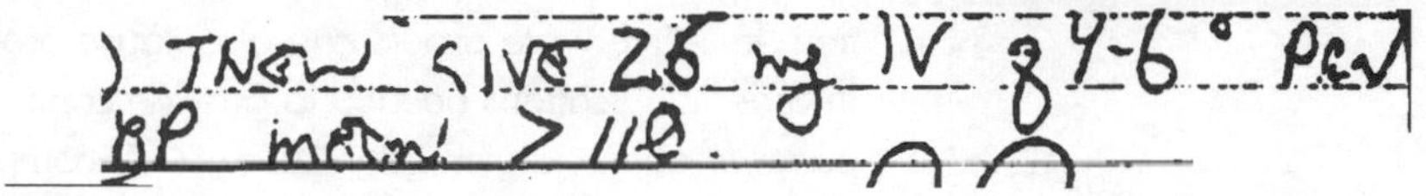

This order for 2.6 mg of hydralazine was misread as "26 mg."

Pharmacists and nurses should be responsible for independently double-checking the calculation. This entails recalculation, not just "eye-balling" the mathematics. The child in this example weighed 57 pounds (25.9 kg). If the doctor had written the dose as "2.6 mg (0.1 mg/kg)," the mistake may have been recognized.

Prescribers must ensure that clinical personnel understand the order before they leave the floor or hang up the phone. They should look over what has been written and request that all verbal orders be repeated. Completing patient charts one at a time, rather than in batches, ensures that the pre-scriber is on hand to answer the transcriber's questions.

Errors such as that just described are more likely to occur when floor per-sonnel have access to medications before the order has been reviewed by a pharmacist. Therefore, it is important that institutions develop guidelines that define what types of medications will be available to clinical areas with-out pharmacist review. Hospitals should define situations in which pharma-cists and nurses should not dispense or administer certain drugs without allowing time for expert review by a peer group.[31]

Establishment and enforcement of institutional, therapy-specific dose limits can reduce the possibility that an improper dose will reach a patient. Dose limits could be established, for example, for the maximum amount for a single dose, per 24-hour period, per cycle of therapy, and for a lifetime amount of a certain drug (e.g., anthracyclines). Drugs and limits should be communicated to all personnel involved in ordering, dispensing, and administering medications. An easily retrievable list should be made available for referral. Where software allows it, maximum doses should be entered into pharmacy computer systems. Pharmacists and nurses should be aware that any dose exceeding the limit may not be dispensed unless it undergoes an independent review that includes input from clinicians other than the involved prescriber, nurse, and pharmacist. Such a review would outline steps to be followed to ensure that all necessary information is available to guide in decision making.

Failure to Write Orders

Although writing orders provides many opportunities for miscommunication, failing to write orders can also cause problems. An example is failing to order medications needed to provide continuous therapy at the time of a patient's admission or after surgery. A complete drug history should be taken upon admission of every patient. When medications are resumed postoperatively, or whenever a patient is transferred from one hospital area to another, all previous medication orders should be reviewed. Specific orders should be written. Orders to "resume all previous medications" are not acceptable.

Verbal Orders

Verbal (spoken) orders should be avoided whenever possible. Only physicians, pharmacists, and nurses should be permitted to dictate and receive verbal prescriptions and orders.[8]

Many of the precautions that apply to written orders apply to verbal orders as well. Care must be taken to ensure that the prescription or order is heard correctly. Many drug names sound alike. Some of these products have overlapping dosage ranges, which increases the risk for error. For example, one woman in premature labor with twins had received various tocolytic agents, including magnesium sulfate. A perinatologist told the attending physician to order 100 mg of indomethacin by saying the words *two fifty milligrams* (meaning two 50-mg suppositories) if other agents were not effective in suppressing labor. The next day, when the magnesium sulfate was no longer effective, the attending physician called in a verbal order for "250 mg of indomethacin." The nurse hesitated to administer five suppositories. However, in communicating her concerns to the prescriber, she became intimidated and decided to give the medication. The perinatologist later confirmed that the order should have been 100 mg. Fortunately, no injury occurred.

Stating the words *one hundred milligrams* instead of *two fifty milligrams* would have been clearer. Had this dose been expressed in writing, this error would not have occurred. This incident makes a strong case for avoiding verbal orders. It also shows that error prevention entails more than removing problem products from patient care areas, reading labels three times, or implementing medication administration protocols. Rather, error prevention is a state of mind—an attitude of collaboration and cooperation.

Numbers in the teens can sound like multiples of 10, from 30 to 90, which can be mistaken for 13 and 19, respectively. A case in point occurred when a discharged patient was readmitted to the hospital and the admitting physician wrote a prescription for "olanzapine 50 mg q h." The nurse questioned the high dose, but the physician insisted that the patient had been discharged on that dose. Upon checking, the pharmacist found that the patient had been taking 15 mg of olanzapine during a previous hospital stay. In the medical record, the oral discharge summary had been misunderstood by the transcriptionist, who recorded "50 mg" instead of "15 mg."

Dictated medical records must be checked by the prescriber, and verbal orders should be stated in the way that pilots state numbers (e.g., say "one-five mg" instead of "fifteen mg"). Practitioners cannot assume that medical records are correct. When medical records staff return dictations to practitioners for double-checking, they should mark the drug doses in boldface type as a signal to practitioners to verify them.

Verbal orders should be enunciated slowly and distinctly. Difficult drug names should be spelled out, and complete and nonambiguous information should be relayed. The recipient should transcribe the order and immediately verify it by reading it back to the prescriber. In the institutional setting, provisions should be made to place the order in the patient's chart. The prescriber should countersign the order as soon as possible (preferably within 24 hours, although a longer period may be necessary in long-term care facilities).[8]

Verbal orders that specify the dose in number of tablets, ampules, or vials, as well as those that state a volume without also expressing the concentration, have led to serious errors because many medications are available in several package sizes and strengths. These errors underscore the importance of expressing doses by unit of weight. In addition, the person preparing the dose should call out exactly what was prepared.

Verbal orders may be necessary in an emergency. Despite the need for haste, precautions such as those just described are essential. The following two cases of errors that occurred in conjunction with emergency verbal orders also illustrate how important these factors are.

In the first case, a physician ordered "naloxone one-half amp i.v. stat" for an elderly patient experiencing respiratory depression from meperidine. The nurse took a 10-mL, 1-mg/mL vial of naloxone from an automated dispensing unit and administered half of the vial, a total dose of 5 mg of naloxone. The physician meant half of a 1-mL, 0.4-mg/mL vial, or 0.2 mg.

In the second case, a physician ordered "0.1 of flumazenil i.v., repeat every 30–60 seconds," to reverse the effect of midazolam in an elderly patient. The nurse administered four doses of flumazenil 0.1 mL, and the patient's status remained unchanged. A second nurse noticed that the first nurse was drawing up 0.1 mL instead of 0.1 mg (1 mL). The correct dose was administered, and the patient was aroused.

A final concern with verbal ordering of medications that applies to the outpatient setting is the possibility of fraud. In such cases, a layperson may attempt to call in a prescription (often for a controlled substance). The responsibility for preventing such occurrences is borne by the pharmacist who takes the order. If all the appropriate information is given correctly by the caller and the pharmacist still suspects that the verbal prescription may be an attempt at fraud, the prescriber should be called to verify the prescription.

Electronic Order Transmission

To avoid verbal orders, many institutions now use electronic communications, such as e-mail and facsimile transmission. Faxes, however, may present problems. The Institute for Safe Medication Practices was recently informed of an incident involving an order for bleomycin. The order asked for a test dose of the drug and then, if no acute reaction was observed, the administration of 8.2 units of bleomycin. Because the amount of the test dose was not specified, the pharmacist called the nursing unit. After the nurse received the order for the test dose, she faxed it to the pharmacy, noting that the original order would follow. A copy of the fax appears in Figure 8–6.

The pharmacist prepared to fill the prescription, which would have totaled

13.2 units. Since he found only one vial, containing 15 units, in the refrigerator, he asked the pharmacy buyer to place a stat order. At this point,

another pharmacist commented that it was odd that the test dose (believed at this point to be 5 units) should be almost the same size as the therapeutic dose (8.2 units). Further preparation of the doses was halted until the original order was received.

Figure 8-6

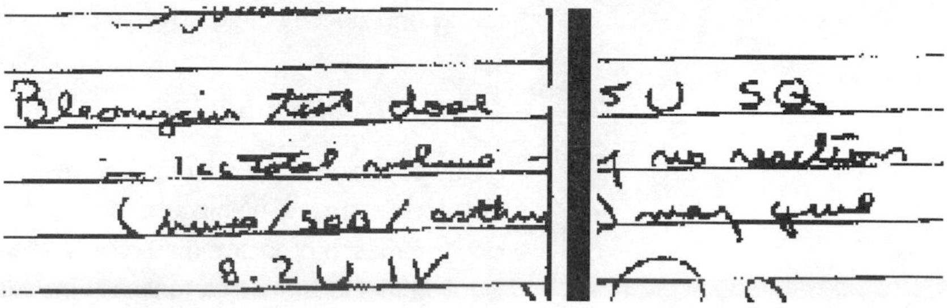

A vertical streak, caused by "noise" during a facsimile transmission, interfered with the readability of this order for bleomycin.

When the original order arrived in the pharmacy, it became evident that the physician wanted a test dose of 0.5 unit. An extraneous vertical line on the fax transmission fell in exactly the right place to obscure the decimal point and cause confusion.

Several measures can be taken to reduce the possibility of error when orders are transmitted by fax. Equipment that produces copies with streaking should be immediately repaired. Routine maintenance is essential. Ideally, no order faxed to a pharmacy should be filled until the original copy has been received. However, this approach obviates the chief benefit of fax transmission, which is speed. A compromise is to review each fax order carefully. If the copy contains blackened or faded areas, or if there is significant phone line "noise" appearing as small, random, black marks or streaks on the paper, the pharmacist should carefully inspect the copy to ascertain whether such marks appear in the area where the order has been written. If there are extraneous marks in this area, the pharmacy should verify the order before dispensing the drug or wait for the original to arrive. Even if the copy is clear, the order must be checked against the original or verified before the medication is dispensed.

Conversion to electronic prescribing by entering orders on a computer could correct many of the problems described in this chapter. Poorly handwritten prescriptions would be eliminated. Proper terminology could be ensured. Ambiguous orders and omitted information could be prevented. Vital patient and drug-specific information, such as overdose warnings, drug interactions, and allergy alerts, could be presented electronically to the prescriber at the moment of order entry so that potential adverse drug events that would otherwise go unrecognized can easily be avoided. Schiff and Rucker[32] have observed that virtually all prescriptions written in the United States are still handwritten. They also noted that a recent investigation of

245 pharmacies revealed that more than 30% filled simultaneous prescriptions for potentially lethal combinations! The use of computers would not only help prescribers avoid dosing mistakes; they would also help in monitoring and documenting adverse events and therapeutic outcomes.[32]

Drug Formulary System

Many physicians are under the impression that a drug formulary is a cost control mechanism and nothing more. In truth, an effective formulary system is first and foremost a proactive medication safety feature. When drugs and administration methods are systematically included (or deleted) in a controlled drug formulary, there are numerous benefits in addition to cost control. First, each new drug added through a formulary system undergoes a peer review process that uncovers any safety concerns with the drug. As a result, drug protocols or other specific policy or practice issues can be implemented before, rather than after, use of the drug. Examples include restricting the use of a chemotherapy agent to medical oncologists or determining the maximum dose of a drug that can be safely dispensed. In addition, when drugs are systematically added to the formulary, there is adequate time available to educate the staff before the drug is used. An organized formulary also ensures that the number and variety of drugs is kept to a minimum. Staff will use a limited number of drugs, with which they are familiar. When a nonformulary drug is ordered, pharmacists will know to provide special instructions and appropriate hazard warnings to all who will be involved in the medication use process. Drug formularies are pivotal tools for delineating and directing prescribing to the "drugs of choice." An excellent discussion of the drug formulary and associated misconceptions has been authored by Rucker and Schiff.[33]

Resolving Conflicts in Drug Therapy

Many serious medication errors involved a drug order that at least one practitioner believed to be unsafe. In some of these cases, practitioners did not question the order because they were intimidated by the prescriber. More often, practitioners questioned the order by discussing it with a supervisor, pharmacist, or physician. Nevertheless, the practitioners' concerns were not addressed, the order was not changed, and the medication was administered in error. The missing link in preventing these errors is a clear process for handling concerns about drug therapy. This process should conclude only when all practitioners are satisfied that no harm will come to the patient. Although each process may vary to meet the unique needs of the organization, the following guidelines are recommended for handling concerns and conflicts with drug therapy orders.[24]

If a nurse is concerned that physician-ordered drug therapy may not be safe, he or she should contact the pharmacist. This step is critical, especially when the drug ordered will be removed from unit stock or a patient's medication supply from home. The pharmacist must take an active role in determining the safety of the drug order and must not delegate clarification of the order to nursing staff. Rather, he or she should investigate the safety of the order and contact the practitioner as needed.

If the pharmacist suspects that a drug therapy is potentially harmful, he or she should pursue the matter until satisfied that the therapy will not harm the patient or until the order is changed. The issue should be completely researched before contacting the ordering physician so that concerns can be clearly communicated and based on facts, not only on opinion. The safety of the order may be confirmed by reviewing the medical record, talking with the patient, researching the matter through reputable drug resources, consulting with other pharmacists or physicians, or discussing the order directly with the prescriber. Supporting documentation (protocols, journal articles, etc.) should be requested from the prescriber to verify the safety of the order, but these should be read carefully. Many errors begin with the physician misinterpreting published information, misprints in texts, or ambiguous statements in the reference.

If the pharmacist is not satisfied that the patient will not be harmed and the prescriber will not change the order, he or she should consult with the prescriber's chief resident, chief attending physician, department chairperson, or a specialist in the area of the drug therapy ordered. If the individual consulted agrees that the order may be unsafe, he or she should contact the ordering physician.

If concerns about drug therapy persist despite these efforts, it should be considered whether more significant harm would result from administering the drug than from withholding it. Clinicians should refuse to dispense (or administer) a drug if they are reasonably sure that withholding the drug is the safest action. The issue should be referred to an ad-hoc group for peer review to determine the order's safety.

The physician should be neither requested nor allowed to give the drug himself or herself when a concern for patient safety remains unanswered. Patient safety is not served by attempting to transfer responsibility to the physician for any patient harm resulting from drug administration. There is likely to be little legal or emotional absolution for the pharmacist or the nurse if the patient is injured. Finally, the clinician should document his or her actions objectively on a standard incident report.

••••
References

1. Lesar TS, Briceland L, Stein DS. Factors related to errors in medication prescribing. *JAMA.* 1997; 277: 312–17.

2. Anonymous. A study of physicians' handwriting as a time waster. *JAMA.* 1979; 242: 2429–30.

3. Feldman H. Analyzing the cost of illegible handwriting. *Hospitals.* 1963; 37: 71, 74, 77, 80.

4. Vitillo JA, Lesar TS. Preventing medication prescribing errors. *Ann Pharmacother.* 1991; 25: 1388–94.

5. Brodell RT, Helms SE, KrishnaRao I, et al. Prescription errors: legibility and drug name confusion. *Arch Fam Med.* 1997; 6: 296–98.

6. Long KJ. The need for obligatory printing in medical records (letter). *Hosp Pharm.* 1991; 26: 924.

7. Cabral JD. Poor physician penmanship. *JAMA.* 1997; 278: 1116–17.

8. American Society of Hospital Pharmacists. ASHP guidelines on preventing medication errors in hospitals. *Am J Hosp Pharm.* 1993; 50: 305–14.

9. *Recommendations to Correct Error-Prone Aspects of Prescription Writing.* Enclosure to news release #96C03. Rockville, Md: National Coordinating Council for Medication Error Reporting and Prevention.

10. Rappaport HM. Consistency in prescription writing (letter). *Ann Intern Med.* 1992; 117: 1059.

11. Cohen MR, Davis NM. Avoid dangerous Rx abbreviations. *American Pharmacy.* 1992; NS32: 112–13.

12. Jones EH, Speerhas R. How physicians can prevent medication errors: practical strategies. *Cleve Clin J Med.* 1997; 64: 355–59.

13. Cohen MR, Davis NM. Expressing strengths, doses, and drug names properly. *American Pharmacy.* 1992; NS32: 216–17.

14. Cohen MR, Davis NM. The health sciences need a controlled vocabulary. *American Pharmacy.* 1993; NS33(9): 24.

15. United States Pharmacopeial Convention. Move to metric: apothecary system no longer recognized by USP. Drug Product Quality Review No. 37. 1993; 1–2.

16. Cohen MR, Davis NM. Who needs the apothecary system? *American Pharmacy.* 1992; NS32: 482–84.

17. Hoffman RS, Smilkstein MJ, Rubenstein F. An "amp" by any other name: the hazards of intravenous magnesium dosing (letter). *JAMA.* 1989; 261: 557.

18. Ward C. Medication errors: what's a dose? *Pharm-Fax of Fairfax Hospital.* 1989; 5: 19, 24.

19. Davis NM, Cohen MR. More look-alike and sound-alike errors. *American Pharmacy.* 1993; NS33(10): 32.

20. Davis NM, Cohen MR. Purpose of medication will reduce errors. *American Pharmacy.* 1992; NS32: 878–79.

21. Cohen MR, Davis NM. Drug name suffixes can cause confusion. *American Pharmacy.* 1992; NS32: 301–02.

22. Cohen MR. Medication error reports. Naming drug products is serious business. *Hosp Pharm.* 1990; 25: 747–48.

23. Institute for Safe Medication Practices. A novel way to prevent medication errors. *ISMP Medication Safety Alert!* Warminster, Pa: Institute for Safe Medication Practices; 1997.

24. Davis NM, Cohen, MR. *Medication Errors: Causes and Prevention.* Huntingdon Valley, Pa: Davis Associates; 1981.

25. Institute for Safe Medication Practices. Designing preprinted order forms that prevent medication errors. *ISMP Medication Safety Alert!* Warminster, Pa: Institute for Safe Medication Practices; 1997.

26. Cohen MR, Davis NM. Developing safe and effective preprinted physicians' order forms. *Hosp Pharm.* 1992; 27: 508, 513, 528.

27. Perlstein PH, Callison C, White M, et al. Errors in drug computations during newborn intensive care. *Am J Dis Child.* 1979; 133: 376–77.

28. Institute for Safe Medication Practices. Preventing death by decimal. *ISMP Medication Safety Alert!* Warminster, Pa: Institute for Safe Medication Practices; July 31, 1996.

29. Rieder MJ, Goldstein D, Zinman H, et al. Tenfold errors in drug dosage (letter). *Canadian Medical Association Journal.* 1988; 139: 12–13.

30. Lesar TS. Errors in the use of medication dosage regimens. *Arch Pediatr Adolesc Med.* 1988; 152: 340–44.

31. Cohen MR, Anderson RW, Attilio RM, et al. Preventing medication errors in cancer chemotherapy. *Am J Health Syst Pharm.* 1996; 53: 737–46.

32. Schiff GD, Rucker TD. Computerized prescribing. *JAMA.* 1998; 279: 1024–29.

33. Rucker TD, Schiff G. Drug formularies: myths-in-formation. *Hosp Pharm.* 1991; 26: 507–14, 519–21.

9.

Preventing Dispensing Errors

Michael R. Cohen, MS, FASHP

Institute for Safe Medication Practices
Huntingdon Valley, Pa.

Pharmacies are responsible for dispensing medications accurately. To this end, pharmacists must develop and follow policies and procedures to prevent dispensing errors and to ensure that drugs are distributed safely to patients. To do so, they must alter the way in which they view the causes of medication errors.[1] Rather than blaming the individual who was most directly involved with an error, they must identify and correct systems failures. Policies and procedures must be continually updated in response to newly identified areas of failure in the system of drug distribution.

Types of Dispensing Errors

In this chapter, the term *dispensing errors* refers to medication errors linked to the pharmacy or to whichever health care professional dispenses the medication. These include errors of commission (e.g., dispensing the wrong drug or dose) and those of omission (e.g., failure to counsel the patient or screen for interactions). Dispensing errors can be categorized as mechanical errors (those occurring in the preparation and processing of the prescription) and judgmental errors (those involving patient counseling, screening, or monitoring).[2] Additionally, an error can be classified as a slip (failure to achieve goals through reliance on automatic behavior after a distraction has occurred or due to poor system design) or a mistake (choosing inappropriate goals through conscious deliberation, perhaps because of lack of knowledge).[3] Finally, errors may be potential (i.e., detected and corrected prior to the administration of the medication to the patient) or actual.[4]

Most dispensing errors involve the dispensing of an incorrect medication, dosage strength, or dosage form. The second most common cause is a mis-

Table 9-1

1. Lock up or sequester drugs that could cause disastrous errors.

2. Develop and implement meticulous procedures for drug storage.

3. Reduce distractions, design a safe dispensing environment, and maintain optimum work flow.

4. Use reminders such as labels and computer notes to prevent mix-ups between "look-alike" and "sound-alike" drug names.

5. Keep the original prescription order, label, and medication container together throughout the dispensing process.

6. Perform a final check on the contents of prescription containers.

7. Compare the contents of the medication container with the information on the prescription label.

8. Enter the manufacturer's identification code into the computer and on the prescription label.

9. Perform a final check on the prescription label. When possible, use automation, such as bar coding.

10. Provide patient counseling.

calculation of dose. The third is failure to identify drug interactions or contraindications.

Acknowledging the causes of an error is the first step in preventing future errors. Once the cause of an error is identified, measures can be taken to institute the appropriate policies or procedures and educate staff.

Common Causes of Dispensing Errors

It is essential to screen new employees for their knowledge of medication error prevention methods, hire well-trained pharmacy personnel, and help staff keep their knowledge current through continuing education opportunities and professional publications. However, employers and supervisors can take additional steps toward the goal of an error-free work environment. Ten of the most important measures are summarized in Table 9–1. A discussion of these and other issues follows.

Work Environment

Workload. Pharmacists in community and institutional practice settings rank work overload as the most significant cause of dispensing errors.[5] Pharmacists in both of these settings are under great strain as departments and companies are forced to downsize. Compounding the potential for error is the stress placed on the pharmacist by the imposition of a maximum time allowance for the dispensing of prescriptions. These limits are put in place by misguided supervisors or companies who value timeliness over accuracy.

The most obvious solutions to work overload are to have sufficient personnel available and to eliminate time limits on dispensing. One state pharmacy association has issued an Employee Model Contract stating that no pharmacist should routinely dispense more than an average of 15 prescriptions per hour and that pharmacists should be required to take rest breaks every 2 to 3 hours and meal breaks of at least one half-hour every day.[2] Although profession-wide acceptance of these recommendations is unlikely, employers have been disciplined by state boards of pharmacy, as well as courts of law, when errors have been caused by unreasonable pharmacist workloads.[2]

Distractions. Pharmacists are often distracted from one task to attend to another. Although not all distractions can be eliminated, some may be reduced. For example, ringing telephones may break the pharmacist's concentration. Solutions that may reduce this distraction include using a fax machine for order transmission and a telephone answering machine for routine refill requests and for those times when a critical task cannot be interrupted. Another option is to employ trained support personnel to answer the telephone.[6] It is important to ensure that training of these personnel includes guidance on which calls they are permitted to handle and which must be referred to a pharmacist.

Errors may be avoided by reducing or eliminating the distraction caused by unnecessary conversation among pharmacy personnel while prescriptions are being processed. Just as pilots are in a "sterile cockpit" and are not permitted to engage in non-flight-related conversation when the plane is below 10,000 feet, pharmacists and others should not be permitted to engage in idle chatter when performing critical functions. These critical steps[7] include

- review and assessment of the prescription,
- computer data entry,
- review of patient profiles,
- assessment of computer alerts,
- selection of the proper medication
  (both in the computer and from the shelf),
- verification of the product expiration date,
- counting or measuring the medication,
- affixing the label,
- double-checking the prescription,
- returning the stock container to its proper location,
- taking the patient's history,
- patient counseling, and
- verification of any questions regarding the prescription
  with the prescriber.

Work Area. A poorly designed work area can contribute to dispensing errors. A well-designed work area has proper lighting, adequate counter space, and a comfortable temperature and humidity. It facilitates smooth work flow from one task to the next throughout the prescription dispensing process. It is removed from areas of heavy traffic.[6] The work area should be kept as free of clutter as possible. When a container is no longer in use, for example, it should be returned to its proper storage area or discarded.[8] Consideration should also be given to the placement of telephones; they must be close enough for convenience without being a source of distraction.

Adequate space should be allotted for each medication and each strength; crowded medications are more prone to being interchanged or returned to an incorrect location.[5] All prescription bottles should be stored with the label facing forward.[6] Medications should not be stored on shelves or in bins, cabinets, or drawers that have external storage labels, because medications in similar packaging can be mistaken for one another if only the storage label is used for identification.[6]

Separate areas should be assigned to medications administered by different routes. That is, oral medications should have a designated area, as should injectables, products for inhalation, topical products, otic preparations, ophthalmic preparations, and rectal preparations. Some pharmacies prefer to separate oral liquids from other oral medications. Auxiliary labels indicating the route of administration should be available in the area in which the products are stored and should be used to further differentiate products when a prescription is dispensed. For example, amoxicillin oral suspension is available in dropper bottles for pediatric use. When the suspension is used for an ear infection, parents have been known to inadvertently place it in the child's ear rather than give it by mouth. An auxiliary label reading "For oral use only" would help prevent this error.

Efforts should be made to call attention to "high-alert" medications and pairs of medications that are frequently confused (see Chapter 5). High-alert medications, which include oral warfarin, injectable potassium chloride, lidocaine, heparin, and controlled substances, should be specially marked and placed in an isolated or locked area.[6] If this is not possible, auxiliary reminder labels may be used to draw attention to the product and warn the dispenser to use additional caution when dispensing.

It may also be beneficial to separate frequently confused pairs (such as thiamine 100-mg and thioridazine 100-mg tablets) or strengths of drugs (especially medications that are available in strengths that vary by a factor of 10, such as 2.5-mg and 25-mg Compazine® suppositories).[9] Again, auxiliary labels should be used to draw attention to the products and encourage added caution.

Many pharmacies post lists of drug names that have frequently been confused. One such list is available from the U.S. Pharmacopeia (USP) (800-227-8772). The Safety Briefs feature in the *ISMP Medication Safety Alert!* from the Institute for Safe Medication Practices (ISMP) (215-947-7797) is also helpful. Although such lists can assist in identifying problem name pairs, their utility is somewhat limited because it is impossible for practitioners to memorize them in order to know when to check on questionable orders.

Computer warnings can prevent mix-ups between products with similar names and strengths. Many systems have a "clinical flag" or "formulary note" screen or field that can be adapted to show important information prominently on the computer monitor. Like a road sign that warns about a dangerous intersection ahead, this feature can alert the person entering the order when a look-alike or sound-alike danger is present. For example, when Norvasc® is entered into the computer, a formulary note screen can appear alerting the pharmacist that it often looks like Navane® when hand-written.[7] The pharmacist can then confirm the order if necessary.

Use of Outdated and Incorrect References

The ISMP frequently publishes accounts of medication errors that can be traced to the use of outdated texts. Because new and important information is constantly surfacing, the use of expired medical texts is dangerous. It is well worth the cost to discard old references as soon as more recent editions are available. Certain computerized resources, such as *Facts and Comparisons* on monthly CD-ROM or *Micromedex,* are ideal for patient care areas because they are constantly being updated.

For example, on the basis of information from the 8th edition of the *Handbook on Injectable Drugs*, published in 1994,[10] sterile water was used to prepare 3000 mL of 5% albumin from 25% albumin during a critical national shortage of 5% albumin. Albumin can be diluted with sterile water, sodium chloride 0.9%, or dextrose 5% in water, but large volumes of sterile water or dextrose cause a substantial reduction in tonicity. When such a solution is infused into a patient, hemolysis occurs. In the 9th and 10th editions of the same text (published in 1996 and 1998, respectively),[11,12] the monograph for albumin was changed to note that if sterile water for injection is the diluent, the tonicity of the diluted solution must be considered because hypotonicity can cause hemolysis. Unfortunately, the ISMP learned of several cases in which information from the 8th edition led to the preparation by a pharmacy of a large volume of 5% albumin diluted with sterile water for plasma exchange. As a result, several deaths occurred.

This is but one of many examples in which confusing or incorrect statements in texts led to problems. In Chapter 15, on chemotherapy, a case is described in which a journal inadvertently used an incorrect or ambiguous statement or term that led to a serious medication error. In this case, the journal indicated that the dose of vincristine sulfate was 1.4 mg/m^2 on "days 1–8" instead of "days 1 *and* 8." An overdose resulted when the patient received vincristine daily rather than weekly.

Mistakes are often made on charts, in books, and in journal articles. Suspicious situations need appropriate follow-up. Utilization of the various checking systems described throughout this book, including the many recommendations in Chapter 15, is imperative.

Solutions to Dispensing Errors

Workplace Management

Inventory. Pharmacies can help reduce errors by selecting their brands and supplies carefully. This strategy is especially helpful in overcoming confusion caused by look-alike labels. Pharmaceutical manufacturers design their labels to be recognized across their product line, and this may lead to errors.[13] This is especially true for generic injectable medications that are manufactured by more than one pharmaceutical company.

Many manufacturers of generic medications have introduced label changes that make it easier to distinguish one product from another. These companies should be preferred over those that have not introduced such features. Pharmacists and pharmacy purchasers must remain vigilant for look-alike packaging within a manufacturer's product line or between products from different manufacturers and warn all personnel to send products back, separate them, or mark them with auxiliary labels to distinguish between them.

For example, continuing significant errors have been reported stemming from confusion between lipid-based drug products and their conventional counterparts. Specifically, confusion between three pair of drugs has been reported: (1) lipid-based forms of amphotericin B (Abelcet®, Amphotec®, Ambisone®) and conventional amphotericin B for injection (available generically and as Fungizone®); (2) the pegylated liposomal form of doxorubicin (Doxil®) and its conventional counterpart, doxorubicin hydrochloride (Adriamycin®, Rubex®); and (3) a liposomal form of daunorubicin (DaunoXome®, daunorubicin citrate liposomas) and conventional daunorubicin hydrochloride (Cerubidine®). Dosages of lipid-based products differ greatly from those of their conventional counterparts. Thus, confusion concerning dosing, or substituting one product for the other, has resulted in serious injuries and deaths. Separate storage for conventional and lipid-based products and cautionary labels on products would be excellent methods to prevent errors. In addition, the need for formulary control and systematic educational processes when introducing these new products should be stressed. Adequate warnings and reminders, including computer warnings, can reduce the potential for confusion. It is strongly recommended that prescribers refer to lipid-based products only by their brand names.

Inventory should be inspected at least quarterly, and outdated products should be removed from the shelves. Dangerous chemicals should not be stored in the pharmacy.[6,14] If such substances are required for compounding, they can be obtained at the time they are needed. To prevent accidental ingestion, standard containers for oral medications should not be used to store substances that are not meant for systemic use. Departments and individuals should not be permitted to requisition empty prescription containers or blank pharmacy labels, because the pharmacy will no longer control what is stored in the containers or written on the labels.[14]

Keeping track of outdated items is difficult, even within the pharmacy. Monitoring in clinics and private practice areas may be even harder because there may not be an individual who is specifically assigned this duty. Most problems are caused by manufacturers' samples in ambulatory areas (e.g., items with poorly marked expiration dates and short-dated items received from suppliers). Publicizing specific dates will remind everyone of the importance of this review.

Hours of Operation. Twenty-four-hour pharmacy service is strongly recommended in hospitals. When 24-hour service is not available, a limited supply of medications should be accessible to authorized nonpharmacists for use in initiating urgent medication orders. The list of medications available after hours, as well as the policies and procedures governing their use (including a provision for subsequent pharmacist review of all after-hour access), should be developed by the pharmacy and therapeutics committee. Items made available for after-hour access should be selected with safety in mind. The number, types, quantities, dosage forms, and container sizes of the medications should be limited.

A system such as this eliminates the need for nonpharmacists to enter the pharmacy. An additional recommendation for institutions that do not provide 24-hour pharmacy service is to have a pharmacist on call around the clock for questions and emergencies.[4]

Pharmacy departments that do provide 24-hour service must select the pharmacists and support staff for the evening and night shifts carefully to ensure provision of quality pharmaceutical care during off-peak and potentially error-prone hours.

Computer Systems. Many serious adverse drug events are absolutely preventable with well-designed computerized systems. For example, one recent situation involved a massive overdose of colchicine. A physician called for 2 mg to be given intravenously every hour "until diarrhea (develops) or symptoms are relieved." A pharmacist recognized the error (standard texts note that fatalities have occurred after as little as a 5-mg cumulative intravenous dose) and attempted to contact the prescriber, withholding the dose until the order could be clarified. However, the prescriber could not be reached. Later, when informed by a nurse that therapy had not yet begun, the physician demanded that it be initiated immediately. Due to a lack of communication, two different pharmacists sent enough colchicine ampuls to last for several doses. Nurses who administered the drug were unaware that an overdose was being given. The patient developed diarrhea after 12 mg was given, and the drug was stopped. Despite supportive efforts, the patient died soon thereafter.

There is no clear distinction among nontoxic, toxic, and lethal doses of colchicine. Although gastrointestinal symptoms are often used as a guide to dosing, these symptoms rarely occur with intravenous administration and therefore should not be used as an indicator of impending toxicity. A well-designed computer system could easily establish that the maximum cumulative intravenous dose per 24 hours is not to exceed 4 mg, and that no more colchicine is to be dispensed by any route for at least 7 days afterward. Thus, label processing and dispensing of massive, accidental drug overdoses could be prohibited. Unfortunately, it has been my observation that few hospitals or pharmacies utilize such a system, even if the capability exists.

The pharmacy computer system should be capable of supporting and assisting pharmacists in their work. The system should be chosen for its ability to maintain patient profiles and to check for and alert the dispenser to medication overdoses, underdoses, duplicate therapy, overuse, potential allergic reactions, and interactions with concurrently prescribed medications.[2] It should also be configured such that the alert functions cannot be disabled and serious warnings cannot be easily or mistakenly overridden. A quality assurance system should be an integral part of any system that does allow an override. Such a system should then generate lists of overrides for retrospective review by management. Additional features to look for in a computer system include the neatness, clarity, organization, and understandability of the labels and reports that are generated, as well as of the display screens showing patient profiles and order entries.

Pharmacy computer software should screen for the following:

- Dose limits: Computer screening for the predetermined dose limit of a medication can help prevent pharmacists from entering a prescription order that could inadvertently result in an overdose. In situations where "stat" or one-time orders are often written, these systems alert pharmacists when the accumulated amount of a drug would be excessive. These functions require computer records of the patient's weight and height; in some cases, they rely on calculations of body surface area.

  Three types of dose checks are needed: (1) cutoff for a single dose, (2) cutoff for total amount of drug allowed in a 24-hour period, and (3) cutoff for an entire course of therapy.

Screening the dose cutoff by ingredient is also needed because the use of various multiple-ingredient products can yield an excessive amount of a particular drug. Such an event may occur, for example, if plain acetaminophen is given to a patient receiving Darvocet-N 100®.

- Allergic reactions: Many software packages do not flag ingredients to which the patient has reported an allergy. Worse, many pharmacists do not screen for allergies because allergy information has not been entered or has been inconsistently entered into the patient database. Information on allergies is essential.

- Cross-allergies: Screening for cross-allergies, such as allergies to codeine and oxycodone, codeine and morphine, and penicillin and cephalosporins, is a must.

- Duplication of drug ingredients: Screening for similar ingredients in different products is necessary to prevent drug duplication.

- Duplication of therapeutic classes: Screening is needed to prevent duplications of therapeutic drug classes (e.g., giving omeprazole and an H_2-antagonist to the same patient).

- Drug interactions: Fast and effective screening to detect drug interactions requires a significance level that catches major interactions but does not flag minor interactions. Even when the proper significance level is set, there is a risk that pharmacists may override the interaction and miss a dangerous situation. A system that flags important interactions but merely prints out less urgent messages without interrupting work flow might be more effective. Having to justify an override would be more likely to make the pharmacist think critically about interactions. Regular review by a clinical supervisor of all overridden interactions is recommended as a quality control measure.

- Contraindicated drugs or drugs that need dosage modifications in specific diseases: A database organized by patient diagnosis should be available from software vendors. This system could incorporate International Classification of Diseases (ICD) codes or, at a minimum, track a few important diagnoses. Such a system could, for example, prevent a patient with renal failure from receiving nephrotoxic drugs or alert the pharmacist when a dosage of a highly metabolized drug is too high for a patient with liver disease.

- Prescriber order entry: Computer entry of prescriptions is effective in reducing medication errors. It eliminates problems with poor handwriting as well as the need for transcription. Computer entry removes a step that is frequently tied to medication errors: incorrect interpretation of the order by the person transcribing it. Through on-line prompting, computerized order entry can provide information on the drug and the patient at the time the order is entered, which further reduces the potential for error (see Chapter 8, page 8.19).

An additional precaution that may be taken to avoid selecting the wrong medication or the incorrect dosage strength or form is to create vastly different computer mnemonics for potentially problematic drug pairs.[9] Mnemonics are not recommended, however, for high-alert medications such as cancer chemotherapy agents, neuromuscular blocking agents, and controlled substances.

An error that illustrates the problems associated with mnemonics occurred in a children's hospital when a physician wrote an order for buspirone (BuSpar®) 10 mg for a child with a seizure disorder. A pharmacist typed the mnemonic "BUS10" to bring buspirone 10 mg onto the computer screen. However, that mnemonic had already been assigned to busulfan (Myleran®) 10 mg, an antineoplastic agent. The pharmacist dispensed busulfan in error. Another example of confusion involves the mnemonic "AZT100," which has been used for both azathioprine (Imuran®) 100 mg and zidovudine (Retrovir®; formerly named azidothymidine) 100 mg. If a patient with acquired immunodeficiency syndrome (AIDS) were to receive an immunosuppressant instead of an antiretroviral, the error could be fatal.

Work Performance

Pharmacy personnel must focus on the task at hand, keeping interruptions to a minimum and maintaining their workload at a safe and manageable level. Each pharmacist and technician must accept the responsibilities inherent in his or her position, including staying current on medications and their indications, interactions, and adverse effects, as well as medication errors. Confirmation bias (i.e., seeing what one expects to see or what is more common, rather than what is really there) must be avoided by recognizing and working to prevent the factors that contribute to it on prescriptions, manufacturer's labels, and dispensing labels[9] (see Chapter 13, page 13.2).

Assessing Prescriptions. Pharmacists must assess each medication order before dispensing it, never second-guessing the prescriber. It goes without saying that illegible handwriting, nonstandard abbreviations, or incomplete information must be clarified with the prescriber before continuing to process the prescription. This clarification should then be documented in writing.[1]

After analyzing the patient's profile and all other information and reviewing drug interactions and allergies, the pharmacist must verify the appropriateness of the medication and its dosage. Any computer alerts must also be considered at this time. An additional precautionary step that is useful when a more common strength or form of a medication is dispensed in place of the less common form prescribed is to highlight anything unusual (e.g., strength or dosage form) to call attention to it.[13]

Look-Alike and Sound-Alike Drug Names. Medications with names that are spelled similarly can easily be mistaken for one another (see Chapter 12). For example, the ISMP has repeatedly warned about the potential for confusing amrinone (Inocor®), an inotrope, and amiodarone (Cordarone®), an antiarrhythmic with negative chronotropic effects. Despite these warnings, errors still occur.

Recently a physician ordered amrinone as a last-ditch effort for a woman with a history of myocardial infarction and stroke. The patient was severely hypotensive from bradycardia, with a heart rate of 20 to 30 beats per minute. A nurse phoned the order to the pharmacy but had trouble pronouncing "amrinone." The pharmacist asked to speak with the physician, and again there was confusion in pronouncing the drug name. Finally the pharmacist switched to the brand name and asked whether it was Cordarone® (amiodarone) that was being requested. The physician said yes and changed the order to Cordarone®. The patient died soon after receiving the wrong drug. Milrinone (Primacor®) has now replaced amrinone at this hospital.

Accidents will continue unless action is taken to avoid the problem. Among other strategies, health professionals should independently confirm the patient's diagnosis before dispensing certain medications. Figures 9–1 through 9–8 are examples of orders that led to errors because of look-alike drug names.

Hospitals and other practice sites must establish policies stating that, except in emergencies, nurses' verbal (i.e., spoken) requests for medications will not be accepted until the pharmacy has reviewed a copy of the order. Pharmacists are more likely than nurses to be aware of newly marketed drugs with names similar to those of familiar drugs. Facsimile machines on each nursing unit and in the pharmacy can facilitate pharmacist review.

Drug orders that are spoken rather than written are often misunderstood, misinterpreted, or transcribed incorrectly; for this reason, they should be avoided whenever possible. For example, "Seldane®" and "Feldene®" sound alike, as do "amrinone" and "amiodarone," as well as many other pairs. All have been confused at one time or another, resulting in a medication error. In many cases, serious injuries have occurred because of misinterpreted verbal orders. When uncertainties exist, the pharmacist must contact the prescriber for clarification.

When it is necessary to use a verbal prescription order, the order should be transcribed immediately and the information written should be carefully verified. This may be done most effectively by requiring that the person taking the order clearly repeat all the information back to the transcriber.[15]

Labeling. The labeling process starts during computer order entry, with the selection and entry of the correct medication, dosage strength, dosage form, quantity, complete directions for use, number of refills, and prescriber name. The purpose of the medication should be printed on the dispensing label if possible. This provides the patient with an additional means to verify and distinguish among prescriptions.

The ISMP is often asked about label placement after intravenous admixtures are prepared. To improve the likelihood that a labeling error will be recognized, some hospitals place labels for intravenous admixtures on the front side of the bag. In this way, both the title (base solution and/or drug name), as listed by the manufacturer, and the pharmacy additive label can be easily scrutinized to make sure that they match. Some practitioners believe that placing the additive label on the reverse side reduces the chances of administration mix-ups because the container is identifiable in any position. Although there is no research indicating which method of labeling is safer, I believe that placing the additive label on the front of the bag, without covering the title, is the safer choice. Manufacturers are asked to label bags containing intravenous solutions on both sides. In addition, applicable auxiliary labels should be used in both inpatient and outpatient settings.

For example, the USP currently requires specific caution labeling with the vinca alkaloid products vincristine (Oncovin®) and vinblastine (Velban®). These two products require warning labels on extemporaneously prepared syringes, stating "FATAL IF GIVEN INTRATHECALLY. FOR IV USE ONLY." In addition, the syringe must be placed into an overwrap (which accompanies the manufacturer's container), which also carries this labeling. Such labels and overwraps are available in the packaging of vincristine products. The package insert for vinorelbine (Navelbine®), the other vinca alkaloid available in the United States, requires only a warning label that states "FOR IV USE ONLY."

The ISMP recommends that other extemporaneously prepared syringes of potentially hazardous substances utilize similar label reminders. For example, oral syringes (with tips that will not accommodate a needle) should

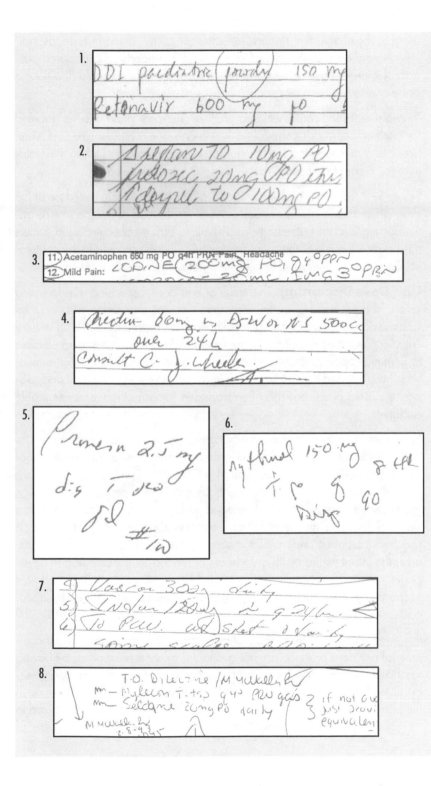

1. Ritonavir (Norvir®) mistaken for Retrovir® (zidovudine) shortly after Norvir® was marketed.

2. Is this a prescription for Prozac® (fluoxetine) or Prilosec® (omeprazole)? During live educational programs, when asked for a show of hands, about 20% of attendees incorrectly see Prozac®. In other words, this particular prescription would be filled with the wrong drug about 20% of the time!

3. A Lodine® (etodolac) prescription incorrectly dispensed as codeine 200 mg.

4. Aredia® (pamidronate) mistaken for "Adria," a nickname for Adriamycin® (doxorubicin). Abbreviating drug names is a dangerous practice.

5. It's almost impossible to tell whether this is Provera® (medroxyprogesterone) 2.5 mg or Premarin® (conjugated estrogens) 2.5 mg.

6. Rythmol® (propafenone) 150 mg or Synthroid® (levothyroxine) 150 mcg? The outcome of a such a mix-up would be disastrous.

7. Imdur® (isosorbide mononitrate) 120 mg or Inderal® (propranolol) 20 mg? Inderal® is also frequently confused with Isordil® (isosorbide dinitrate).

8. Although no longer marketed, Seldane® (terfenadine) prescriptions were often mixed up with Feldene® (piroxicam). When Seldane® was first marketed, its manufacturer sent a national mailing about the potential for a mix-up.

carry an auxiliary label stating "FOR ORAL USE ONLY." Some industrious individuals who have confused oral syringes as improperly manufactured parenteral syringes have actually fashioned them so that they could fit a needle or be connected to an intravenous line.

To avoid switching containers and placing one medication in a vial labeled for another, pharmacists should work with only one container at a time when possible. When working with more than one container and label, they must take extra care to ascertain that the correct label is affixed.[16]

Figure 9–9 shows a label for paregoric that led to a massive overdose of the drug when a nurse misunderstood instructions. Instead of adding just 10 mL, the nurse added the entire bottle, or 60 mL, to 500 mL of enteral fluid. Labels must state the name of the drug, its strength, and the amount in the container. Care must be exercised to prevent ambiguous statements on labels.

Unit Dose Dispensing. The value of unit dose dispensing in preventing errors should not be underestimated. Current standards of the Joint Commission on Accreditation of Healthcare Organizations (JCAHO) require "medications to be dispensed in the most ready-to-administer form possible to minimize opportunities for error."[17] Yet, often due to cost-cutting maneuvers, hospitals and nursing homes often allow systems in which unit dose dispensing is not practiced. This often translates into an otherwise preventable accident.

For example, in a neonatal intensive care unit, a 7.4-mg loading dose of aminophylline was ordered for a premature infant who had episodes of apnea. Instead of 7.4 mg (0.3 mL of a 250 mg/10 mL solution), 7.4 mL (185 mg) was administered to the baby girl. Her theophylline level was markedly elevated, and she developed tachycardia and other significant signs of theophylline toxicity. Her condition deteriorated and she soon required intubation and ventilator support. Despite these and other measures, the infant expired within 36 hours of the incident. According to newspaper reports, aminophylline was available as a floor stock item and was prepared by the nurse who gave it, without an independent check by a second individual.

It is reasonable to interpret the JCAHO standard to mean that, when commercial unit dose products are not available, safety is maximized by having the hospital pharmacy department prepare and dispense non-emergency parenteral doses. In this way, internal mechanisms for quality assurance in the pharmacy, as well as pharmacist–nurse check systems, can be utilized to reduce the potential for error. This process is important in the care of neonates, especially with high-alert drugs such as aminophylline, for which the consequences of errors are great and even minor dose miscalculations could prove disastrous (see Chapter 5).

Despite the JCAHO standard, in many hospitals where ISMP has evaluated medication systems, it has been found that nurses are solely responsible for reconstituting or diluting parenteral doses taken from floor stock, even in a neonatal critical care unit. Worse, this is often done in the absence of a policy stating that medications prepared for neonates must be independently checked by at least two individuals to ensure that the order has been properly interpreted, that the correct medication has been used, and that dosage calculation, preparation, and labeling is accurate. Unfortunately, hospital accreditation agencies, state departments of health, and state boards fail to focus greater attention on this issue, even though it is called for in the JCAHO standards.

Merely asking whether a unit dose system exists, which is often done, is not enough. Although medications and methods of administration available to patients today have dramatically improved outcomes, they can constitute a double-edged sword. Some hospitals, in their quest to minimize costs, have not responded by ensuring that adequate systems and staff are in place to promote safe use of the new medications and delivery techniques. High-level hospital administrators are strongly urged to thoroughly examine medication practices in their own institutions.

Independent Checking

To facilitate checking of the prescription label and the medication being dispensed, the original prescription order, label, and medication container should be kept together throughout the dispensing process, including prescription counseling. When this technique is used, errors made during computer order entry are more likely to be detected.[6]

Pharmacists, doctors, and nurses are taught to avoid errors involving dispensing an incorrect medication by reading labels three times: when taking the drug container from a drug bin or the shelf, when preparing the drug or placing it in the container to dispense, and when returning the stock container to the shelf or discarding it. For additional safety, the National Drug Code (NDC) number on the stock container may be compared with the NDC number in the computer and on the dispensing label.[2,5]

Prescriptions prepared by a pharmacy technician should be verified by a pharmacist, who should compare the label with the original prescription order, the original prescription order with the label on the stock container,

Figure 9-9

Label for paregoric that led to a massive overdose of the drug when a nurse misunderstood instructions. Instead of adding just 10 mL, the nurse added the entire bottle, or 60 mL, to 500 mL of enteral fluid.

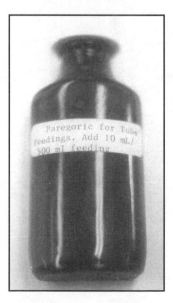

and the medication in the stock container with that being dispensed. The pharmacist should also ensure that appropriate auxiliary labels are used.

A final check should be performed to verify that the patient's name; the drug name, strength, and dosage form; and the directions on the label match those on the original order.[6] When possible, all prescriptions should be double-checked by a second person (pharmacist or technician). This is especially important for medications with the potential to cause serious harm to a patient if given erroneously.

The chance of making an error in dosage calculation or measurement is minimized by check systems. A check might be required for all calculations or measurements or only for those within specific categories. For example, checks could be mandatory for medications prescribed for any patient under 12 years of age; in certain situations (e.g., in critical care settings when a drug infusion requires a dose in micrograms per kilogram per minute); and for insulin infusions, chemotherapy, and compounding of patient-controlled analgesia. Calculators and computer programs may improve accuracy, but they do not eliminate the need for an independent review of calculations and concentrations of solutions.

It may be possible to avoid dose calculations in a number of ways. Examples are using the unit dose system exclusively; using commercially available unit dose items, such as premixed parenteral solutions used in critical care; and standardizing doses and concentrations, especially of drugs used in critical care. The use of standard dosage charts on the floors and standard formulations in the pharmacy minimizes the possibility of error. For example, in critical care units, physicians need only to order the amount of drug they want infused and to list the titration parameters. No one has to perform any calculations, because dosage charts provide the information needed to select appropriate flow rates on the basis of the patient's weight and the dose ordered.

Standard concentrations for frequently prepared formulations should be recorded and made accessible for reference in the parenteral preparation area in the pharmacy. All calculations must be double-checked independently by a second staff person and documented by the pharmacist. Diluents as well as active drugs must be checked. To facilitate checking, the stock container of each additive and its syringe should be lined up in the order in which they appear on the container label. The final edge of the plunger piston should be aligned with the calibration marks on the syringe barrel indicating the amount to be used.

In many hospitals, automated compounders are used for preparing large- and small-volume parenteral solutions. Automated equipment has been known to fail. Some accidents have occurred because solutions were placed on the wrong additive channel. Furthermore, the software that drives automated equipment is so complicated that errors sometimes occur because the person using it does not recognize that the information he or she is placing in it is incorrect. Therefore, it is important that the pharmacy have an ongoing quality assurance program for the use of automated compounding equipment. This program should include double-checks and documentation of solution placement within the compounder, final weighing or refractometer testing of the solution to ensure that proper concentrations have been compounded, and ongoing sampling of electrolyte concentrations. Pharmacists who prepare special parenteral solutions (e.g., total parenteral nutrition base solutions or cardioplegic solutions) in batches should have additional quality assurance procedures in place, including sterility testing and quarantine until confirmation.

Extemporaneous compounding of intravenous solutions occasionally results in improperly mixed solutions. Administration of hypotonic or superconcentrated solutions of dextrose, for example, has resulted in brain injury and death. Contributing factors include the use of poorly trained individuals to compound solutions, inadequate supervision, arithmetic errors, misuse or malfunction of an automated compounder, look-alike labeling on manufacturer-supplied dextrose containers, and lack of an adequate quality assurance process.

Extraordinary quality assurance must be undertaken when compounding intravenous solutions. Personnel must ensure that all calculations are independently checked by at least two individuals, and these persons should also confirm that the correct solutions are being used. Automated equipment with bar-code capability can contribute to safety. Pharmacists should always calculate the expected weight of the final product on the basis of the specific gravity of the ingredients and the final volume. Each bag should be within 5% of the calculated weight. Another technique is to mark the beginning volume of each container before mixing and at the end of the filling cycle and to check each container to determine whether final volumes are appropriate. These processes require an investment of less than 5 minutes per patient.[1] Another way to perform a final check is to place a drop of solution in a refractometer to determine the approximate dextrose concentration.[2]

Patient Counseling

Patient counseling has a critical role in ensuring accurate dispensing. Studies have demonstrated that 83% of errors are discovered during patient counseling and corrected before the patient leaves the pharmacy.[6]

Pharmacists should employ a "show and tell" technique during patient counseling by opening the container to take a final look at the medication themselves and show it to the patient. An error may be caught at this point if the patient has been prescribed the same medication in the past and does not recognize the medication in the container.[2,13]

The pharmacist should also ask the patient questions during the counseling session. The patient's responses reflect how well the pharmacist interpreted the prescription order. Specific questions may include the following:

- What did your doctor tell you this medication is for?
- How did your doctor tell you to take this medication?
- What directions did the doctor give you for using this medication?
- Do you have any questions?[2,13]

An educated patient is the final safety check in the prevention of medication errors.[15] Patients should be instructed to question medications or effects that are out of the ordinary and to contact the pharmacist or the prescriber if they have concerns. Oral counseling should be supported by written information regarding the medications dispensed.

Medication Error Prevention and Monitoring Systems

Pharmacy departments should lead multidisciplinary efforts to examine where errors arise in the drug use process. All dispensing procedures must be examined regularly and the cause of breakdowns identified so that preventive measures can be designed. Pharmacy technicians need to tell their pharmacist supervisors what they need, in terms of personnel, training, facility design, equipment, drug products and supplies, computer systems, and quality assurance programs, in order to do their jobs effectively.

Pharmacists and pharmacy technicians must work together to design quality assurance programs that produce the information needed to identify problems and make appropriate changes. For example, joint reviews of the accuracy of unit dose cart fills are of great help in detecting reasons for missing or inaccurate doses and in changing the dispensing system accordingly. Programs can be established to monitor the accuracy of pharmacy computer order entry. Quality improvement efforts that include a review of medication error reports enhance understanding of the system and the behavioral defects being experienced and provide a basis for introducing improvements.

Medication errors will never be eliminated. Nonetheless, pharmacists and pharmacy technicians can share their expertise to address safety issues and thus ensure the safest environment possible.

••••
References

1. Davis NM, Cohen MR. Changing how pharmacists think about errors. *American Pharmacy.* 1995; NS35(2): 11, 46.

2. Abood RR. Errors in pharmacy practice. *US Pharmacist.* March 1996: 122–30.

3. Davis NM, Cohen MR. Slips and mistakes in dispensing. *American Pharmacy.* 1994; NS34(4): 18.

4. American Society of Hospital Pharmacists. ASHP guidelines on preventing medication errors in hospitals. *Am J Hosp Pharm.* 1993; 50: 305–14.

5. Davis NM, Cohen MR. Ten steps for ensuring dispensing accuracy. *American Pharmacy.* 1994; NS34(7): 22–23.

6. Ukens C. Deadly dispensing: an exclusive survey of Rx errors by pharmacists. *Drug Topics.* March 1997: 100–11.

7. Davis NM, Cohen MR. Sterile cockpit. *American Pharmacy.* 1995; NS35(12): 11.

8. Medication Error Reports. Error 361—Keep work areas cleared of unnecessary items. *Hosp Pharm.* 1987; 22: 1251.

9. Davis NM, Cohen MR. Learning lessons from dispensing errors. *American Pharmacy.* 1994; NS34(5): 27–28.

10. Trissel LA. *Handbook on Injectable Drugs.* 8th ed. Bethesda, Md: American Society of Hospital Pharmacists: 1994.

11. Trissel LA. *Handbook on Injectable Drugs.* 9th ed. Bethesda, Md: American Society of Health-System Pharmacists: 1996.

12. Trissel LA. *Handbook on Injectable Drugs.* 10th ed. Bethesda, Md: American Society of Health-System Pharmacists: 1998.

13. Davis NM, Cohen MR. A sample of dispensing errors reported. *American Pharmacy.* 1993; NS33(11): 22.

14. Cohen MR, Davis NM. Confusing name: tips for storing drugs. *American Pharmacy.* 1994; NS34(2): 20–21.

15. Davis NM, Cohen MR. More look-alike and sound-alike errors. *American Pharmacy.* 1993; NS33(10): 32.

16. Cohen MR, Davis NM. Pharmacy label mix-ups. *American Pharmacy.* 1992; NS32(1): 26–27.

17. Joint Commission on Accreditation of Healthcare Organizations. *Comprehensive Accreditation Manual for Hospitals—The Official Handbook.* Oak Brook Terrace, Ill: 1998 TX.3.5-TX.3.5.2.

10.

Effective Use of Dispensing Automation

Mark Neuenschwander

Chief Executive Officer
The Neuenschwander Company
Bellevue, Wash.

This chapter focuses on what automation can do to limit or increase opportunities for errors associated with the distribution, dispensing, and administering of medications. The discussion is divided into two parts. The first part covers dispensing technologies for filling inpatient orders. The second concerns outpatient dispensing technologies. Technologies in both categories are divided into centralized and decentralized systems.

Inpatient Automated Dispensing Systems

Automated dispensing technologies for filling patient orders are increasingly common in hospitals. They include pharmacy-based devices that assist in unit dose patient cassette filling for 24-hour exchange or "just-in-time" delivery as well as ward-based devices. The latter range from systems that manage limited lines of medications (e.g., narcotics, as-needed medications, and some floor stock items) to those that manage full lines of medication and essentially eliminate the need for cassette exchange. Most decentralized technologies use stationary cabinets. Some employ portable carts.

Centralized Systems

Pharmacy-based automated dispensing systems can be divided into two kinds: (1) those that repackage bulk medications and (2) those that use over-packaged, manufacturer-wrapped units of use.

Repackaging Systems. Many hospitals and institutional pharmacies employ repacking and labeling machines for solid oral medications (Table 10–1,

Table 10-1

Inpatient Centralized Systems	
Function Performed	**Names of Devices**
A. Pack and label unit dose	AutoPak
	Euclid Cadet
	Odessa MediPack
	UniPak
B. Pack and label blister cards	MTS 500 and MTS 1500
	Rx Systems
C. Pick, pack, and label unit dose	ATC 212 and ATC Profile
	AutoMed 250 and 520
	Envoy
D. Pick, pack, and label multidose	ATCPlus and ATC Profile
	AutoMed
	Envoy
E. Pick, pack, and label blister cards in unit and multidose	AutoPack BPM
F. Over-package	Automated Packaging Systems
	Exper Calypso
	Pyxis 1-Pak
G. Robotically pick over-packages and fill patient cassettes	APS RxOBOT
	American BioRobotics
	Pyxis Homerus 1-Star
	Exper Hyperion

A and B). Because these machines use bulk medications from containers packaged by the manufacturer, the term "repackaging," rather than "packaging," is used.

Bulk medications are identified by staff and manually loaded into the machines. Running one drug at a time, the machines then package the medications into unit dose packets or blister cards. Some of the more advanced devices stock multiple lines of bulk tablets in numerous canisters (Table 10–1,

C and D). These canisters must also be hand filled; once filled, however, the machine automates picking as well as packing and labeling.

The manufacturers of these devices have built various safeguards into their systems' hardware, software, and recommended operational procedures. For example, bulk medication canisters typically require pill-specific calibration. This ensures that only one pill is released at a time. Mechanical, electrical, and/or optical sensors verify that the pill has been released. Additionally, each canister will fit only into its appropriate slot in the machine. Some systems have bar code labeling on the canisters. To verify accuracy, technicians scan the bulk supply of medication (i.e., the manufacturer's bottle) and the canister they intend to fill. One machine scans the bar code on newly filled canisters to verify that they are in the correct location before dispensing.

As a rule, the greater the number of human functions that can be automated, the greater the potential for reducing error. Nevertheless, whenever a machine picks from canisters filled by humans, there are still opportunities for errors and for mislabeled medications to make their way to patients. A single error in filling a canister has the potential of multiplying substantially: if 400 pills are put in a wrong canister, there are 400 opportunities for error.

Some systems automate compliance pack production (see Table 10–1, C, D, and E). For subacute, long-term, and ambulatory patients, packages are produced with several days' medications. Patient name, drug, dose, and time to be administered are printed on each administration pack. This reduces opportunities for errors of omission, redundancy, and mistaken identification. These systems are also capable of producing multidose packages (e.g., three different drugs for a single administration). It could be argued that this feature offsets some of the potential gain of compliance packaging. For example, if one drug in the multidose pack is discontinued, compliance might be more complicated for the patient or caregiver than otherwise.

Errors may arise from cross-contamination. Some picking and packing devices have a common chute through which all doses pass before being wrapped. This means that amoxicillins, for example, cannot be run through the machines unless they are coated. Some pharmacists will not take the risk even if the medications are coated.

Systems That Use Over-Packaging. Hospitals and other institutional pharmacies carry out their repackaging operations under state regulation. Manufacturers are subject to the Food and Drug Administration (FDA) Code of Federal Regulations (CFRs) and the Current Good Manufacturing

Practices (CGMPs) outlined therein, which are more stringent than state laws. For this reason, of all the unit dose medications a hospital uses, the least likely to be mislabeled are those wrapped by the manufacturer.

Many unit doses today are processed by repackaging houses, and the number stands to increase. The accuracy of repackagers may or may not be as reliable as that of the manufacturer, depending on how conscientiously the company approaches the task. Although repackagers are subject to a portion of the CFRs (e.g., packaging, labeling, cleaning, and training), some are not put through the same inspection paces as are the manufacturers. The trend, however, is toward tighter scrutiny and enforcement from the FDA (and, when narcotics are involved, the Drug Enforcement Administration).

What about the re- and over-packaging practices of hospitals? Although the FDA has drafted a document outlining standards for hospitals, there is little evidence that they are being enforced. As hospital pharmacies become "repackagers" for other hospitals in their network, the FDA may be expected to increase its involvement in this area.

Some pharmacy-based systems "roboticize" the processes of picking medications and placing them in patient cassettes (Table 10–1, G). Rather than packing or labeling medications, they require special "robot-ready" packaging from three source options:

1. Hospitals may over-package manufacturer-wrapped unit doses.

2. Repackagers may over-package manufacturer-wrapped unit doses.

3. Manufacturers or repackagers may wrap "naked" unit doses in robot-ready blister packages.

The labeling accuracy of over-packaging by technicians varies from hospital to hospital. Depending on how conscientious the hospital is, the potential for errors may be large or inconsequential. It could be argued that hospitals that use over-packages prepared by CGMP-compliant repackagers are least likely to experience mislabeling errors. Even though more repackagers are processing greater lines of robot-ready medications for their customers, there will always be a need for some over-packaging by hospitals. Good policies and procedures and quality assurance to ensure pharmacy packaging accuracy are of utmost importance. There is opportunity for a double-check with over-packaging. An alert pharmacy person or nurse, in observing the manufacturer's inside packaging, may catch an occasional errant over-package.

Assuming that the over-packaged medications are correctly labeled, incorporating robotic handling in the distribution process can do much to help lower error rates. First, in the dispensing functions, robots are capable of flawlessly scanning, picking, and delivering the right package to the right patient's cassette. Second, there is even greater opportunity for error elimination at the point of administration. Uniform bar-coded over-packaging enables a hospital to use bedside scanning for verification and documentation. For verification, the benefit is obvious. When a patient's arm band and medication are scanned, there is little opportunity for confusing bed A for bed B, a nurse's left pocket for her right pocket, or patient McDonald for patient MacDonald.

As for documentation, assume that a medication is charted "as given" when it is taken from an automated cabinet at the nursing station. Then suppose it is administered much later, and that the "charted by exception" record in the cabinet is never reconciled. Or perhaps the medication is never administered, and the nurse forgets to inform the cabinet. In such circumstances, utilization data are inaccurate. Reliable monitoring and measuring of outcomes are at risk. Redundancies and the dangers of inappropriately adjusting therapies are more likely.

Buried in fine print in the April 1, 1995, issue of the *American Journal of Health-System Pharmacy* are some germane thoughts from the minutes of the American Society of Health-System Pharmacy Council on Professional Affairs[1]:

> *The Council believed, for example, that arrangements to allow "charting by exception" for drugs may pose significant risks to both patients and providers. Charting by exception is an approach to patients' medical records sometimes used in patient-focused-care systems and in which it is assumed that all ordered medications have been administered and that they have been administered according to medication orders unless a record to the contrary is made. The Council was highly skeptical about the safety of such an arrangement and believed that substantial safeguards would have to be in place for it to be acceptable. Unless this could be devised, overt charting of all doses of medications administered was seen as a safer procedure.*

Automation has the greatest chance of reducing the incidence of errors when it incorporates point-of-administration scanning for documentation as well as for verification. Although manufacturers could easily provide a scannable drug number, lot number, and expiration date, they do not. They should be encouraged to do so, however, and such a demand would not be out of order. Until then, over-packaged medications bring this possibility closest to a reality.

Decentralized Systems

There are a number of decentralized (ward-based) automated dispensing systems, with varying degrees of potential for limiting or increasing opportunities for error (Table 10–2). Decentralized automated dispensing devices can be said to be to pharmacists and nurses something like what automated teller machines (ATMs) are to banks and customers. The statement is more or less true, depending on the device.

Some of today's systems incorporate "swipe" cards; all require users to enter identification and personal identification numbers. Some provide software that ties each transaction to a patient profile. Like an ATM, this configuration keeps nurses from mixing up patients' drugs, just as cash machines keep clients from mixing up their checking and savings accounts. Ideally, these dispensing devices provide quicker access with fewer mix-ups.

To date, most of these devices have been used to handle limited lines of medication (e.g., narcotics, as-needed medications, and limited floor stock). Some hospitals, however, are now using them to handle 80% to 95% of the medications used in a given care area.

Although these devices are similar to ATMs, there are some noteworthy differences, as can be seen from the following discussion.

Most like ATMs are dispensers that offer strict, single-item access and limit the operator's access to a single dose of medication. This is analogous to an ATM from which a customer selects "withdraw" and from the next menu selects "$20." In response, the ATM machine delivers one $20 bill.

Less like ATMs are drawers that offer single-line access to multiple doses of a medication. The nurse is instructed to count and verify the number of medications in the drawer or pocket with the number showing on the screen and then to take one. This is unlike an ATM in that the latter does not open a drawerful of $20 bills and ask the customer to verify the count on the screen before taking one.

Least like ATMs are drawers that offer multiline access, granting nurses access to multiple doses of multiple lines of medication. These are less like cash machines and more like cash drawers, from which the operator has access to $1, $5, $10, and $20 bills.

| Inpatient Decentralized Systems | Table 10-2 |

Type	Names of Systems
A. Stationary for limited lines	Access[a,b,c]
	Acudose[a,b,c]
	ApotheSystem[a,b,c]
	Controlled Drug Module[a,c]
	Omni Rx[a,b,c]
	MediTROL 80[a]
	MedSelect-Rx[a,b,c]
	MedServ FS[b,c]
	MedStation 500 and 1000[b,c]
	MedStationRx 1000[a,b,c]
	SureMed[a,b,c]
	PyxisStation[a,b,c]
B. Stationary for full lines	ApotheSystem[a,b,c]
	Envoy[a,c]
	OmniSupplier Pharmacy Module[b,c]
	MediTROL 160[a]
	MedSelect-Rx[a,b,c]
	MedStationRx 1000[a,b,c]
	MedStationRx 2000[a,b,c]
	SureMed[a,b,c]
	Homerus and Hydra[a]
C. Portable	MedServ EMAR[a,b,c]
	Medispense[b,c,d]
	Autros[b,c]
	American BioRobotics[a,d]

[a] Single-item access. [b] Single-line access. [c] Multiline access. [d] Patient-specific access.

Proper packaging does not guarantee that technicians and pharmacists will place a medication in its proper place in an automated dispensing device, nor does it guarantee that nurses will retrieve the correct medication. What about safety issues when it comes to stocking, retrieving, and returning medications to these various devices?

Stocking. The right medications have to be picked from the pharmacy and then hand placed in the proper compartment of the dispensing device. Should not the same safety precautions required in filling patient cassettes in the pharmacy be taken in stocking these devices (e.g,. adequate lighting, lack of interruptions, careful concentration, meticulous checking) and, even more so, at the dispensing device? Suppose that a 40-dose dispenser is filled with the correct medication but the wrong dose. The next 40 transactions involving that medication are in danger of resulting in administration errors.

New replenishment programs emerging from cooperative efforts between wholesale distributors and automation vendors offer promise toward error-free stocking of decentralized cabinets. These programs require bar coding of medication packets and cabinet compartments. Persons who restock the cabinets must have matching scans of bar codes of each medication and its proper location in the cabinet.

Retrieving. There is some evidence that nurses tend to "lean on" automation: in other words, they are less likely to check medications retrieved from an automated box than those removed from a manual exchange cart.

Moreover, it is commonly agreed that opportunities for error diminish when access is narrowed. This was proven as hospitals moved from open floor stock to unit dose delivery. Instead of picking one patient's four medications from 100 bottles on the shelf, the nurse picked them from the few medications in the patient's cassette. The Pyxis Corp. demonstrated safety-added benefits early on in automating the narcotics box. Instead of picking the right medication from 40 line items in a double-locked box, the nurse was given access to a carousel pocket containing only the medication needed, even if it was in multiple doses.

What are the risks, however, when multiple-line (matrix) drawers or, even worse, dividerless bins are employed? Has safety been compromised? Now the nurse has to find the correct pocket, sometimes out of 60 options. To obtain three drugs, a nurse might have access to 180 drugs.

There is a spectrum of opinion among advocates of automation systems. At one end are those who are satisfied with using matrix drawers for all but Schedule II drugs and dangerous medications. At the other end are those who insist that all medications be dispensed as single items. In the middle are individuals with various comfort levels with the different applications of these drawers. Most vendors offer combinations of single-item, single-line, and multiple-line (matrix) access configurations.

Two omens suggest that the future will usher in stricter regulation of decentralized devices. An indication of the first may be found in a document entitled *Automated Medication Storage and Distribution System Guidelines*, issued by the Minnesota State Board of Pharmacy.[2] The eighth guideline of this document states: "The use of multiple medication drawers or bins must be limited to non-legend drugs or medications properly packaged and labeled for an individual patient." Although these are not yet regulations, they provide a hint as to the direction in which boards will gravitate as they are called on to address the impact of automation on pharmacy practice.

The second omen may be found in a procedure that has been implemented at the University of California at San Diego Medical Center, a fully decentralized facility. They use matrix drawers only for over-the-counter products. They use single-line access drawers for all legend drugs. Additionally, surveys indicate that the majority of customers want at least single-line access for legend drugs and that they strongly prefer single-item access for Schedule II products.

When matrix drawers are used, devices that electronically highlight the proper bin are an added safety feature. Adding lids over each matrix compartment is even better, because it helps ensure that medications do not fall into the wrong place. Safer still are devices whose lids light up to indicate the proper bin. If the operator lifts the wrong lid, an alarm sounds and the incident is recorded.

When systems handle only bar-coded medications and require verification scanning upon retrieval of each medication, drawer configuration is not as critical to the process from a safety standpoint. This final dispensing check redeems otherwise risk-prone devices.

Systems that tie the transaction at the box to patient profiles further promote safety. They limit access to medications ordered for a given patient. Some limit access to a certain time frame. Some prompt nurses when medications are due. These options help avoid omission errors as well the administration of redundant or wrong medications. However, all the systems allow for nurse override. More than a few in the profession insist that safety calls for pharmacies to be increasingly restrictive in allowing overrides.

Returning Versus Restocking. Hospitals and departments within hospitals vary with respect to procedures for returning drugs to decentralized boxes. Some require the nurse to return them only to the return bin. Others allow some nurses to return some drugs to stock.

At least one device will not allow any nurse to return any drug to stock. As a rule, single-item dispensers cannot accept returns, whereas single-line and matrix drawers can. Even though hardware might permit returns to stock, software can be configured to prohibit returns. Again, risk will be greatly diminished when cabinet medications are bar coded and systems require match scanning of both item and bin when a medication is returned to stock.

Administration. Even if the nurse retrieves the correct and properly labeled medication for a patient at the right time, there is still a gap between the device and the bedside. In general, the closer the decentralized device is to the bedside, the smaller is the potential for error. This is one advantage of an automated mobile cart that transports the medications and dispensing functions to the bedside, if not the door of the patient's room (Table 10–2, C).

Most cart technologies use manufacturer- or pharmacy-packaged medications. One device houses small cassettes of bulk oral solids and automatically dispenses the tablets into soufflé cups for the patient whose profile is on the screen. Dispensing the medications one patient at a time, at the point of administration, stands to reduce incidence of error.

The Minnesota Board of Pharmacy recognizes the gap between box and bedside in its seventh guideline: "A policy and procedure must define how the drugs will be delivered from the automated device to the patient."[2] The main area of concern is the potential for mix-ups when multiple drugs are being dispensed and delivered to multiple patients.

Procedural questions must be addressed: Are nurses allowed to remove more than one patient's medications in a single transaction? If a drawer is open for one patient's transaction and a nurse sees a medication she knows another patient will be needing, may she take it at that time? Where does the nurse put the medications to be dispensed? Are her pockets good enough?

There are a number of options for retrieving routine or scheduled medications from dispensing cabinets in a decentralized system. They include retrieving

1. all the medications for a single patient for a single administration,
2. all the medications for more than one patient for a single administration,
3. all the medications for a single patient for a single shift, and
4. all the medications for more than one patient for a single shift.

Approach 1 is safest because it poses the least danger of interchanging one patient's medications for another. Approaches 2 and 4 may present problems when a medication is discontinued.

Approaches 2, 3, and 4 require an additional system for keeping one patient's medications separate from those of others. One way is to place them in a plastic self-sealing bag, along with a receipt. Placing them in various pockets is inappropriate unless they are in patient-specific, sealed bags.

Another option is to fill patient cassettes one at a time. They may be placed in a small hand-carried tote or on a medication cart. This, however, is little more than cart fill. The fundamental question is: Which personnel and filling environment are most conducive to an accurate cassette fill? Pharmacists and pharmacy technicians, who work in a controlled environment, or nurses on the wards?

It will be interesting to see which decentralized system, if any, will be the first to incorporate bar-coded envelope production for all medications dispensed from the cabinet. Why not, when the medication is dispensed from the cabinet, have a patient-specific envelope simultaneously issued into which the medications could be immediately placed by the nurse? This would prompt the nurse to give the medication, remind the nurse if he or she has forgotten, and prevent administering medications to the wrong patient.

Patient-specific labeling is not essential for electronic point-of-administration verification, provided that the medication shows up at bedside with its own readable and uniform bar code and the system's scanner is tied into each patient's medication profile. If a hospital were going to decentralize virtually all of its medications in ward-based cabinets, the safest approach, though it would be costly, might be to stock the cabinets entirely with over-packaged, scannable medications.

When it comes to safety in the medication process, the most important gap where errors can occur is the least addressed by automation at this point. The gaps between ordering and dispensing are certainly critical, and most systems have made progress in closing some of these. But the crucial gap is between dispensing and administering. This is where progress is needed.

No matter how many medications are stored in decentralized cabinets, there will always be a need for patient-specific cassettes for handling multiple-use medications and other miscellaneous items. The safest approach may be to designate an electronically controlled drawer on the dispensing cabinet for each patient who has need for such medication.

Outpatient Automated Dispensing Systems

Outpatient technologies, like those in inpatient areas, can be divided into centralized and decentralized systems. Centralized outpatient systems are used to fill prescriptions from retail or consolidated pharmacy sites. Decentralized systems fill patient prescriptions from doctors' offices, clinics, and, perhaps someday, from stand-alone dispensing cabinets in nontraditional settings.

Centralized systems include technologies that fill strip packages, blister cards, and bottles from bulk oral solids. Decentralized systems use prefilled bottles and manufacturer-packaged items.

Centralized Systems

Strip Packaging and Envelope Packagers. Some of the technologies already discussed that dispense individual unit dose packages are also employed to dispense envelopes and strip packs (compliance packs) of medication. For example, instead of a 30-day bottled prescription containing 30 tablets (one per day), a 30-pack compliance strip contains one pill per pack. Each packet bears the name of the patient, the drug and its dose, and the date and time to be administered. Pack-specific labeling helps avoid redundancy and omissions; it also provides a better means for promoting and monitoring compliance. Automated dispensing devices used in centralized outpatient systems are listed in Table 10–3.

Most strip packagers use multiple canisters. When operators are filling these canisters, systems should require that they match scans of manufacturers' bottles and the dispensing canister to be filled. This practice can virtually eliminate filling errors.

Blister Card Packagers. Blister card fillers can be categorized into those that fill cards from a hopper containing a single line of pills and those that fill cards from multiple drug canisters (Table 10–3, C and D).

When the blister card backing has each dose marked with administration time, redundancies and omissions are more easily avoided. They are not, however, without problems. Suppose that multiple drugs are placed in a single blister for a single administration. Then one of the pills is discontinued. A patient who has to sort strips and eliminate the discontinued drug midway through a 30-day cycle may present higher risk than a patient who is instructed to discard a single bottle.

Bottle-Filling Devices. The category of bottle-filling devices includes large devices used by consolidated pharmacies that have large walk-in populations or that provide mail order services. Smaller devices may be found in community pharmacies. They range from devices that automate only pill-counting to those that automate the entire filling process. Some pick the proper vial, robotically transport it to the proper location for automatic filling, and apply the computer-produced label. Some even cap the bottle and send it to the proper mailing tote.

Opportunities for error occur at the time of canister filling. It is no small error when a canister is filled with the wrong medication. This possibility is minimized in most systems, because they involve pill-specific calibration for each canister. In addition, most systems require matching scans of bar codes on manufacturers' bottles and the cassettes into which they are going. Others require matching scans of bar codes on canisters and the position in the machine where the cassette belongs. Others depend on mechanical devices that will not allow a cassette to be placed in a wrong location. One robotic system actually scans the bar code on the cassette with each filling to verify that the vial is at the proper filling station. Thorough and redundant scanning reduces chances for error.

Generally, the more fully a system is automated, the less potential there is for error. For example, some systems require the worker to manually locate the correct dispensing bin. Computers find the bins more accurately. When humans have to take a labeled bottle to the dispensing bin, even if the computer has selected the correct bin, they may inadvertently take in hand a

Outpatient Centralized Systems		Table 10-3
Function Performed	**Names of Systems**	
A. Pick, pack, and label compliance strip packs (single or multidose)	ATCPlus and ATC Profile AutoMed	
B. Pick, pack, and label compliance envelopes (single or multidose)	Envoy	
C. Pack and label blister cards	MTS 500 and MTS 1500 Rx Systems	
D. Pick, pack, and label blister cards in unit and multidose	AutoPack BPM	
E. Pick and count for bottles	Baker Cells PharmASSIST	
F. Pick, count, fill, and label bottles	Quick Script OptiFill Auto Script III Script Pro 200	

wrong bottle on the way to the right filling spout. Robotics does a more accurate job of taking the right vial to the right filling station.

Some systems require a final human check by asking the pharmacist to look inside the bottle before capping it. She or he must verify the appearance of the tablet with an image of the correct medication as shown on the computer screen. Other systems do not have this final check. It could be argued that the final visual check by a pharmacist is a safer practice.

It is not too difficult to demonstrate that fully automated bottle-filling machines produce fewer filling errors than those involving human action. When a machine error does occur, it is associated with under- or overfilling vials by a few tablets, not with filling the vial with the wrong drug.

Cross-contamination is a concern with some of these systems. If all pills must pass through a common hopper on their way to the bottle, the system cannot run some medications (e.g., unless they are coated). Even then, some pharmacists argue that cross-contamination is too much of a risk.

Decentralized Systems

The area of decentralized systems is less well developed when it comes to dispensing automation than others (Table 10–4). Nonetheless, there are companies that provide prefilled, low-cost bottles of commonly used medications to doctors for dispensing to patients before the office visit concludes. Some use computer software-operated automated dispensing cabinets. These cabinets range from open-shelved "dumb cupboards" with electronically operated remote latches to secure cabinets that dispense each prescription singly. The latter, by eliminating human hunting, are safer. When bar code scanning and human-read verification of labels are required before the dispensing process is completed, the opportunity for errors is reduced even more.

There are two schools of thought about outpatient dispensing programs. Both argue that they can improve the quality and lower the cost of providing pharmacy care. Both insist that compliance is promoted when patients receive their medications at the point of care. However, one school seems bent on avoiding or going around pharmacists, while the other seems determined to bring better pharmacy services into the doctors' offices and the entire process.

It is important to distinguish between pharmacy information and pharmacists. The safest systems are those that proactively bring electronic pharmacy information into the physician's decision-making process before he or she writes a script. Drug databases, as well as screening for allergies, conflict-

Table 10-4

Outpatient Decentralized Systems (Clinic Based)

ADDS[a]
AllScripps[c]
MedStation[a,b,c]

[a] Single-item access.
[b] Single-line access.
[c] Multiline access.

ing therapies, redundancies, inappropriate doses, and other risk factors, ensure safer script filling. The safest systems require the doctor, when necessary, to have a pharmacist review and approve the order before dispensing the medication. In some instances, live consultation is required. Some systems facilitate this consulting via video conferencing. All of this stands to provide safer medication practices, not only in rural areas where there is no pharmacy nearby, but also in urban areas where the pharmacist on duty can interact with another pharmacist across the country who specializes in the therapy at issue.

It should be understood that neither doctors nor their office associates are doing any counting. They simply dispense pre-packs. Systems that dispense single bottles or require bar code scanning to verify that the right bottle is being used for the right label are safest.

Some believe the day is coming when pharmacies will remotely operate dispensing cabinets in nontraditional, highly accessible areas, much as ATMs provide bank services in grocery stores. Identification cards, personal identification numbers, and interactive screens will enable patients to pick up a doctor-prescribed, pharmacist-approved medication at their local supermarket at midnight. These systems will provide patients with printed instructions and warnings. They may also require patients, when necessary, to have a video conference with a pharmacist before the cabinet will dispense their medication. It is arguable that such delivery systems could be safer than over-the-counter pick-ups. On occasion, humans mistakenly give a patient someone else's medications. Sometimes customers deceptively retrieve orders belonging to someone else. It is not so easy to fool an ATM-like machine. Videotaping transactions will undoubtedly be a feature of these systems.

Summary

Automation has great potential for decreasing medication errors. It does not, however, automatically reduce chances of error; in some instances it might even increase the opportunity for errors. Thus, automation should be carefully evaluated and even more carefully applied. Where automation stands to reduce opportunities for medication errors, pharmacies and pharmacists should take advantage of it to ensure the safest possible medication distribution practices.

• • • •
References

1. American Society of Health-System Pharmacists, Council on Professional Affairs. *Am J Health Syst Pharm.*, 1995; 52: 743.

2. Automated Medication Storage and Distribution System Guidelines. Minneapolis, Minn: Minnesota Board of Pharmacy Rule 6800.7520; January 1995.

11. Errors Associated with Medication Administration

Michael R. Cohen, MS, FASHP

Institute for Safe Medication Practices
Huntingdon Valley, Pa.

During their training, nurses are introduced to the "five R's"—right drug, right route, right dose, right time, and right patient. This dictum is useful in clinical practice as a check for accuracy during drug administration. At the same time, this advice can be problematic because it may imply that responsibility for accurate drug use lies solely with the person administering it.

Not only is this idea false, it also places enormous pressure for perfection on the person administering medication. Medication use is a multidisciplinary process. Responsibility for accurate drug administration lies with multiple individuals and, more important, the organizational systems in place to support safe medication administration.

Necessity for Independent Double-Checking

Because there are many opportunities for error, the ideal medication administration system is one in which there is more than one practitioner between the drug and the patient. Persons who prescribe, dispense, and administer drugs must rely on one another to detect and prevent errors. For example, while screening orders, a pharmacist may detect a prescribing error such as an inappropriate dose, duplicate therapy, or a drug interaction. When checking medications prior to administration, a nurse may detect a pharmacy dispensing error. While reviewing a daily computer printout of a patient's current medication regimen, a physician may detect the inadvertent discontinuation of a drug by nursing or pharmacy staff.

Every health care institution must develop and monitor procedures to govern the ordering, dispensing, and administration of medications. When such procedures are not followed, the system of checks and balances is bypassed and errors are more likely. Such unsafe conditions exist when nurses or others who administer medication prepare doses from floor stock, borrow doses meant for one patient and administer them to another, or obtain doses from an automated dispensing cabinet before a pharmacist has screened the order.

Consider this example of what can go wrong when this double-check system is violated. A nursing staff development director was asked to fill in as a staff nurse on the intensive care unit. One of her patients was supposed to receive pentobarbital. She misread the medication administration record (MAR) and thought that the patient was to receive phenobarbital intravenously. When she could not find phenobarbital in the patient's medication bin, she assumed that the pharmacist had forgotten to put it there. She retrieved a supply from floor stock and administered the drug. Had the nurse called the pharmacist to double-check about the "missing dose," this error could have been detected.

Double-checking is also vital at the time of order transcription. The nurse or unit clerk may be less familiar with medications and dosage forms than the pharmacist. It is less likely that the wrong drug, dose, or dosage form will reach a patient when both pharmacy and nursing staff have reviewed it.

For example, a physician wrote an order for "Rocephin 1 gm IVPB q12." Because of the poor handwriting, the unit clerk and nurse interpreted the "q12" as "qid." The nursing staff was unaware that Rocephin is usually given only once or twice daily. Following procedure, a copy of the order was sent to the pharmacy. The pharmacist recognized the error and immediately called the nursing unit. Had this intervention not occurred, the patient may have received twice the prescribed amount. Dose omissions are also less likely under a system that requires double-checking, because an order that is missed on the nursing unit has a chance of being recognized in the pharmacy, or vice versa.

Most hospitals have adopted the unit dose drug distribution system. Medications arrive in ready-to-use, single-dose form. The nurse can check each dose to make sure it matches the order transcribed in the MAR. The greatest safety advantage of the unit dose system is that the pharmacist and the nurse can independently interpret, transcribe, and verify each dose before dispensing or administering it. When a pharmacist dispenses a dose of medication that does not correspond to the MAR, it is a signal that something may be incorrect. A pharmacist or nurse may have misinterpreted the order, a mistranscription or an error in computer order entry may have occurred, or the wrong drug may have been selected. The process is halted until the situation is investigated and corrected if necessary. In contrast, when a single nurse interprets, transcribes, prepares, and administers the dose, it is unlikely that the system will provide adequate checks to capture errors.

Pharmacists maintain records of each patient's allergies, chronic conditions, and current diagnosis. They screen each order to ensure that contraindicated drugs are not dispensed. This safety feature is eliminated when pharmacist screening is bypassed.

For example, a patient admitted to a hospital emergency room stated that he had an aspirin allergy. A doctor ordered ketorolac (Toradol®), failing to realize that both aspirin and ketorolac are nonsteroidal anti-inflammatory drugs and have cross-allergy potential. The nurses removed ketorolac from an automated dispensing cabinet and gave it intravenously. The patient developed anaphylaxis and died. Had the order been screened through the pharmacy computer system, this event probably would not have happened.

Processing Medication Orders

Medication orders may be written by hand, entered directly into a computer system, or spoken aloud (generally referred to as "verbal" orders). Regardless of how the order is communicated, it must be correctly transcribed into the MAR. Information that must be transcribed includes the drug name, dose, route, dosage form, and time of administration. If a "stop time" is indicated in the order, this should also be recorded.

Written Orders

Order Forms. Most hospitals use NCR (no-carbon-required) forms to document physician orders. The original is placed in the patient's chart, and a copy is sent to the pharmacy. The two-part form allows for separate interpretations of the orders by nursing and pharmacy personnel. In hospitals with computer ordering systems, the physician enters an order and an MAR is printed to signal nursing staff that a new drug has been prescribed. Simultaneously, a label is printed in the pharmacy to start the dispensing cycle. The use of NCR forms and direct computer entry both reduce the potential for errors.

Printed lines are necessary on the first page of NCR order forms because they make it easier to write neatly. Unfortunately, these lines may also obscure portions of a drug order. They may hide the top of a numeral seven (7) and make it look like a one (1), or they may obscure decimal points and other marks.

For example, a physician who intended to order 0.5 mg of terbutaline failed to place a zero before the decimal point. The transcriber failed to see the decimal point because it was obscured by the line. As a result, the patient received 5 mg instead of 0.5 mg of the drug. In another instance, an unnecessary decimal point and a zero were added to an order for 1 mg of warfarin (i.e., the order was expressed as 1.0 mg), and a patient received 10 mg instead of the intended 1 mg.

Errors such as these can best be prevented by adding a zero before a decimal point and by eliminating trailing decimal points and zeroes. An additional aid would be to eliminate the lines on the back copy of the NCR form. The person receiving it could then clearly see decimal points or other marks that might otherwise be inadvertently obscured by lines on the top copy.

Other errors are possible with NCR forms. Writing on one NCR form with an additional NCR form underneath, for example, may cause the same set of orders to appear twice. Depending on the patient identity stamp that is placed on the form, a pharmacist could receive and process a set of such orders for the wrong patient or process a second set of orders that is several days old for the original patient.

Prescribers should be sure that no additional forms are directly below the one on which they are writing. If they are writing on a stack of forms, they should place a manila folder or other heavy paper between the top form and the forms beneath it.

Incomplete Orders. The nurse has the responsibility to question all incomplete or unclear orders before administering any medication. Even if the course of action seems obvious, the nurse must not make any assumptions about the prescriber's intent.

For example, a physician ordered "Mycostatin® (nystatin) suppository, one at bedtime" for a woman recovering from a cerebrovascular accident. The route of administration was not noted. A nurse working the night shift prepared the tablet according to the package insert instructions and placed it into the patient's vagina. The following morning, the nurse learned that the physician had intended that the patient dissolve the drug in her mouth to treat an oral yeast infection, an acceptable practice with this dosage form.

In another case, a physician wrote the following order for a 12-year-old patient with asthma: "Theodur® 300 mg 1½ tablets bid." The nurse was not sure whether the physician wanted her to administer 1½ x 200-mg tablets (a 300-mg dose) or 1½ 300-mg tablets (a 450-mg dose). The nurse called to clarify the order and learned that the physician had intended for the patient to receive a total dose of 300 mg and was unaware that Theodur® was even available in a 300-mg tablet. By questioning, the nurse prevented an overdose.

Drug Indications. One of the most effective ways to prevent administration of the wrong drug is to make sure that it is appropriate for the patient. For this reason, the prescriber should include the indication for the drug with the order whenever possible. This precaution is most essential for medications ordered to be taken as needed.

Brand Versus Generic Names. Because there may often be many brand names for a single generic drug, it is best to refer to medications by their generic names. Because many prescribers order medications by brand name, pharmacies that make available computer-generated MARs can provide an important service. These records are usually produced every 24 hours from orders entered into the computer. To reduce confusion, they contain both the brand names and the generic names of products. Such a system can also enhance patient safety because it provides consistency (e.g., in spelling and dose documentation) and allows nurses to compare their transcriptions with those of the pharmacist. Computer-generated MARs can also provide consistent drug messages and warnings and information on patient allergies, diagnosis, and chronic conditions.

Abbreviations. Abbreviations of drug names, dosage units, and references to timing of medication administration are commonly used. Institutions should maintain a list of dangerous abbreviations that should never be used. Misunderstandings caused by the use of unapproved abbreviations have caused many errors. For example, in one instance a physician ordered "heparin 5000 units sub q 2 h prior to surgery." The order was interpreted as "heparin 5000 units subcutaneously every 2 hours prior to surgery"; the prescriber had actually intended that the patient receive a *single dose* subcutaneously 2 hours prior to surgery.

Abbreviating drug names also often causes problems. For example, "HCTZ 50 mg," used as an abbreviation for hydrochlorothiazide 50 mg, can easily be mistaken for hydrocortisone 250 mg if the "Z" looks like a "2."

It is recommended that abbreviations and acronyms not be used in drug orders. If they are used, readers must be sure to clarify all orders bearing unapproved or confusing abbreviations. Abbreviations should not be carried forth onto the MAR.

Apothecary Versus Metric Symbols. Only the metric system should be used in orders or on the MAR. Apothecary symbols are often misinterpreted or used incorrectly. For example, when a nurse mistook the dram symbol (one teaspoon) for "oz" on an order for Donnatal® Elixir, a patient was given a sixfold overdose. The U.S. Pharmacopeia now requires that prescriptions written for compendial articles state the quantity and strength in metric terms. Terms such as *grains, drams,* and *minims* are not acceptable. Physicians who continue to write orders using apothecary terms and symbols should be reminded of this requirement and helped to understand that use of the metric system can help prevent errors.

Verbal Orders

Orders that are spoken aloud—in person or by telephone—rather than written down are more error-prone than written orders, because the only record of the transaction is in the memories of those involved. When a verbal order is recorded by the recipient, the prescriber assumes that the recipient understood correctly. No one except the prescriber, however, can verify that the recipient heard the message correctly.

The interpretation of what someone else says is inherently problematic because of different accents, dialects, and pronunciations. Background noise, interruptions, sound-alike drug names, and unfamiliar terminology compound the problem.

For example, an emergency room physician gave a spoken order for "morphine 2 mg iv." The nurse, however, heard "morphine 10 mg iv." The young patient received a 10-mg injection and developed respiratory arrest. In another instance, a physician called in an order for "15 mg" of hydralazine to be given intravenously every 2 hours. The nurse, thinking that he had said "50 mg," drew up two 20-mg vials and one half of a third vial, which she administered to the patient. Within a few minutes, the patient developed tachycardia and had a significant drop in blood pressure. The nurse called the doctor. Fortunately, a rapid infusion of fluids restored the patient's blood pressure to a safe level. Repeating spoken orders to prescribers and pronouncing each digit of a number (i.e., "one five" mg instead of "fifteen" mg) can help prevent misinterpretation.

When a nursing home telephones medication orders to a pharmacy, the pharmacist must rely on the nurse to ensure that the order is accurate. If the nurse misreads an order, the pharmacist rarely has enough information at hand to detect the error. If the order were faxed to the pharmacy rather than telephoned, both the nurse and the pharmacist would have an opportunity to interpret what was written, and the potential for accurate order interpretation would be doubled.

Faxes, electronic mail, and computer order entry are reducing the need for spoken medication orders. To ensure that orders are properly directed, fax machines used for ordering should not have programmed speed dial buttons. If the wrong button is pushed, the order can reach an incorrect location. This may not only delay therapy but may also violate patient confidentiality.

The following guidelines may reduce the possibility of errors associated with spoken orders:

1. Limit spoken orders to emergent or urgent situations.

2. Do not allow spoken orders when the prescriber is present and the patient's chart is available, unless it is impossible for the order to be written down (for instance, when a physician who is in the middle of a procedure needs to prescribe a medication).

3. Do not accept spoken medication requests in the pharmacy unless a written order is simultaneously faxed or otherwise seen before the medication is dispensed.

4. Require prescribers to limit spoken orders to formulary drugs, because names of other drugs are more likely to be misheard and their uses may be less familiar to staff than those of formulary products.

5. Limit the number of personnel who may receive spoken orders.

6. Whenever possible, have a pharmacist receive all spoken orders. When spoken medication orders are received by pharmacists, or when order changes are directed to pharmacists in the course of clarifying drug orders, have a mechanism by which the pharmacist can transcribe the order directly into the medical record.

7. Be sure that the person receiving a spoken order is familiar with the caller. This is important because cases of fraudulent spoken orders have occurred. Make sure that the person receiving the message has the caller's telephone number in case it is necessary to call him or her back.

8. Have a second person listen to the conversation whenever possible. If the person taking the message is inexperienced, this should be required. A speaker phone may be used in some areas, providing that the need for confidentiality is recognized. Some receivers may want to record telephone orders for documentation.

9. Record the order directly onto the order sheet of the patient's chart. Transcription from a scrap of paper to the chart introduces another opportunity for error.

10. Do not use abbreviations.

11. Enunciate clearly. Spell drug names, especially those that are unfamiliar. If names are unfamiliar or abbreviations are used, say, "T as in Tom," "C as in Charlie," and so forth. Pronounce each digit of numbers: for example, say "one six" instead of "sixteen" to avoid confusion with "sixty."

12. Require that the receiver read back the transcription to the caller. This step is absolutely essential.

13. Ensure that the order makes sense in the context of the patient's treatment plan.

14. Have the order signed, dated, timed, and noted according to hospital procedure. It must then be processed and eventually placed into the patient's chart.

15. Have the prescriber read and sign the order within a predetermined time frame.

Identification of Patients

Errors in patient identification often occur because of distractions and interruptions. Nurses often must simultaneously prepare doses for more than one patient. If they are interrupted while preparing the medications, they may confuse one patient's medications with those of another when they return to their task. In other cases, orders are written for the wrong patient or transcribed onto the wrong patient's MAR.

Identification with arm bands is a simple means of ensuring that the right drug is administered to the right patient. Even if the nurse greets the patient, the arm band must be checked before the medication is administered. Nurses routinely care for several patients, and because most patients are scheduled to receive their medications at the same time, it is possible for a nurse to give the wrong medication to the wrong patient. When a nurse is caring for two patients in the same room, the risk of a mix-up is even higher.

A spoken affirmation of the patient's name does not replace the need for arm band identification. For various reasons, patients may respond in a positive manner when asked to verify their names. For example, when a nurse asked a patient if he was "Mr. Thomas," the patient replied "Wright." Assuming that the patient had given an affirmative reply (i.e., "right"), the nurse gave Mr. Wright medications that were intended for his roommate, Mr. Thomas. Another example involved a patient who was tired of waiting for his oncology appointment. When a nurse entered the waiting room and asked for "Mr. Smith," a patient got up and entered the treatment area. Fortunately, the patient's spouse reported that "Mr. Smith" was actually "Mr. Brown." The patient assumed that all the oncology clinic patients received the same chemotherapy, and in an effort to speed up his appointment, he pretended to be Mr. Smith.

In clinics and other places where arm bands are not used for identification, consideration should be given to applying temporary identification bands at registration. Up-to-date photographic images may also be used to aid in accurate patient identification. The nurse can at least check the patient's driver's license or ask for the patient's address to match against information already in the medical record.

Some hospital computer systems place a bar code on the patient's identification band. The bar code identifies the patient and verifies that the medications, when scanned prior to administration, are appropriate for that patient.

Patient Education

If patients are aware of the medications they should be receiving, they can alert their nurses to potential errors in medication administration. If a patient questions a dose of medication, that dose should not be administered unless the reason for the refusal can definitely be determined to be invalid.

For example, when a patient with diabetes insisted that a dose of 85 units of NPH insulin was too much, the nurse checked the order and the MAR. Both indicated that the 85 units was correct; however, she took the patient's concern seriously and called the attending physician. She learned that the patient was correct; the dose had been ordered in error because another physician had relied on medical records from the patient's prior admission.

In health care facilities where unit dose packaging is used, the nurse compares the medication package with the MAR before administering a dose. Ideally, the nurse takes the unit dose packages into the patient's room and gives the unit doses to the patient. In this manner, patient education can take place at the time of drug administration, and the patient has the opportunity to verify that the medication is correct.

A well-educated patient is a strong defense against errors. Educating patients and querying them before administering any drugs may help. If the nurse speaks with the patient about what the medication is and what it is for, the patient will have the opportunity to object if something is wrong.

Timing of Medication Administration

Doses are supposed to be administered within a specific time frame. Acceptable limits for the timing of drug administration are defined by each institution; usually, it is within 30 to 60 minutes of the scheduled time. Use of the unit dose system has improved the timeliness of medication administration because it reduces medication preparation time.

The morning medication administration time is the busiest. More medications are administered in the morning than at any other time, and the potential for errors is therefore the highest. For this reason, many hospitals have adopted standard alternate times for the administration of certain medications that require laboratory monitoring or specific patient assessment before administration. For example, in many institutions, warfarin is given at bedtime so that the international normalized ratio (INR) for anticoagulant monitoring can be checked earlier in the day and the daily dose can be adjusted if necessary. Digoxin is frequently given at noon, when few medications are given, so that the nurse will have time to check the patient's apical and radial pulses as indicators of digoxin level.

Nurses must consider the timing of administration of each medication in relation to that of any others the patient is receiving. For example, oral antacids should not be administered with quinolone antibiotics, such as ciprofloxacin, because the antacid will bind to the quinolone. Incompatibilities among intravenous medications must be checked before medications are combined in the same infusion container or run together at a Y-site. At the time that medications are ordered and added to the MAR, drug interactions or incompatibilities should be noted and appropriate timing of medications should be scheduled in cooperation with the pharmacy.

As-needed medications present a special concern. Because they are not administered at routine times, the nurse must make sure that the appropriate time interval has passed before the next dose is given.

Medication Preparation

Labels must be read three times: (1) when obtaining an item from the storage area or the patient's supply; (2) when preparing the dose for administration; and (3) after administration, when discarding the empty package or replacing a partially used container. Some nurses give the patient the unit dose package to open, showing the unit dose wrapper to the patient and discarding the wrapper in the patient's room. This gives the patient an opportunity to verify the accuracy of what is being administered.

In settings where a unit dose system is used, medications should not be removed from their containers in advance of the time they are to be administered. Although it may seem more convenient, this practice defeats the purpose of the unit dose system. Once medications have been removed from their packaging, it is difficult to identify them. The loss of identity of each dose means that a drug cannot be returned if an order is changed or if it is unused. An unlabeled dose is at far greater risk of being mixed up with another drug than is a labeled dose.

The following example illustrates the importance of keeping medications in their packaging until at the bedside. A night-shift nurse was preparing medications for three patients when a female patient with Parkinson's disease requested aspirin. After confirming the order, the nurse placed two aspirin tablets into another cup. She then picked up all four cups, into which she had opened each patient's medications, and headed for the patients' rooms. Remembering that the patient who requested the aspirin frequently complained about getting her medications late, the nurse administered that patient's medication first. She soon realized that she had switched the cups and given the woman who had requested aspirin the morphine sulfate tablets intended for another patient with cancer.

Crushing oral solid medications can destroy the effect of some drugs and, in some cases, cause an adverse reaction. For example, long-acting medications such as Procardia XL® and medications with enteric coatings should not be crushed. Precautions need to be taken for crushing drugs with cytotoxic potential to prevent exposure to airborne dust created when crushing. The American Society of Health-System Pharmacists recommends placing each unit-of-use package in a small plastic bag and crushing the medication with a spoon or pestle, taking care not to tear the bag.[1] A list of drugs that should not be crushed is published annually in *Hospital Pharmacy*.[2] It should be made available in the pharmacy and nursing units. The pharmacist should always be asked whether it is safe to crush any medication or open any capsule before its administration.

Patients should be observed during medication administration. Medications should not be left at bedside unless this is specifically ordered or they are placed there according to hospital policy. Leaving medication for a patient to take later could lead to any number of problems. For instance, medications may be hoarded by a depressed patient and used for a suicide attempt, or they may be taken intentionally or accidentally by a visitor or another patient.

Dosing Considerations

It is unusual for a single dose to be composed of more than two dosage units, and nurses should question all such orders. If the dose is indeed found to require several tablets or capsules, pharmacists can often formulate it into a single dosage unit to make it easier for the patient to swallow.

For example, a nurse in an intensive care unit prepared what she believed to be a 25 mg/250 mL infusion of phenylephrine. The vials of phenylephrine stated, in bold print, "1%." The drug name and "10 mg/mL" appeared in smaller print that was partially obscured by a colored band. The nurse thought that each vial contained 1 mg and prepared the infusion using 25 vials (250 mg). The infusion was hung by another nurse on the next shift. Shortly thereafter, the patient's systolic blood pressure rose to 208 mm Hg. The nurse suspected that something was wrong with the infusion; after she remade and hung the infusion, the patient's systolic blood pressure decreased to 100 mm Hg. Upon investigation, the 25 empty vials were found in the trash can.

When a patient who has been receiving nothing by mouth (NPO) becomes able to ingest oral medications, or when a patient previously taking oral medication is placed on NPO status, medication doses may change because the bioavailability of most medications is higher when they are given intravenously. For example, levothyroxine is only 50% bioavailable orally; a patient who is switched from the oral to the intravenous route with no change in dosing will, in effect, receive double the necessary dose. The pharmacist and nurse must double-check all medications whenever changes in NPO status occur.

Pediatric and chemotherapy doses must be independently double-checked before administration, because there is little room for error with dosages of these agents. When a physician orders a pediatric or chemotherapy drug, the designation "milligrams per kilogram" (mg/kg) or "milligrams per meter squared" (mg/m^2) should be part of the order. This will enable a second practitioner to recalculate the dose and independently confirm it before dispensing and administration. In addition, the nurse should make sure that the measuring devices used with pediatric solutions and suspensions are calibrated correctly for the medication.

An error took place with a cyclosporine oral solution when a nurse used the supplied oral syringe to measure a 30-mg dose for a baby. The product is supplied in a solution of 100 mg/mL, but the syringe supplied with the product has a scale that starts at 0.5 mL (50 mg). The nurse drew 3 mL (300 mg) into the syringe, thinking that she was drawing 30 mg. The child received this overdose for several days.

When administering intravenous medications, nurses must make sure that the dose and infusion rate are correct. Prescribers may not always include the infusion rate, assuming that the nurse will be aware of it. This has led to serious errors. For example, many patients have died as a result of receiving concentrated potassium chloride (KCl) as a bolus instead of as a diluted infusion. Aggravating the situation is the fact that some physicians have prescribed it as "KCl 40 mEq iv bolus." To some people, "bolus" means "at once."

Medication Devices, Delivery Systems, and Intravenous Equipment

Today's intravenous infusion devices accurately regulate the amount infused. This is a great improvement over earlier methods of gravity control, both in terms of therapeutic outcome and patient safety. Some devices, however, allow free flow of intravenous solutions after the tubing set is removed. If the nurse does not close the gravity flow control clamp before removing the tubing set from the device, the solution will continue to flow. This design flaw has led to many patient injuries and even deaths. Devices that are protected against free flow are available, but not every institution uses them. The nurse administering intravenous medications should check to see whether the device is protected against free flow. If it is not, the nurse must be very careful when disconnecting the infusion from the device and must ensure that the clamp is closed.

Regardless of whether the device is protected against free flow, however, the pump settings should be independently checked when "high-alert" drugs are administered (see Chapter 5). The likelihood of a pump setting error or line mix-up is increased when more than one pump is in use or when dual-channel pumps with the capacity for multiple rate settings are used. The additional time required to have another practitioner check pump settings on high-alert drugs and tubing placement is well spent.

Medications meant to be given by nasogastric tube have been given intravenously. The mistake often occurs when the practitioner does not accurately identify the tubing before the administration. Most at risk are patients who have intravenous lines and small-bore polyurethane nasogastric feeding tubes or percutaneously inserted gastric tubes in place. Unfortunately, these small-bore tubes have distal ends that accommodate parenteral Luer connections such as those on the end of an intravenous set. This makes it possible to connect, for example, an enteral feeding solution or an oral drug solution to an intravenous line.

To give medications via nasogastric tube, nursing unit personnel may place liquids into parenteral syringes. Another technique is for the nurse to attach plastic Luer adapters to the tips of otherwise incompatible oral syringes. Even with adapters, having the pharmacy prepare doses in oral syringes is safer than having nurses draw up medications extemporaneously; however, the risk of inadvertent intravenous injection exists whenever Luer connectors are attached.

To make oral syringes safer, manufacturers provide special labels printed with the word "ORAL" in large, red, upper-case letters. When using oral syringes, health care workers should always use these labels. These labels should be affixed to the syringe plunger before the syringes are dispensed, because the syringe cannot be used unless the label has been removed. This practice makes it hard for anyone to fail to recognize that the syringe is for oral use.

The best solution to this problem is to make the connectors on nasogastric tubes and intravenous lines incompatible. A new standard for enteral feeding set connectors and adapters implemented by the Association for the Advancement of Medical Instrumentation (ANSI/AAMI ID54-1996) should help accomplish this.

Whenever a patient has an intravenous line and any other type of tubing in place, a quality assurance process must be followed to ensure that nurses label the distal ends of all catheters to help identify the type of tube or catheter being accessed. Precautions should extend to labeling of epidural catheters, because inadvertent epidural administration of fluids intended for intravenous use has also occurred and can be harmful.

The sooner that tubes or catheters that are no longer needed are removed, the safer it is for the patient. Staff should be told to remove lines as soon as possible, especially in patients who simultaneously have intravenous lines, feeding tubes, or other lines in place.

In the past, it was sometimes possible for health care workers to overcome potential confusion by remembering that only sterile, clear liquids were suitable for intravenous administration. That changed with the introduction of intravenous lipid products in the 1970s and, more recently, with intravenous lipid emulsions such as lipid-based amphotericin and doxorubicin. These drugs make it important to reemphasize what liquids can and cannot be given intravenously. If given in a large enough dose, suspensions not intended for intravenous use will lodge in the pulmonary capillaries as emboli and possibly cause death (see note, next page). Oral solids should never be crushed and injected for the same reason. These medications are also not sterile.

Case Example

A part-time pharmacist received an order for 29,000 units of "penicillin G (aqueous crystalline) IV q 8 hours" to treat congenital syphilis in a neonate.[3] Because he was unfamiliar with the term "aqueous crystalline," the pharmacist referred to a standard reference text. While looking at the monograph for penicillin G procaine, entitled "PENICILLIN G PROCAINE, AQUEOUS (APPG)," he noted a sentence that read: "When high sustained serum levels are required, use aqueous penicillin G, either IM or IV."

The pharmacist did not realize that this meant penicillin G potassium, which is also referred to as an aqueous or crystalline form of penicillin. Associating the terms *aqueous* and *IV* with the written order, and not realizing that the text actually contrasted penicillin G potassium with penicillin G procaine (which is used only for sustaining low penicillin levels), the pharmacist incorrectly dispensed penicillin G procaine for intravenous use. The patient received two doses of the drug intravenously before the error was recognized. Fortunately, no harm occurred.

Pharmacy references often refer to penicillin G procaine by its synonym, *penicillin G procaine, aqueous* because it is an aqueous suspension. The example just described has occurred more than once. Although this patient survived, Galpin et al.[4] reported that administering penicillin G procaine intravenously may form potentially fatal pulmonary or cerebral emboli. Toxicity from the procaine component also may occur. Although there is no specific warning against intravenous injection on the syringe itself, it does state that the drug is for deep intramuscular use only.

The word *aqueous* should not be used in conjunction with penicillin G products. Ordering penicillin G simply as "penicillin G potassium," "penicillin G sodium," "penicillin G procaine," or "penicillin G benzathine" would eliminate confusion.

Documentation of Drug Administration

Once a dose of drug has been administered, it must be immediately recorded on the MAR. Recording drug administration before it actually takes place runs the risk that, in the event that the nurse is called off the floor before all doses are administered, the nurses remaining with the patient may assume that the medication has been administered. This may lead to a dose omission. On the other hand, if a nurse elects to chart doses for all of her patients later, rather than immediately after administration, and is called off the floor before this is accomplished, the remaining nurses will not be aware that the medications have been given. In this case, double dosing is likely.

All medications should be documented consistently in one place. Special drug administration records, usually reserved for anticoagulants, cardiac medications, and insulin, are useful because they provide extra space for recording monitoring variables. If these records are kept separately in the patient's chart, however, the MAR will not give a complete picture of the drug therapy.

For example, a nurse administering aspirin to a patient was surprised when the patient indicated that he was told not to take aspirin while he was taking Coumadin®. The nurse had not seen an order for Coumadin® on the patient's MAR, because the record of anticoagulants was kept separately in the patient's chart. Had the patient not intervened, the nurse would not have known to question the order for aspirin.

When patients refuse doses, the prescriber must be informed and an explanatory note should be left in the patient's bin to alert the pharmacist of

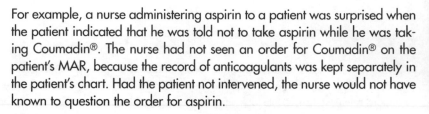

Note !

Reporting Medication Errors

All errors should be recorded in the patient's chart. An admission of an error need not be documented. An incident report should be filed so that a quality assurance check can be conducted (see Chapter 19).

the situation. When unadministered doses are returned to the pharmacy without adequate explanation, follow-up should take place to learn the reason for the returned dose. This helps ensure that drugs are not accidentally discontinued prematurely.

In some cases, a pharmacist may learn that pharmacy records do not properly indicate that a drug has been discontinued. Should this happen, follow-up can prevent medication errors stemming from the availability of a discontinued medication in the patient's bin.

••••
References

1. American Society of Hospital Pharmacists. ASHP technical assistance bulletin on handling cytotoxic and hazardous drugs. *Am J Hosp Pharm.* 1990; 47: 1033–49.

2. Mitchell JF, Pawlicki KS. Oral solid dosage forms that should not be crushed: 1998 update. *Hosp Pharm.* 1998; 33: 399–415.

3. Cohen MR. Inadvertent IV injection of penicillin G procaine. *Hosp Pharm.* 1977; 12: 142.

4. Galpin et al. "Pseudoanaphylactic" reactions from inadvertent infusion of procaine penicillin G. *Ann Intern Med.* 1974; 81: 358.

The Role of Pharmaceutical Trademarks in Medication Errors

Dan Boring, PhD

Chair, Labeling and Nomenclature Committee
Center for Drug Evaluation and Research
Food and Drug Administration
Rockville, Md.

George Di Domizio

Gemini Trademark Services
Green Lane, Pa.

Michael R. Cohen, MS, FASHP

Institute for Safe Medication Practices
Huntingdon Valley, Pa.

Pharmaceutical trademarks that look or sound alike play a major role in medication errors, as illustrated in many of the examples provided in Chapter 9. Why do such errors occur? Some would say that prescribers are too careless when they write an order. Others would maintain that pharmacists do not take appropriate measures to interpret the order correctly. Hospitals and other health care institutions may not establish and maintain adequate safety protocols. The Food and Drug Administration (FDA) and other regulatory organizations can be cited for not doing a better job of preventing look-alike and sound-alike names from entering the market. Pharmaceutical manufacturers may also be partly at fault, because it is they who develop trademarks.

As we seek to create an environment with fewer medication errors, it is helpful to examine the sources of trademark-related errors. It is also helpful to understand the process used by the FDA to evaluate the names proposed by manufacturers for new products. Finally, it is instructive to discuss the role of the pharmaceutical industry and individual practitioners in minimizing errors associated with trademarks.

Sources of Errors Associated with Trademarks

Ad Hoc Abbreviations

A physician treating a patient for a urinary tract infection intended to prescribe Noroxin®, the trademark for Merck & Co.'s (West Point, Pa.) brand of norfloxacin.[1] He wrote the prescription using "norflox," a self-styled abbreviation for the generic name of the drug. The community pharmacist interpreted the order as "Norflex®," which is the trademark for McNeil's (McNeil Consumer Products Co., Fort Washington, Pa.) brand of orphenadrine citrate, a muscle relaxant. The patient received Norflex®. The error was discovered when the patient's spouse contacted the pharmacy to report that the patient felt weak and was hallucinating.

In this case, the physician increased the probability for error by using an unapproved abbreviation. No one knows how often this kind of prescription shorthand is used, but it occurs frequently enough to cause significant concern. An informal survey of 41 hospital-based physicians conducted in 1992 at the University of Michigan revealed that about half of them routinely used "norflox" as an abbreviation for norfloxacin on prescriptions.

Look-Alike and Sound-Alike Trademarks

Even when physicians write the correct name, errors can happen. Patients for whom Levoxine®, a thyroid preparation, had been prescribed, inadvertently received Lanoxin® after a pharmacist misread the prescription (Figure 12–1).[2] The fact that these medications have the same dosage form (tablet), route of administration (oral), frequency of administration (daily), and tablet strength (0.125 mg) contributed to the likelihood of this error. After similar errors involving this trademark pair were reported, the manufacturer of Levoxine® changed the name of its product to Levoxyl®.

Another example of a medication error is drawn from a report received by a drug manufacturer from a hospital pharmacist. A nursing unit clerk was

Figure 12-1

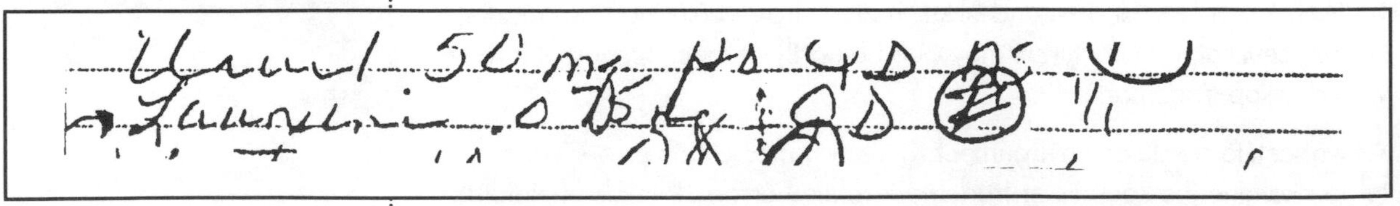

Levoxine® on line two of this prescription order was read Lanoxin®.

transcribing information from the medical chart of a patient who was supposed to be receiving Lasix®, a diuretic, and Losec®, then a newly released anti-ulcer product. Since each product was prescribed at 20 mg and the names appeared quite similar in handwritten form, the unit clerk thought there was a duplicate notation on the patient's record. She "corrected the error" by deleting Losec®. The error was detected when the patient's condition deteriorated and charts were reviewed.

Merck & Co., which at the time licensed Losec® in the United States, thereafter changed the product trademark to Prilosec® to avoid further confusion. The decision came after the company received a number of reports of actual errors, near misses, and practitioner concerns from both the hospital and retail sectors of the drug market.[3]

A list of 645 look-alike and sound-alike drug pairs has been published elsewhere.[4] The U.S. Pharmacopeia (USP) has also published a list of look-alike and sound-alike drugs.[5] These compilations have limited usefulness, however, because it is impossible for practitioners to memorize them in order to know when to check on questionable orders.

The Institute for Safe Medication Practices has suggested ways in which computerization can help prevent look-alike and sound-alike mix-ups.[6] Computers can be programmed to display a "clinical flag" or "formulary note" on the monitor that alerts the user to potential mix-ups. Similar to a road sign that warns about a dangerous intersection ahead, this feature can alert the person entering the order when a look-alike or sound-alike danger is present. A current list of name pairs is available from the USP (12601 Twinbrook Parkway, Rockville, Md., 20852-1790).

Brand Names with Suffixes

Another problem with pharmaceutical trademarks stems from the use of letter or number suffixes to designate specific properties of a drug or dosage form.[7] Such errors are particularly common just after the launch of a new product, when some health professionals may not yet be aware of the meaning of the newly coined suffix and may confuse it with prescription abbreviations or other medical terms. For example, the suffix "XL" is used to indicate a once-daily form of nifedipine (Procardia XL®). Some health professionals initially confused "XL" with the roman numeral 40 (XL) and dispensed 40 mg of the immediate-release version of the drug. Others heard "SL" (sublingual) rather than "XL" when they received a spoken order. Some patients received the immediate-release version of nifedipine sublingually and developed abnormally low blood pressure.[8]

The trade name "Percocet-5®" was coined to indicate that 5 mg of oxycodone was contained in this tablet. When doctors ordered "Percocet 5," some inexperienced nurses thought the dose was supposed to be five tablets, which resulted in overdoses. The manufacturer soon dropped the "-5" suffix.

Pharmaceutical companies should exert care when developing suffixed trademarks and consider the possibility of mix-ups with existing terms.

Brand-Name Extensions

Manufacturers sometimes apply a slight variation of a popular brand name to a newly marketed, over-the-counter drug that contains active ingredients that are quite different from those in the preexisting product.[9] For example, "Mylanta" is a brand name used for many years for an aluminum and magnesium hydroxide suspension. In 1996, Mylanta AR®, which contains famotidine, was launched. The new product does not contain aluminum and magnesium hydroxide, yet the names are very similar.

It is essential that product names make it as easy as possible for consumers to differentiate products. Some pharmacists have warned colleagues and consumers about the possibility for mix-ups resulting from the use of brand-name extensions and have called for an end to it.[10]

Role of the FDA

Review of Proposed Names

The FDA's Center for Drug Evaluation and Research has developed a system of coordinating committees to provide guidance on a variety of technical subjects and other topics. One of these is the Chemistry, Manufacturing, and Controls Coordinating Committee (CMC CC), which supervises several technical committees and working groups. The CMC CC technical committees develop and update policies and provide guidance for these policies. The committees also provide advisory services to internal constituencies in the Center for Drug Evaluation and Research.

One of the technical committees of the CMC CC is the Labeling and Nomenclature Committee (LNC), which provides recommendations to reviewing divisions on labeling statements and evaluates the acceptability of proposed proprietary and established names.[3] The LNC is a voluntary group whose members are selected on the basis of their broad experience in health care and the regulatory arena. It includes members from the Office of New Drug Chemistry; the Office of Generic Drugs; Compendial Operations Staff (FDA's liaison with the USP); the Division of Drug Marketing, Advertising, and Communications; and the Center for Biologics Evaluation and Research. One member of the LNC serves as FDA liaison to the U.S. Adopted Names (USAN) Council.

The authority for the establishment of the LNC resides in the U.S. Code of Federal Regulations, regulation 21 CFR 201.10(c) (available through the U.S. Government Printing Office and revised annually). This regulation lists five reasons for misleading labeling, two of which are commonly used during LNC review of a proprietary name:

1. 21 CFR 201.10(c)(3) states, "The employment of a fanciful proprietary name for a drug or ingredient in such a manner as to imply that the drug or ingredient has some unique effectiveness or composition when, in fact, the drug or ingredient is a common substance, the limitations of which are readily recognized when the drug or ingredient is listed by its established name." This by itself is not sufficient justification to reject a name, but the name may suggest elements that are difficult to support. For example, it may imply that the product has superior effectiveness or a unique benefit over related products when this is not the case.

2. 21 CFR 201.10(c)(5) states, "Designation of a drug or ingredient by a proprietary name that, because of similarity in spelling or pronunciation, may be confused with the proprietary name or the established name of a different drug or ingredient."

The evaluation of a proprietary name begins with submission of a drug application to the reviewing division with authority over that product. An applicant may ask for an LNC review at that time or leave it to the division's discretion to ask for a review. Divisions are not required to use the LNC, but most do. The division prepares a Request for Trademark Review and sends it to the chair of the LNC. The chair assigns the request to an LNC member, who presents it at the monthly LNC meeting. The agenda is given to each committee member in advance of the meeting so that all members are acquainted with each name that will be presented. The proprietary names are discussed until all members are satisfied. A vote is taken, and a decision is made on the basis of majority rule.

The chair combines the members' commentaries into a consult and sends it to the reviewing division within 30 days. The division sends the consult to the applicant, either verbatim or in edited form. If this time frame is too long, the LNC may conduct the evaluation by electronic mail and can respond within 48 hours.

The applicant is encouraged to prepare a rebuttal if it has an alternative opinion on an LNC consult. The information in the rebuttal often clarifies points that the LNC found to be unsatisfactory and may result in a reversal of the original recommendation.

On the basis of years of experience, the LNC has developed a sense of what makes an acceptable proprietary name. It has identified the following problem areas:

- Sound-alike and look-alike names;

- Misleading, incorrect, or unsafe elements encoded into a name;

- Claims that are not supported by clinical data;

- Prefixes or suffixes that may be confused with a common medical abbreviation;

- Inclusion of a dosage form or regimen in the proprietary name;

- Suggestion of an unapproved use;

- Similarities in storage environment (two products with similar names will cause the committee less concern if they are physically separated in pharmacy storage areas and will always remain so—for example, if one is a topical product and the other an oral solution); and

- Unacceptable similarity between the generic and brand names (the USAN Council discourages the use of USAN syllables in a trademark because it bars the subsequent generation and adoption of other names for similar products; therefore, the LNC generally does not approve of names that contain too much of the USAN name or any of the USAN "stem").

The LNC is concerned with letters that are easily blurred or confused when handwritten (e.g., W, M, N, C, L, and O). The committee is especially sensitive to similar syllables in the first part of a proprietary name (e.g., Dynacin®, Dynacirc®), because the prescriber's handwriting may become even less legible at the end of the name.

Although a proprietary name may be evaluated at the Investigational New Drug (IND) stage, a majority of review requests (about 90%) are submitted at the New Drug Application (NDA) stage. A name that has been reviewed at the IND stage is re-evaluated at the NDA stage because the collection of pending names may have changed since approval of the IND submission.

The LNC does not approve proprietary or established names. It is the responsibility of the LNC to evaluate these names by consultation from the reviewing division and to relay its recommendations regarding the suitability of submitted names to the appropriate review division.

Postmarketing Surveillance

FDA's Medication Errors Committee (MEC) focuses on trademarks that create problems after a product has been marketed. The MEC has three core members and four ad hoc members, including a physician, a pharmacist, and a nurse. It serves primarily as an internal surveillance group that monitors reports of medication errors, but it can also make recommendations to the reviewing divisions at the FDA that have primary responsibility for decisions on possible regulatory action.

At its monthly meetings, the MEC evaluates medication error reports submitted to FDA's MedWatch Program and to the USP Medication Errors Reporting Program. It categorizes these error reports as follows:

- Reports that require no further action because they involve issues such as professional practice errors that go beyond labeling and packaging.

- Recurring errors, which are forwarded to the reviewing division to grant them higher visibility. MEC maintains a "watch list" of multiple reports of errors associated with a single trademark.

- New and significant errors, for which MEC requests a consultation with the reviewing division that approved the product. This consultation generally involves discussions with the division's consumer safety officer and other reviewers.

The reviewing division may respond to committee action in a variety of ways. In some cases, a change in the product labeling or packaging may help solve the problem; in others, a "Dear Health Professional" letter is requested. In extreme cases, the company is asked to rename the product.

Role of the Pharmaceutical Industry

In recent years, the pharmaceutical industry has assumed a more proactive role in supporting efforts to prevent or minimize medication errors. Many companies are taking explicit measures to predict the likelihood of medication errors linked to visual or phonetic similarities in brand names. Pharmacists are increasingly involved in these evaluation processes.

Trademarks are important corporate assets, and companies make significant investments in them. Many in the industry believe that a great name can salvage a mediocre product and that a poor name can destroy the chances of a potential "blockbuster." An effective trademark can

- distinguish a seller's product from a competitor's product;

- distinguish a product from related products;

- identify a common source of goods, thereby unifying brand preference;

- convey an impression of product quality or of another desirable feature;

- generate brand-name loyalty;

- imply an association with a market leader; and/or

- provide marketing exclusivity for a product in countries with weak or nonexistent patent laws.

Hoping to adopt a trademark that will carry as much recognition and recall value as possible, manufacturers use a variety of methods to select brand names. Some hold contests in which the employee who submits the winning name is rewarded. Others use electronic random-name generators. Some hold brainstorming sessions within their marketing department. Still others engage the services of a trademark development firm.

Searching for Error-Prone Trademarks

Many companies enlist the assistance of pharmacists, directly or through a vendor, to identify potential problems with visual or phonetic similarities between a proposed name and existing names. One model used for this purpose is Error Potential Analysis (Safe Medication Practices Consulting, Inc., Huntingdon Valley, Pa.). Under this model, pharmacists and nurses review proposed trademarks that appear as handwritten physicians' orders to detect visual similarities with products currently on the market. Proposed trademarks are also presented in spoken form to help the practitioners uncover phonetic similarities between the names under consideration and existing products. The proposed trademarks are also evaluated against a number of factors associated with medication errors (e.g., similar dosages, dosage strengths, dosage forms, dosage regimens, clinical indications, storage requirements, and trade packaging). This service is offered to the pharmaceutical industry under the name "Error Index" (Wood Worldwide, New York, N.Y.).

The Errors Recognition and Revision Strategies (ERRS) model, offered by Medical Errors Recognition and Revision Strategies, Inc. (Med-ERRS), a subsidiary of the Institute for Safe Medication Practices, is a similar error identification service. It performs a computerized preliminary evaluation of trademark candidates using phonetic algorithms and psycholinguistic principles developed at the University of Illinois.[11] The ERRS model also uses the Internet to include products marketed worldwide in its evaluation.

The method incorporates failure mode and effects analysis to uncover potential problems arising from look-alike, sound-alike, and other kinds of nomenclature problems, such as confusion with medical terminology or equipment. The clinical environment (intensive care unit, pharmacy, etc.) in which the product will most likely be used (stored, ordered, transcribed and computerized, dispensed, etc.) is part of the evaluation process. The goal is to simulate the environment to bring problem areas to the surface so that actions can be taken to minimize or eliminate possible errors. Health care professionals—a mix of community and hospital-based pharmacists and physicians and nurses in each country—are located around the world because projects are often international in scope. An acceptability check of the trademark among the physician and pharmacist respondents is also performed. As part of the Med-ERRS trademark evaluation methodology, each candidate is reviewed from the perspective of the FDA LNC, the European Medicines Evaluation Agency, USAN, and the Japanese Authority.

Among other services aimed at detecting potential problems in trademarks is the Brandtest methodology, used by the Brand Institute, Miami, Fla.

Role of Practitioners

Practitioners can reduce the chance of medication errors caused by products with similar names. Davis et al.[4] describe problems with brand and nonproprietary names and emphasize the need for physicians to write legible, complete orders and to speak slowly and clearly when giving spoken orders. They recommend that the person receiving the order repeat it to the person who has given the order.

Pharmacists and nurses must read prescription orders carefully. Knowing what conditions have been diagnosed in patients and coupling this information with the ordered medication can help prevent errors. Communication with patients is an important way to prevent errors. Physicians should educate the patient or family member about the names and purposes of all their medications. Nurses and pharmacists should reinforce this information. If the patient knows what to expect, he or she is better prepared to question a misinterpreted order.

Physicians can contribute to error reduction by including the purpose of each medication on the prescription. This helps with patient education and can contribute to accurate identity of the medication (see Chapter 8, page 8.8). Physicians should also include the strength of the medication on the prescription. This information can be valuable when the need arises to distinguish between look-alike or sound-alike names. Pharmacists and nurses who maintain good prescription records and keep up with new drug products are more likely to recognize errors in interpretation than those who do not.

Bar coding and computerization of prescription ordering can help prevent errors caused by misinterpretation. Use of these systems should be encouraged. Lacking computerization, physicians should print the names of drugs in block letters. This would be especially helpful in reducing errors associated with newly marketed or otherwise unfamiliar drugs.

Summary

The processes by which pharmaceutical products are named are complex, expensive, and time consuming. Manufacturers invest a great deal of money in selecting a name, in the belief that a good name can influence sales and minimize the potential for legal liability. Nonetheless, a substantial portion of medication errors can be attributed to confusing names, and problem names still manage to get approved. All involved in nomenclature must be aware of these problems and collaborate to eliminate or reduce them.

••••
References

1. Pincus JM, Ike RW. Norflox or Norflex? Letter. *N Engl J Med.* 1992; 326: 15.

2. Cohen MR. Medication error reports: Levoxine could be read as Lanoxin. *Hosp Pharm.* 1992; 27: 906–07.

3. Boring DL, Homonnay-Weikel AM, Cohen MR, et al. Avoiding trademark trouble at the FDA. *Pharmaceutical Executive.* 1996; 16: 80–88.

4. Davis NM, Cohen MR, Teplitsky B. Look-alike and sound-alike drug names: the problem and the solution. *Hosp Pharm.* 1992; 27: 95–98, 102–05, 108–10.

5. US Pharmacopeia. Stop, look, and listen. *Drug Quality Review.* 1995; 49.

6. Institute for Safe Medication Practices. A novel way to prevent medication errors associated with drug mix-ups. *ISMP Medication Safety Alert!* 1996; 1(15): 1.

7. Cohen MR. Medication error reports: naming drug products is a serious business. *Hosp Pharm.* 1990; 25: 747–48.

8. Cohen MR. Medication error reports: name "Procardia XL" is problem for pharmacists. *Hosp Pharm.* 1990; 25: 403–04.

9. Hussar DA. "Name games" should no longer be tolerated (editorial). *Pharmacy Today.* 1997; 3: 4.

10. Rupp MT, Parker JM. Drug names: when marketing and safety collide. *American Pharmacy.* 1993; NS33: 39–42.

11. Lambert BL. Predicting look-alike and sound-alike medication errors. *Am J Health Syst Pharm.* 1997; 54: 1161–71.

13.

The Role of Drug Packaging and Labeling in Medication Errors

Michael R. Cohen, MS, FASHP

Institute for Safe Medication Practices
Huntingdon Valley, Pa.

At one time or another, each of us has purchased the wrong product because of similarities in packaging between the item we intended to select and another one. For example, many people accidentally purchase regular Pepsi Cola rather than diet because the containers are similar in color, print, size, and shape.

Similar mix-ups occur with medications. Poor labeling and packaging frequently contribute to medication errors. The consequences are far greater than those associated with choosing the wrong beverage. Choosing the wrong medication may cause a life-threatening or fatal event.

The person who administers a medication is responsible for selecting the correct drug and dose. This is done by reading the label. Most professionals are taught to read labels at least three times: when obtaining a drug package, when using a drug package, and when returning a drug package to stock or discarding an empty package. Most health providers claim that they do this routinely; however, the evidence is often to the contrary. In some cases, oversights stem from poor training. In others, the cause may be careless work practices or lack of knowledge that product-related problems have already surfaced.

Although proper training and increased alertness are undeniably important, attention to a third factor—drug packaging and labeling—is also essential. "Look-alike" packaging can result in confusion. Errors occur when information appears in an obscure position on the label or when it is presented in very small print. The size, boldness, and contrast of printing on labels are not always ideal. Complicating the situation is that the labels are often read under less-than-ideal conditions. Errors have been associated, for example, with the accidental administration of lidocaine instead of IV dextrose by a team of paramedics working on an embankment at night.[1]

This chapter examines the problems associated with drug labeling and packaging and suggests techniques for overcoming them.

Confirmation Bias

Before beginning to study drug labeling and packaging, it is helpful to examine the human factor. Errors are often induced by familiarity with procedures and materials, coupled with the innate tendency of humans to perceive confirming evidence more readily than disconfirming evidence.[2]

We often see what is familiar or what we want to see, rather than what is actually there. For example, ask someone to glance at the words in Figure 13–1 and tell you what they see. Most people reply "Paris in the spring," because it is a familiar phrase. Close reading, however, reveals that the word *the* appears twice.

How does this apply to medication error prevention? Recent pharmacy graduates read labels carefully because new pharmacists have yet to become familiar with medications. After a while, people begin to work more rapidly, often picturing a sought-after item in their mind's eye. They are no longer as careful as they were. If a drug has distinctive packaging, the potential for mix-ups is slight. If several drug products have similar packaging, or if labeling is hard to read, the potential for error increases. Drug look-alikes, especially when combined with suboptimal working conditions, can cause health professionals to overlook important information. This phenomenon, known as "confirmation bias," contributes to errors involving drug packaging and labeling.

It is not enough to caution health providers to be more careful. We must recognize that it is human nature to identify items by color, shape, type of font, symbols, and similar characteristics. The health care community, and especially the pharmaceutical industry and regulatory authorities, must recognize the problems presented by confirmation bias and collaborate to overcome them.

An example of how a product label can contribute to confirmation bias appears in Figure 13–2 (see color plates). The original packaging is shown on the left; redesigned packaging appears on the right. The labeling was changed after reports of delays in treatment that had occurred because of the similarity in packaging between topical Adrenalin®, used to stop

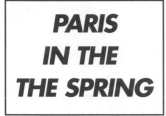

Figure 13-1

PARIS
IN THE
THE SPRING

This phrase illustrates how an error can be induced by familiarity.

bleeding, and injectable Adrenalin®, used to treat emergencies such as cardiac arrest and asthma attacks. Some medical personnel had unknowingly stocked their emergency supply kits with the topical agent. It was not until an emergency occurred and the box was opened that they discovered that their kit contained the topical product.

In this example, both the individuals replenishing emergency supplies and those removing the vials from storage exhibited confirmation bias. They wanted the injectable form; however, they identified the item by its appearance, including the title (Adrenalin® Chloride Solution), the distinctive white and dark-red design, the shape of the box, the horizontal bands at the bottom of the label, and the "1:1000" concentration. The distinguishing words (i.e., "Nasal Solution" and "Topical Application," versus "Injection" and "Hypodermic Use") were relatively small and not seen.

The new packaging is distinguished by a sharp contrast in color. The words "For Hypodermic Use" appear in white letters in a red box. Since this packaging was introduced, no mix-ups have been reported to the U.S. Pharmacopeia Medication Errors Reporting Program (USP MERP).

Mix-ups have also occurred between premixed heparin bags and DuPont Pharma's Hespan® (hetastarch, sodium chloride) in McGaw's Excel® bags. The main problem seems to be that the names Hespan® and heparin share the characters "H-E," "P-A," and "N" in the same order. In addition, both products are supplied in premixed bags with similar coloring (Abbott's heparin also has red and blue type similar to Hespan®), and they are often stored near one another due to their similar spelling. In one case, a nurse inadvertently took a bag of heparin 25,000 units from unit stock and infused it over an hour. The patient's activated partial thromboplastin time (aPTT) became markedly elevated, but no adverse outcome occurred. In another case, a physician wrote a prescription for Hespan® for a patient who had become hypotensive after a bilateral hip replacement. A nurse retrieved heparin from an automated dispensing cabinet, where it was stored beside Hespan®. Despite an elevated aPTT, this patient also was not harmed. In a third case, however, a patient died after receiving heparin in error and then hemorrhaging. The Institute for Safe Medication Practices (ISMP) has communicated with DuPont, the manufacturer, and McGaw, Inc., the packager, to suggest better background for the title area of the Hespan® container. ISMP also recommended enhancing the letter "S" in the name to highlight the primary character in "Hespan" that differs from the letters in "heparin," as well as enhancing the appearance of the generic name "hetastarch" on the Hespan® container.

Improving the Readability of Drug Labeling and Packaging

Manufacturers can use a variety of techniques to improve the readability of drug labeling and packaging. Some of the most important are discussed here.

Reducing Label Clutter

In 1991, three premature infants died in a hospital nursery after receiving erroneously prepared heparin flushes through umbilical-line catheters.[3] The problem began in the pharmacy, where heparin for catheter flushes had been prepared by adding 250 units of heparin to 250 mL of 5% dextrose injection. Syringes of heparin 2.5 mL, 1 unit per mL, were prepared from the admixture; labeled; and sent to the neonatal intensive care unit. The fatal errors occurred because an employee pulled a 250-mL, 15% (2-mEq/mL) container of potassium chloride concentrate that had been placed in the bin intended to hold 250 mL of 5% dextrose injection. The heparin was diluted with the potassium chloride instead of dextrose. Each infant received about 5 mEq of potassium via intravenous push.

The containers were correctly labeled. Had they been properly read, the error would not have occurred. The problem was linked to similarities in appearance between containers of 5% dextrose and 15% potassium chloride.[3] Dextrose 5% injection is used directly as an intravenous infusion and as a vehicle for other drugs. Fifteen percent potassium chloride 250 mL is a pharmacy bulk package meant only for use in diluting potassium in preparation of intravenous admixtures. Nonetheless, the packaging of the two products was nearly identical (Figure 13–3). Both had the same aluminum bails for hanging the bottle on an intravenous pole. They also had the same shape and contained equal volumes of clear liquid.

For years, pharmacy employees had gone to the same bin for dextrose. They had correctly prepared thousands of syringes. This time, the potassium bottle rested in a bin labeled "Dextrose," and its label was partially obscured because the container was turned on its side. Even though the name of the drug was printed in red, it was not visible. Similarities in shape and size of the bottle contributed to the product's being placed in the wrong bin.

After this error occurred, the manufacturer redesigned the packaging for potassium chloride (Figure 13–4). The name is now more prominent, and it appears on a side panel as well as on the front. It is also easier to determine that the product is a pharmacy bulk package that must be diluted before intravenous use. The peel-off cap and bottle ferrule have been modified. The statement "Dilute before IV use" appears in contrasting print.

Many words commonly used on prescription drug labels (e.g., "Brand of," "Tabloid," "Preparation of," "Mix-O-Vial") serve the manufacturer more than the user and therefore should be eliminated. Figure 13–4 illustrates how label clutter can be reduced. Essential information should

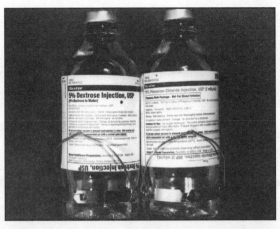

appear in a prominent position on the front label. This includes the brand and generic names, strength or concentration, and warnings, if any. Less important information, including the manufacturer's name and logo, National Drug Code (NDC) number, package size, USP designation, control number, expiration date, bar code, and needle length and size (or needleless designation), are best placed on the side panel or in the package insert, unless noted otherwise in the Code of Federal Regulations (21 CFR 201 10).

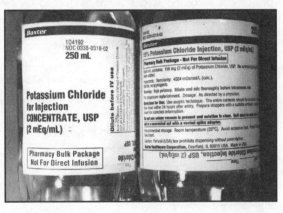

Figure 13-4

Relabeled bottle containing potassium (left), contrasted with the old labeling (right).

In 1992, the Committee to Reduce Medication Errors of the Pharmaceutical Manufacturers Association submitted to the USP and the Food and Drug Administration (FDA) recommendations for the design of labels for small-volume parenteral products. The committee recommended eliminating the words "sterile," "nonpyrogenic," and "pyrogen-free," as well as the phrases "May be habit forming," "Federal law prohibits dispensing without prescription," and "For usual dose, see accompanying package insert" (or other words to that effect). A USP–FDA advisory panel on label simplification adopted these recommendations and added some of its own, including the elimination of controlled-substance designators (e.g., CII) and of lists of storage requirements when an article can be stored at room temperature in normal light.[4] The implementation of some of these recommendations required changes in federal law.

The FDA Reform Act of 1997 authorizes replacement of the federal legend statement ("Federal law prohibits dispensing without prescription") with an "Rx only" symbol. In addition, the phrase "Warning: may be habit forming" may be eliminated from certain scheduled drugs. FDA has the authority to make other changes called for in the label simplification project.

Color Coding

Color coding is the systematic application of a color system to identify specific products. It may be distinguished from color differentiation, which entails using color to distinguish a single product.

Manufacturers have no research-based evidence on which to make decisions concerning the use of color to code or differentiate products. Nonetheless, it is already used to a limited extent in health care. One example of color coding is a scheme endorsed by the American Academy of Ophthalmology for caps and labels of ophthalmic products (Table 13–1).

Color coding, along with distinctive background patterns or borders, has been proposed as a way to reduce drug administration errors in anesthesia.[5] The American Society for Testing and Materials (ASTM) has developed a standard for user-applied labels in anesthesiology.[6] The ASTM standard calls for each color and border or background to represent a different class of drugs. Induction agents would have labels with yellow backgrounds, benzodiazepines would have orange labels, narcotics would have blue labels, and so forth. Such labels are now available and widely applied in the operating room, but commercial pharmaceutical manufacturers have not embraced the idea.

Although actual color coding schemes may help to differentiate drug classes, the system is scientifically untested and may actually increase the chance of intraclass medication errors, because products of various agents and strengths within a single class would have labels of the same color. With similar corporate logos, fonts, package sizes, and color combinations factored in, dispensing errors have occurred. For example, Bausch and Lomb anti-infective caps and carton labels use a tan background on a large portion of the label. Mydriatics and cycloplegics use a red background, miotics use green, beta-blockers use yellow or blue, and so forth (Figure 13–5; see color plates). CibaVision products are similarly labeled. The ISMP has recommended purchasing ophthalmic products within the same class from different vendors in order to reduce similarities and prevent errors. In many pharmacies, topical products, including ophthalmic agents, are separated

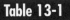

Table 13-1

Color codes for topical ocular medications

Class	Color	Pantone Number
Anti-infectives	Tan	467
Anti-inflammatories/steroids	Pink	197, 212
Mydriatics and cycloplegics	Red	485C
Nonsteroidal anti-inflammatories	Gray	4C
Miotics	Green	374, 362, 348
Beta-blockers	Yellow or blue, yellow C	290, 281
Adrenergic agents	Purple	2583
Carbonic anhydrase inhibitors	Orange	1585
Prostaglandin analogs	Turquoise	326C

from other inventory and stored by brand. In this case, doing so increases the chance of a mix-up, because look-alike products will be stored next to each other.

Efforts to use color must be carefully thought through. For example, an attempt by Cutter Laboratories to color code its small-volume parenteral products resulted in several medication errors in the early 1980s. Individual strengths and concentrations did not receive distinctive colors. As a result, sodium chloride injection in 0.9%, 14.6%, and 23.4% concentrations all bore a yellow label. Confusion among the various concentrations of sodium chloride led to inadvertent injections of the concentrated drug.

When properly used, color can be helpful. Using color to differentiate the three concentrations of sodium chloride would have helped to prevent confusion in the case just cited. For example, solutions of three concentrations of dopamine—40 mg/mL, 80 mg/mL, and 160 mg/mL—are color differentiated red, green, and orange, respectively. Color can also be used to draw attention to specific portions of a label. For example, 500-mL bottles containing 50% dextrose might display the title in red print, and 500-mL bottles containing 5% dextrose feature black print.

Some manufacturers use red to draw attention to warnings on the label. The manufacturers of the three sodium chloride concentrate products shown in Figure 13–6 (see color plates) use red print to warn that the product must be diluted. Some industrial engineers believe that the red provides an especially vivid warning (perhaps because it looks like blood), but this has not been proved.

If all products in a manufacturer's line had identical color schemes and were the same size and shape, reading would be the only way to differentiate products. For example, the Baxter ATC 212 automated dispenser produces 1.5-square-inch, identically labeled unit-dose packages for all the items it dispenses. No errors have been associated with this approach.

Making every product a different color might be effective. The number of colors is finite, however, and without absolute consistency among manufacturers, one manufacturer's product would inevitably be confused with another, either in its own line or in that of another manufacturer. Vendors who frequently switch manufacturers might find this system particularly problematic.

Color coding has other disadvantages; for example, colors may fade when exposed to light. Moreover, despite the existence of standardized Pantone colors, it is not always possible for a manufacturer to exactly reproduce colors from batch to batch. Finally, an estimated 8% of men and less than 1% of women have some difficulty with color vision.[7] Because of problems such as these, the American Society of Health-System Pharmacists (ASHP) opposes the use of color to identify drug products.[8]

Two-Sided Labeling

Two-sided labeling is highly recommended because it can reduce errors resulting from the inability of the user to read the front label.[1] Abbott Laboratories packages many of its premixed intravenous products with two-sided labeling on the plastic minibag foil overwrap. The company implemented such packaging after several errors, and at least two deaths, were reported in 1993. In one case, Mivacron®, a neuromuscular blocker premixed solution, was confused with Zantac® injection; in another, Mivacron® was confused with intravenous metronidazole. (The latter incident is described in Chapter 20.) Part of the problem was that the minibags were impossible to differentiate from one another when stored face down; a second problem was that the products in question were sometimes accidentally stored near one another. Finally, their foil outer wraps did not list the contents prominently. Figure 13–7 shows the old and new packaging of Mivacron® (see color plates).

Containers for intravenous lidocaine from all major manufacturers have been confused with containers for other premixed products, including heparin. In response to requests from ISMP, Abbott now affixes two-sided labeling on both the immediate container and the overwrap of its premixed lidocaine. In addition, labels are placed directly on the intravenous container (Figure 13–8). Marsam Pharmaceuticals places labels on the front and back panels of its entire product line. Once removed from shelf packaging, these products can be identified, no matter how the product is positioned.[9]

Contrast

Problems with contrast are particularly evident on small items. Manufacturers often use ceramic print on clear glass, which has no contrasting background. This violates a 1989 American Society for Testing and Materials standard (D4267-89),[10] which requires manufacturers to provide contrast between the type used for the proprietary and established names of the drug, as well as between the amount of drug per unit and either the immediate drug container or an opaque background. The standard also prescribes a legibility test requiring that the name and amount of the drug be legible in a light of 20 footcandles at a distance of about 20 inches (500 mm) by a person with 20/20 unaided or corrected vision.

Depending on the color of the print, the background, and lighting conditions, a label may be virtually illegible. This has led to serious consequences. For example, in the past Parke-Davis ampuls of Pitocin®, Adrenalin®, and Pitressin® have frequently been mixed up, sometimes with fatal consequences.[11] Wyeth-Ayerst's vials of phenylephrine and heparin (Figure 13–9) have also been confused. The readability of the labels on the two vials (Figure 13–9, bottom) greatly improved after an opaque background was provided.

Expressions of Concentration and Strength

The way in which a manufacturer denotes the strength of a drug may also lead to errors. For example, a number of errors have been reported in which the entire contents of a 20-mL, 40-mg/mL gentamicin container were injected instead of the correct dose (i.e., 40 mg). The original container is shown on the left in Figure 13–10. Because the concentration (40 mg/mL) is listed so prominently, inexperienced users believed that the entire container held 40 mg. They confirmed the 40-mg/mL concentration, but failed to read the additional important label information. The volume does appear elsewhere on the label, but it was overlooked. The concentration is listed more prominently on the redesigned container on the right.

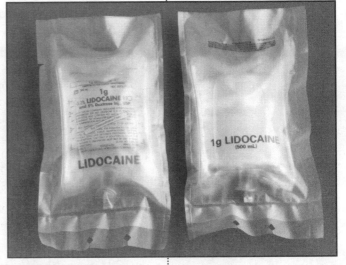

Figure 13-8

Labels for Abbott's lidocaine are now placed directly on both the intravenous container and its overwrap to avoid mix-ups with other premixed products.

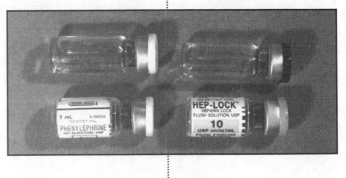

Figure 13-9

Vials of phenylephrine and heparin, before (top) and after (bottom) contrasting labeling.

Figure 13-10

The prominent display of the concentration of gentamicin in this container (left) led many users to mistake it for the total contents of the bottle.

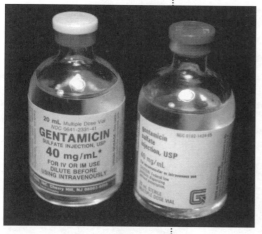

Figure 13-11

The concentration of Cerebyx® has been confused as the total amount of drug in the vial.

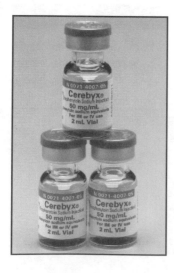

The volume of the Cerebyx® (fosphenytoin) vial is listed in one position and the strength (in milligrams of phenytoin sodium equivalent units [PE]) per milliliter ("50 mg PE/mL") is listed in another position. This makes it appear to some as though only 50 mg PE is in the vial (Figure 13–11).

Recently, a 2-year-old child presented to the emergency room with seizures. Cerebyx® 150 mg intravenous (100 mg PE) was ordered. Since most medications used in the emergency room were drawn from floor stock, pharmacy technicians delivered drugs upon verbal (i.e., spoken) request. A technician misread the Cerebyx® label and delivered three 10-mL vials (total of 1500 mg PE). A nurse also misread the label, assuming that 50 mg was in each vial. She drew up 30 mL (1500 mg PE) instead of 150 mg of Cerebyx® (100 mg PE) and handed it to another nurse, who administered the drug. Assuming the proper dose had been diluted, the second nurse did not question the 30-mL volume. The patient died soon after injection. Excessive amounts of phenytoin were found in the child's blood. Due to confusing labeling, some hospitals have placed restrictions on the prescribing and dispensing of this drug. In February 1999, after another child's death, FDA asked Parke-Davis to redesign the label to better reflect its 500 mg PE/mL contents.

In 1994, Burroughs Wellcome alerted investigators participating in a study of vinorelbine (Navelbine®) of a problem related to product concentration. The company had received reports of users who read the label on the 5-mL container, also saw the concentration (10 mg/mL), and concluded that the entire container held 10 mg. The volume did appear on the label, but these users did not see it. Three patients received a fivefold overdose of vinorelbine, and one patient died. The product is now on the market with an improved label. This incident points to the need for careful design of labels on investigational drugs.

Similar problems have been reported with other products. At one time, both Pronestyl® and procainamide injections listed the per-milliliter concentration in a prominent position on the packaging. The volume appeared elsewhere (Figure 13–12, left). Users repeatedly mistook the per-milliliter concentration as the amount in the vial. After receiving several error reports, the ISMP asked the FDA to require manufacturers to express both per-milliliter and total contents together on the front label panel (Figure 13–12, right). FDA agreed, and no further errors have been reported.

Errors of a similar nature have occurred with Roche's Versed®. Pharmacia and Upjohn's Camptosar® was involved in several errors that were similar to the vinorelbine error. Immediately after the product was marketed, the concentration (20 mg/mL) was mistaken for the total vial contents. The errors led to several injuries and deaths.[12]

FDA does not state how concentration is to be labeled, but it has told the ISMP that it does not normally allow total content labeling with multiple-dose vials greater than 2 mL because of concern that someone might mistake the total content listed on the label as an appropriate single dose. ISMP believes it would be better to list both the per-milliliter concentration and total volume and amount in metric weight side by side on the label, regardless of whether it is a multiple-dose vial. The label should "shout" out the total contents. Moreover, each designation should appear within the same border or within the same shaded background. A USP–FDA advisory panel has made such recommendations.[4]

The labeling of oral solid dosage forms sometimes expresses the amount of drug in a misleading way. For example, UDL Laboratories at one time distributed acetaminophen 650 mg (two 325-mg tablets) in a unit-dose package labeled "325 mg."[13] Pentasa® (mesalamine) 250 mg has been packaged in a two capsule unit-dose package labeled for one capsule (Figure 13–13). How is the user to know whether the entire package or each capsule contains the labeled dose? Manufacturers should stipulate the amount per tablet as well as per package (e.g., "Pentasa® 500 mg [2 x 250-mg capsules]").

Company Name, Logo, and Corporate Dress

Logos and other designs can interfere with product identification, as illustrated by an error that led to an outbreak of severe, unexplained illness on a neonatal ward in a hospital in Canada.[14] Patients were initially thought to

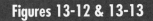

Figures 13-12 & 13-13

13-12: Procainamide before (left) and after (right) label design. The new label displays per-milliliter and total contents together on the front panel.

13-13: Packaging of Pentasa® (mesalamine) does not specify whether contents of "250 mg" refers to each capsule or to both capsules combined.

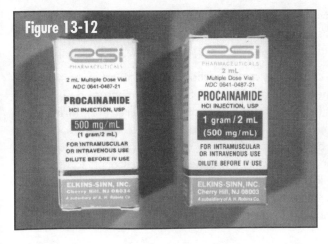

Figure 13-12

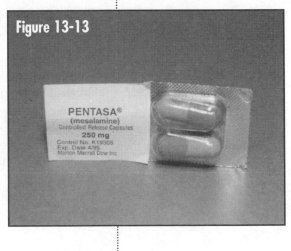

Figure 13-13

have sepsis, but investigations showed that the illnesses were the result of repeated administration of racemic epinephrine to patients who were supposed to receive vitamin E. The packagings of the two products were nearly indistinguishable (Figure 13–14; see color plates). Both were manufactured by the same company in 15-mL screw-cap bottles. Both bottles were amber, and both bore a label with black print on angled, alternating, blue-and-green bands. This style was used for the company's entire product line.

Lines, bars, stripes, and similar visual devices can also interfere with readability. Even the company name may get in the way of the drug name.

The ISMP recommends that the manufacturer's name always be placed at the bottom of the label and that the most prominent information on the label be the name and strength of the product. Ideally, these two pieces of information should appear within the same background or border.

Standardization of Terminology

USP and FDA should standardize the terminology used on labels. Is a single-dose vial different from a single-use vial? Both terms are used. The very same product may use both terms, as shown in Figure 13–6; in other cases, products bear no such designation on the front label.

The term "single dose" means that pharmacists or nurses should withdraw one dose and discard the remainder, prepare several patients' doses at the same time from the same container, or prepare a large-volume parenteral container for infusion over an extended period of time. It does not mean that the package contains a single dose. Unfortunately, this is how some users have interpreted it. For example, a nurse gave a patient an entire 15-mL (45-mmol) single-dose vial of potassium phosphate injection (Figure 13–15). The correct dose was 1 mL (3 mmol).[15]

The USP–FDA advisory panel on label simplification prefers the word *use* over *dose* and has proposed the term *single-use vial* as an alternative for these and other vials now designated *single-dose vial*.[4]

Another example of lack of standardization may be found in the package labeling for magnesium sulfate injection. Six unit-of-measure designations are used: percent (%), milligram (mg), gram (g), milliliter (mL), milliequivalent (mEq), and milliosmole (mOsm). To add to the confusion, some prescribers order the drug in terms of number of vials or ampuls. Because there are so many dosing expressions, it is difficult for practitioners to recognize excessive doses. To further compound the confusion, some laboratories report values in milliequivalents per decaliter (mEq/dL) or Système International (SI) units.

A unique example of nonstandard dose expression has arisen in conjunction with Cerebyx® (fosphenytoin sodium injection), a prodrug that replaced Dilantin® (phenytoin sodium injection) in 1997. FDA and the manufacturer agreed on labeling that calls for fosphenytoin to be prescribed in terms of its phenytoin equivalent (PE). Fosphenytoin sodium 75 mg is equivalent to phenytoin sodium 50 mg; thus, a 100-mg dose of intravenous phenytoin should be ordered as "fosphenytoin 100 mg PE," not as "fosphenytoin 150 mg." In other words, practitioners are being asked to take the unprecedented step of ordering one drug while referring to the dose of another. This creates opportunities for error. The "PE" designation is often accidentally omitted when ordering, transcribing, or dispensing (labeling) this drug. Some prescribers dose the drug by its actual strength, while others follow the suggested method. Underdoses and overdoses have been the result.

Label Reminders and Warnings

In some cases, the best way to reduce the potential for error is to add a warning to the label. In 1988, after learning of numerous deaths caused by the administration of undiluted potassium chloride injection instead of sodium chloride 0.9% injection, bacteriostatic water, or sterile water for injection, Neil Davis and I organized a meeting of practitioners, regulatory authorities, and manufacturers. The group brainstormed methods to prevent the recurrence of this error. As a result, USP eventually imposed new requirements on the nomenclature and packaging of potassium chloride.[16,17] The name was changed to "potassium chloride for injection concentrate," and a boxed warning that reinforces the need for dilution was added to the label (Figure 13–16). Black caps and a ferrule that seals the rubber stopper to the vial are now required. The phrase "Must be diluted" appears in contrasting color on the cap and ferrule. Although potassium chloride injection accidents still occur, no cases involving substitution of sodium chloride traced to misreading the labels have been reported since these actions were taken. Restricting the availability of potassium chloride in clinical areas has been proposed as the best way to eliminate this problem.[18]

Vincristine provides another example of how warning statements can help reduce errors. After a number of reports of fatal intrathecal injections of vincristine, which should be injected intravenously, modifications in labeling and packaging were requested.[19] USP established a new dispensing standard for the drug. The new standard requires health care workers to package vincristine in syringes or vials with a labeled overwrap that states "Do not remove covering until moment of injection. Fatal if given intrathecally. For intravenous use only." All vincristine containers now carry this warning. Since 1995, the FDA has also required manufacturers to include warning

Figure 13-15

The term "single dose," as used on this bottle of potassium phosphate, has been misinterpreted as meaning that a container contains one total dose of medication.

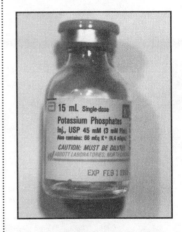

Figure 13-16

After numerous deaths were caused by the administration of undiluted potassium chloride injection, USP now requires a boxed warning that reinforces the need for dilution, a ferrule that seals the rubber stopper, and black cap bearing the phrase "Must be diluted."

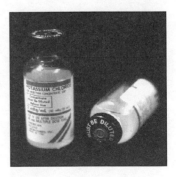

stickers and overwraps in the package. This change was made at the request of the ISMP.

Since the label standard went into effect in 1991, no reports of intrathecal injection have been reported to the USP MERP or to FDA. Unfortunately, accidents continue in other countries. In 1994, the World Health Organization wrote to regulatory authorities worldwide to share the U.S. experience.

Finally, for label warnings, there may be some value in a hierarchy of terminology (e.g., listed in decreasing order of strength, "danger," "warning," "caution," "notice").

Typeface

Clarity can be enhanced by the appropriate use of typeface elements such as serif or sans serif and upper- or lowercase letters.[20] Serifs are the short extenders attached to the tops and bottoms of letters in certain typefaces. Sans-serif (literally, "without serifs") type is plainer than serif type (e.g., serif versus sans serif). Sans-serif letters generally work best for conveying short pieces of information. Letters with serifs take up more space than sans serif letters, and uppercase letters consume more space than lowercase letters. Lowercase letters have characteristics such as ascending and descending strokes that make them easier to read than uppercase letters, which are all the same height. Certain typefaces (e.g., Helvetica, which is sans serif) may provide a bolder warning than others.

Some manufacturers use typeface to enhance distinctive portions of look-alike names on look-alike packages. For example, Wyeth-Ayerst differentiates dimenhydrinate and diphenhydramine by using large and small capital letters for portions of the product name (Figure 13–17).

Small ampuls and vials used for nebulized respiratory medications in the United States and for injectable drugs in some countries present particular problems because the print must be very small. Manufacturers should consider using partially filled ampuls or blister-pack unit-dosing in order to allow adequate space for printing essential information in a legible size. To enhance legibility of essential information on small ampuls, the FDA may sometimes allow exceptions to the information it normally requires on packages and labels.

Package Design

Several serious medication errors involving lidocaine 10% and 20% packaged in intravenous additive syringes can be tied to poor package design.[21]

A customary loading dose of lidocaine for patients with ventricular arrhythmia ranges between 75 mg and 100 mg. Three pharmaceutical companies manufactured this drug in prefilled 100-mg emergency syringes with an attached needle (Figure 13–18). During the decade after the introduction of this product, more than 40 deaths and many serious accidents occurred because practitioners used a syringe containing 1 or 2 g of lidocaine, which was meant to be diluted in a 5% dextrose solution, to prepare a follow-up lidocaine infusion. Lidocaine was repeatedly injected directly into the Y-sites of patients' intravenous lines. Had the syringe been designed so that the needle would fit only an intravenous bag injection port, this could not have occurred.

Practitioners called for the syringe to be redesigned or removed from the market. The premiere edition of *Dateline NBC*, on March 30, 1992, profiled the fatalities associated with misuse of this product. In 1993, the product was withdrawn.

A dual-chamber, heparin partial mix, intravenous container from Baxter has been tied to medication errors that can be related to packaging problems (Figure 13–19). The user must fracture a plastic cannula to mix the contents of the upper chamber, which contains heparin, with those of the lower chamber, which contains a diluent. Some users do not know that the fracture is required, while others forget to do it. As a result, patients have received plain diluent. The product was withdrawn from the market in 1995. The

Figure 13-17

Capital letters distinguish these two product names.

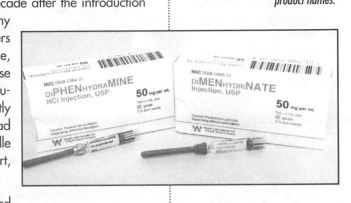

Figure 13-18

Prefilled 100-mg emergency syringes of lidocaine, with attached needle, made by three different manufacturers. Left photo shows how it can be injected intravenously.

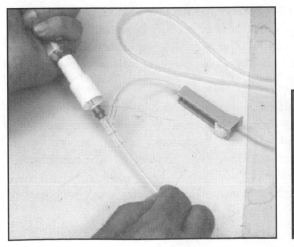

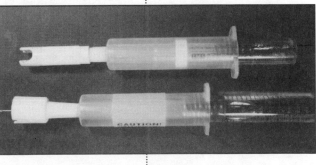

Figure 13-19

This dual-chamber container of heparin plus diluent was designed so that the plastic cannula separating the two chambers must be fractured in order to mix the contents of the bag. The design led to patients receiving only plain diluent.

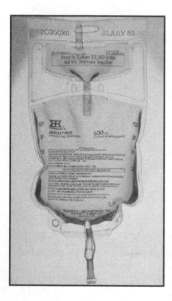

problem could have been resolved by equipping the product with a fail-safe mechanism that prevented administration until the solution had been mixed.

Similar situations exist with Baxter's Viaflex Plus and Abbott's AddVantage, which require that practitioners affix drug vials to intravenous minibags and activate and dilute the drug by crushing a seal (Viaflex®) or removing a diaphragm in the vial (AddVantage®) prior to administration. Problems have occurred when the doses did not reach patients because the user did not take the necessary action prior to administration.[22] In this and many of the other cases cited here, human factors were not adequately taken into account in the product design stage. With monitoring and in-service education, such oversights can be minimized but not eliminated.[23]

The outer packaging used to prevent evaporation of solutions contained in intravenous minibags can increase the possibility of product mix-ups because it reduces label readability. As noted above, foil overwraps used by Abbott presented problems until two-sided labeling was implemented. Baxter minibags wrapped in opaque plastic (Figure 13–20) have been mixed up with one another.[24]

At least 22 cases of Brevibloc® (esmolol) overdoses have been reported since this drug became available in the late 1980s.[25] The overdoses occurred in part because a 2.5-g ampul, rather than a 100-mg vial, was used to prepare a loading dose (Figure 13–21). In evaluating the error, it is apparent that ampuls are normally used for loading doses, since they are always single-dose containers, and that the vials are most often for multiple doses. This is, however, exactly the opposite of the way the product is packaged. The manufacturer did not take into account that loading doses are often ordered in terms of number of ampuls.

The company placed a warning flag on the ampul neck that underscored the need for dilution. However, another accident happened soon after the label change. The company is currently considering making the drug available in a ready-to-use form that would preclude the need for an ampul dosage form.

Five percent hydrogen peroxide developers have been mixed up with ophthalmic products because both are packaged in similar plastic containers. The developer is used to test for occult blood in the stool and is often kept in the bathroom within a patient's room. It has inadvertently been administered into the patient's eye in place of eye drops.[26] Irrigation containers have been mixed up with intravenous containers.[27] Topical nitroglycerin, packaged in tubes, has been used sublingually[28] and as a dentifrice.[29]

Tactile cues can be an important way of differentiating products. For example, in the past, insulin vials had a distinct shape that was related to the insulin type (i.e., regular insulin was packaged in round vials, NPH insulin was in a square vial, and Lente insulin was in a hexagonal vial). This system was discontinued when U-100 insulin products were introduced, even though patients with diabetes, who often have poor eyesight, found it extremely helpful.[30]

In recognition of the extreme consequences of a mix-up, some vials of neuromuscular blocking agents, including Mivacron® (mivacurium) and Tracrium® (atracurium), are packaged in vials with hexagonal necks.

Advertising

Pharmaceutical advertising would greatly benefit from practitioner review. Some advertisements depict poor practices, use dose designations and abbreviations that are in violation of practice standards or regulations, or omit important prescription information. When such practices appear in advertisements, they may stimulate the adoption of bad habits that can result in serious medication errors.

The advertisement for Epogen® in Figure 13–22A is an example. It uses "U" as an abbreviation for the word "unit." The "U" is sometimes misread as a zero (0) and may result in a 10-fold overdose. Amgen, manufacturer of Epogen®, eventually changed the label in response to suggestions from ISMP (Figure 13–22B). Unfortunately, the "U" designation is still used for Eminase® (Figure 13–22C).

An advertisement for Lotensin® (Figure 13–23) uses "q.d." This is often read as "q.i.d.," another dangerous abbreviation, and should not be used.

One advertisement used the abbreviation "MTX" for methotrexate. This abbreviation has been confused with mitoxantrone, a different cancer drug with an overlapping dose. The advertising was changed at the request of ISMP so that "methotrexate" was spelled out.

The Hismanal® advertisement in Figure 13–24A does not state a dose. The advertisement for Glynase® Prestab 3 mg (Figure 13–24B) states that the product

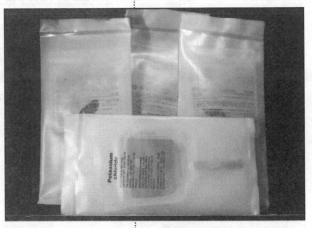

Figure 13-20

Wrapping minibags in opaque plastic prevents evaporation but also reduces visibility of labels.

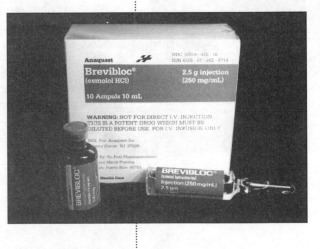

Figure 13-21

Overdoses of Brevibloc® (esmolol) have resulted from using the 2.5-g ampul (right) instead of the 100-mg vial (left) to prepare loading doses.

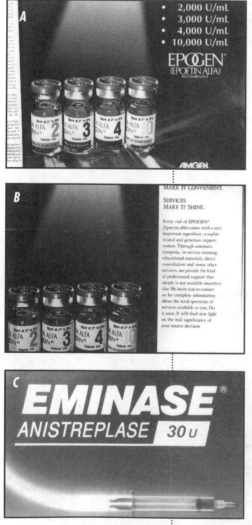

should be "dispensed as written," which is not an appropriate method for expressing directions. Practitioner review could have prevented these mistakes, saved money, and prevented medication errors.

Role of Failure Mode and Effects Analysis in Preventing Labeling and Packaging Problems

Why are there so many labeling and packaging problems? One reason is that decisions concerning labels and packaging are often made without input from practitioners. Package label reviews are often conducted at a desk using proofs rather than the actual label on an actual package. The proofs are often two to three times larger than the actual label or package and are printed on a contrasting background. Compare this method with one in which nurses, physicians, and pharmacists review the actual label and package in an environment similar to that in which the product will actually be used. Practitioners are much more likely to discover potential problems than are designers.

If error is inevitable, it must be anticipated. All pharmaceutical and medical device manufacturers should use failure mode and effects analysis (FMEA) (see Chapter 3). Applied to health care, this analysis entails practitioner review of labeling, packaging, and nomenclature. FMEA was introduced to the health care community by ISMP[31] and is suggested by the FDA.[32] In 1990, the ASHP House of Delegates voted to recommend that FDA require manufacturers to include practitioners in industry discussions concerning drug labeling, packaging, and naming.

All too often, improvements in packaging and labeling occur after errors have been reported. Applied prospectively, FMEA could help the pharmaceutical industry anticipate and avoid problems with labeling and packaging.

The following example, involving Bristol-Myers Squibb Oncology's Platinol®-AQ (cisplatin injection), illustrates how FMEA can be applied in health care.

After the launch of cisplatin injection in the 1980s, overdoses occurred because providers confused daily doses with the total dose for a course of therapy. Moreover, the drug was confused with Paraplatin® (carboplatin) because of similarities in product names. Doses appropriate for carboplatin usually exceed the maximum dose of cisplatin. Severe toxicity and death were associated with cisplatin overdose.

The company decided to use FMEA to resolve this problem. In conjunction with ISMP, an advisory panel of oncology specialists in pharmacy, medicine, and nursing was appointed. The goal of FMEA is to identify problem areas and then take actions to minimize or eliminate the potential for errors. Examination of the clinical environment in which the product will be used (e.g., stored, dispensed, prepared) is part of this analysis.

ERRS™ (Error Recognition and Revision Strategies), a model developed by ISMP for evaluating pharmaceutical products, including trademarks and packages, was used in this effort. Physicians, pharmacists, nurses, and unit clerks were involved in the analysis. Factors such as visibility of brand and generic names; strength, concentration, and volume; differentiation of strengths, forms, and sizes of the same product; presence, prominence, and visibility of required warnings, special instructions, and other label information; and method(s) of assembly and potential for proper use of the package were individually analyzed and scored collectively.

In the case of Platinol®, the potential for confusion with Paraplatin® was discussed, as was the fact that practitioners failed to recognize that the dose they were using was excessive.

As a result of FMEA, several important labeling and packaging changes were proposed, accepted by the company, and approved by FDA, as in the example in Figure 13–25 (see color plates). They include the following:

- The letters "CIS" appear in bold, uppercase, red characters to differentiate this product from carboplatin.

- The word STOP!, written in red within a stop sign, warns the user to verify the drug name and dose.

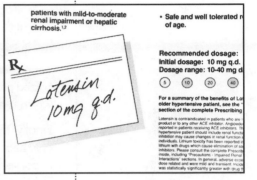

Figure 13-23

This advertisement uses the abbreviation "q.d." (for "every day"), which is often confused with "q.i.d." (four times a day).

Figure 13-24

Examples of inappropriate prescription orders are shown in these advertisements for Hismanal® (A), which does not include a dose, and Glynase® (B), which states that the product should be "dispensed as written."

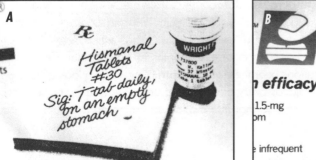

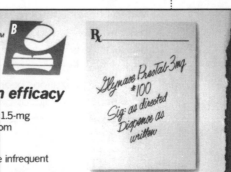

- A boxed warning notes that cisplatin doses of greater than 100 mg/m^2 once every 3 to 4 weeks are rare and advises the user to consult the package insert for further information.

- Information appears on more than one side of the box. No matter how the product is placed on the shelf, the warnings are visible.

- The vial seal and closure call attention to the maximum dose of cisplatin.

- Stickers enclosed in the carton certify that cisplatin has been prepared at the proper dosage.

Lyophilized cisplatin was eventually removed from market and is now available on special notice for chemo-embolism procedures. Only Platinol®-AQ, a solubilized product, remains. This also helps differentiate cisplatin from carboplatin, which is now available only in powder form as a lyophilized product.

Finally, the company conducted an extensive advertising campaign to educate health professionals about the changes and proper drug dose. This step is particularly important. If practitioners are not notified, changes made to improve safety may not be widely understood.

What Practitioners Can Do

This book suggests many actions that practitioners can take to reduce or eliminate medication errors. The most important suggestion is to read labels carefully. Some pharmacists find it helpful to talk to themselves as a double-check. First, they read the prescription or order and decide what is needed. For each item, they repeat to themselves the name of the drug, the strength, and whatever else they need (e.g., "I need thiamine 100-mg tablets"). They obtain the container and confirm it by reading the label to themselves (e.g., "I have tablets of thiamine 100 mg in my hand"). If they accidentally pick up thioridazine 100 mg, they realize the error as soon as they hear themselves saying something different from what they just said earlier.

When pharmacists purchase drugs, they should check ISMP safety alerts to become aware of past errors related to labeling and packaging of these products. It is also important to check these alerts when new drugs are added to a formulary, and again six months to a year later. Group purchasing organizations bear the same responsibility. Known look-alike products should be avoided. Every effort should be made to encourage practitioners to report errors so that information on emerging problems can be disseminated.

International Efforts

Pharmaceutical labeling and packaging speak a universal language. This point was underscored at the 56th Annual World Congress of Pharmacy in 1996. At a workshop sponsored by the ISMP, participants learned that medication errors linked to flawed packaging and labeling were uncomfortably common and strikingly similar throughout the world. With the European Medical Evaluation Agency, FDA, and regulatory authorities of other countries, companies with international operations are being encouraged to involve pharmacists and other practitioners in the design and testing of drug labels and packages.

ISMP encourages international communication about medication errors. It has established an electronic international reporting program on its World Wide Web site (www.ismp.org). Participating countries include Australia, Hong Kong, Israel, Spain, Sweden, the United Kingdom, and the United States. ISMP is represented in Europe by the Spanish ISMP, headquartered in Alicante.

••••
References

1. Cohen MR. Accidental administration of lidocaine premix instead of 5% D/NSS. *Hosp Pharm.* 1992; 27: 142–44.

2. Senders J. Theory and analysis of typical errors in a medical setting. *Hosp Pharm.* 1993; 28: 505–08.

3. Cohen MR. Potassium chloride injection mix-up (letter). *Am J Hosp Pharm.* 1990; 47: 2457–58.

4. Stimuli to the Revision Process. Report and Recommendations of the USP-FDA Advisory Panel on Simplification and Improvement of Injection Labeling. *Pharmacopeial Forum.* 1994; 20: 7885–88.

5. Parr MJ. Labeling drugs. *Anaesthesia.* 1986; 41: 222.

6. American Society for Testing and Materials. Standard D 4774-88. Philadelphia, Pa: 1988.

7. Anonymous. Frequently Asked Questions About Color Blindness. Schaumberg, Ill: Prevent Blindness America; 1999.

8. Report of the Council on Professional Affairs, American Society of Health-System Pharmacists. Use of color to identify drug products. *Am J Health Syst Pharm.* 1996; 53: 1805.

9. Cohen MR. Comments on pharmacy labeling practices. *Hosp Pharm.* 1993; 28: 1039–43.

10. American Society for Testing and Materials. Standard D4267-89. Philadelphia, Pa: 1989.

11. Cohen MR. Dangerous ampul mix-up. *Hosp Pharm.* 1988; 23: 91.

12. Cohen MR. Medication error reports: Camptosar injection labels misread. *Hosp Pharm.* 1996; 31: 1557.

13. Cohen MR. Hazard warning. Acetaminophen unit dose labeling. *Hosp Pharm.* 1988; 23: 695.

14. Solomon SL, Wallace EM, Ford-Jones EL, et al. Medication errors with inhalant epinephrine mimicking an epidemic of neonatal sepsis. *N Engl J Med.* 1984; 310: 166–70.

15. McClure M. Human error—a professional dilemma. *J Prof Nursing.* 1991; 7: 207.

16. Cohen MR. Vials of potassium chloride injection. *Hosp Pharm.* 1990; 25: 191–93.

17. Heller W. USP: of, by, and for the professions. *Am J Hosp Pharm.* 1989; 46: 2522.

18. Cohen MR, Pippis E. Potassium accident in a university hospital ICU. *Hosp Pharm.* 1996; 31: 882.

19. Cohen MR. Hazard warning: deaths due to accidental intrathecal injection of vincristine. *Hosp Pharm.* 1989; 24: 694.

20. Nunn DS. Ampoule labeling—the way forward. *Pharmaceutical Journal* (UK). March 14, 1992.

21. Lidocaine errors. How can they be prevented? *Hospital Pharmacist Report.* July 1990: 1.

22. Cohen MR. Comments on Minibag Plus. *Hosp Pharm.* 1993; 28: 796–98.

23. DeRon MS, Craig SA, Parks NPT. Monitoring system to verify activation of ADD-Vantage system. *Am J Hosp Pharm.* 1989; 46: 702.

24. Cohen MR. Overwrap on Baxter minibags. *Hosp Pharm.* 1995; 30: 439.

25. O'Brien J. Confusing packaging blamed for deaths. Syracuse, NY: *Post-Standard,* May 12, 1997.

26. Cohen MR. Application of nonophthalmics into the eye. *Hosp Pharm.* 1991; 26: 1063.

27. Cohen MR. Hazard warning! Renacidin for irrigation in IV look-alike packaging. *Hosp Pharm.* 1991; 26: 373, 376.

28. Cohen MR. Sublingual nitroglycerin ointment. *Hosp Pharm.* 1981; 16: 351.

29. Cohen MR. Nitroglycerin toothpaste. *Hosp Pharm.* 1987; 22: 195.

30. Cohen MR. Tactile cues for identifying insulin. *Hosp Pharm.* 1996; 31: 87–88.

31. Cohen MR, Senders J, Davis NM. Failure mode and effects analysis: a novel approach to avoiding dangerous medication errors and accidents. *Hosp Pharm.* 1994; 29: 319–28, 330.

32. Vecchione A. War on errors. FDA targets problem names, labeling. *Hospital Pharmacist Report.* 1996; 10: 1, 8.

14. The Patient's Role in Preventing Medication Errors

Stacy A. Wiegman, PharmD, MS
Michael R. Cohen, MS, FASHP

Institute for Safe Medication Practices
Huntingdon Valley, Pa.

Patients can do a great deal to decrease the probability that they will experience a medication error. To do so, they need not spend hours researching medications and diseases. Nor do they have to know everything about the drugs they are taking. They simply need to know what to ask and to insist on answers. An informed patient is one of the best safeguards against medication errors.

After years of frustration over not being able to get physicians and nurses to wash their hands before they touch patients, researchers coordinated a study at four community hospitals to educate patients about the importance of hand washing by staff.[1] Patients were told to ask anyone who came in direct contact with them whether they had washed their hands. For those patients who were hesitant to ask, stickers saying "Did you wash your hands?" were made to wear on hospital gowns. The researchers measured a 42% increase in liquid soap use at the end of the study.

This study showed that patients can have an impact in problem areas and that they are interested in participating. The idea behind it could be applied to patient education about medication error prevention. For example, the Institute for Safe Medication Practices has received reports about errors that occurred because nurses did not check patients' arm bands. To increase nurses' compliance with checking arm bands before medication administration, a hospital could make up buttons for patients to wear that read "Did you read my arm band?" A study released in 1998 by the National Patient Safety Foundation at the American Medical Association in Chicago found that 92% of adults surveyed believe that they can have a positive effect on patient safety. Respondents also believed that providing patients with information on how to ensure their safety would be effective in preventing medical errors. With this in mind, clinicians should take advantage of their patients' interest and willingness to participate.

Patients also need to understand the need for compliance with the drug regimen that has been prescribed for them. Compliance is influenced by a number of factors, many of which can be affected by a knowledgeable and sensitive health care provider.

In this chapter, we discuss the questions that all patients should ask when they receive a medication in the hospital or when they purchase a product at the pharmacy. We also discuss patient compliance, a topic that is closely related to safe and effective medication use. Finally, we present considerations for safe medication use for three specific populations: hospitalized patients, elderly patients, and children.

Table 14-1

Twelve questions concerning safe medication use

Twelve Basic Questions

Most pharmacists, physicians, and consumer advocates believe that to ensure safe medication use, all patients must have the answers to the 12 basic questions listed in Table 14–1.

The answers to these questions provide patients with the tools they need to take responsibility for safe drug use. To be most effective, the answers must be provided at the time the medication is prescribed, whether this is at the patient's bedside in a hospital or in the doctor's

1. What are the brand and generic names of the medication?
2. What is the purpose of the medication?
3. What is the strength and dosage?
4. What are the possible side effects? What should I do if they occur?
5. Are there any other medications I should avoid while using this product?
6. How long should I take the medication? What outcome should I expect?
7. When is the best time to take the medication?
8. How should I store the medication?
9. What do I do if I miss a dose?
10. Should I avoid any foods while taking this medication?
11. Is this medication meant to replace any other drug that I am already taking?
12. May I have written information about this drug?

office. This information must be presented in a form and at a rate that the patient can understand, and it must be periodically reinforced. Patients should be urged to question anything that they do not understand or that does not seem to be in keeping with their understanding.

Sometimes clinicians take for granted that patients fully understand their instructions. Health care providers may assume that what is obvious to them is obvious to their patients, so they omit discussing routine details of proper medication use. Unfortunately, patients often misunderstand the instructions. We recently heard about an asthmatic patient who was not responding to therapy. During follow-up, the patient described how he was using his inhaler. He would get into his car, roll up the windows, release two puffs of medication into the air, and breathe deeply for 15 minutes! At first, he did this in his house. Later he thought it might be more effective to use the inhaler in a confined space. He said he'd been instructed to do this by his doctor, who had picked up an inhaler, held it in the air, and released two puffs to demonstrate its use. The doctor had given the patient no additional instructions.

Clinicians need to be clear and complete in their instructions. Patients may take them literally or may erroneously fill in the gaps when information is omitted. It is important to assume nothing regarding the patient's knowledge base and to leave no room for patients to make erroneous assumptions. Care providers should provide thorough instructions and should always include the obvious.

Patient Record-Keeping

Patients should keep records of all the medications, including over-the-counter products, that they are taking. Such records are especially important for patients who have chronic diseases, who see more than one physician, or who take many medications. Information that should appear on this list is summarized in Table 14–2. Patients should update these lists whenever their medication regimen changes. Many health providers give patients forms to simplify record-keeping.

Safe Drug Use by Patients: Key Points

Name of the Medication

Poor labeling is a major reason for medication errors. Many manufacturers package their products in containers that are virtually identical, as illustrated by the two boxes of lozenges shown in Figure 14–1(see color plates). Only on careful examination does the reader note that one box is labeled "Maximum Strength" and that it contains benzocaine. The other product does not contain benzocaine. Some patients are allergic to benzocaine or could become sensitized to it. Because of the similarity in packaging, patients or health professionals would find it difficult to distinguish these two products.

Brand-name extensions may also cause problems. Popular brand names have become associated with certain ingredients; for example, Tylenol® is associated with acetaminophen and Bayer® with aspirin. Consumers and pharmacists may not realize that, whereas the chief ingredient of Anacin® is aspirin, the chief ingredient of Anacin-3® is acetaminophen. A

- Name, strength, dose, and frequency of dosage of all prescription medications
- Names of all over-the-counter medicines, vitamins, or herbal products
- Known medication or food allergies
- Medications that the patient used to take and the reason why the medication was discontinued

patient taking glipizide for type II diabetes who takes Anacin® instead of Anacin-3® might experience side effects such as dizziness, because aspirin increases the hypoglycemic effect of glipizide.

To prevent errors such as these, pharmacists should advise patients of the differences between ingredients and encourage them to choose single-ingredient products whenever possible. Pharmacists should explain that multi-ingredient products contain medications that are not needed or that may cause side effects. For example, a patient with nasal congestion that is not caused by allergy should take a decongestant only; a decongestant–antihistamine may cause drowsiness.

Readability

The packaging of many over-the-counter products contains a great deal of information; however, the print is often so small that it is virtually illegible. Improving readability has limits because the Food and Drug Administration (FDA) requires that a certain amount of information appear on all labels. The Consumer Healthcare Products Association and FDA have been working to improve label readability. In March 1999 the government announced new requirements for a standard format for nonprescription drug labeling to increase consumer awareness of important drug information.

Some problems with readability stem from physician handwriting. To prevent mix-ups, patients should request that the physician print drug names on prescriptions and indicate the purpose of the drug on the prescription. This will reduce the likelihood of pharmacist misinterpretations of "look-alike" drug names.

Verbal (Spoken) Orders

Many drug names sound alike. When prescriptions are called into a pharmacy, misunderstandings may occur. The solution is to request that the prescriber spell the name of the drug to the nurse or pharmacist taking the order and to require that he or she repeat the name and spelling to the caller. Providing additional information (for example, stating the purpose of the medication) is an additional safeguard. Computerized order processing eliminates the need for telephone orders

Naming the Patient

Medication errors often arise because the nurse gives a drug to the wrong patient. In a hospital, the nurse must read the patient's arm band and check it against the patient's name on the medication. Some hospitals use bar code technology to reduce such errors. Using this technique, the nurse places a bar code scanner close to the patient's arm band and scans it as well as the bar code of the medication. If that medication was ordered for the identified patient, the scanner indicates a match. If not, the scanner flashes a warning light.

A hospital patient should never accept a medication before questioning the nurse to make sure it is the one that has been ordered. In a community pharmacy, the possibility for error can be reduced if the patient insists on counseling and, before leaving the pharmacy, checks to see that his or her name is on the label and that the name of the drug is the same as that provided by the physician. In other situations, the patient's address or social security number may be incorporated into the method of identification.

Medication Storage

The medicine cabinet in the family bathroom is probably the worst possible place to store medications. The heat and humidity of bathrooms may affect the shelf life of the product. For this reason, medications should be kept on a kitchen shelf or in the linen closet, well out of the reach of children and pets.

Storing medications in the bathroom, often next to toiletries, poses a risk of dangerous mix-ups. For example, in one instance a woman reached for the toothpaste and inadvertently grabbed a tube of her husband's nitroglycerin paste. Brushing her teeth with the nitroglycerin, a vasodilator, caused her blood pressure to drop suddenly. Her husband found her unconscious in the bathroom.[2]

Compliance: The Other Side of Safe Drug Use

Noncompliance can be defined as any one of the following:

- Not filling a prescription initially
- Not having a prescription refilled
- Omitting doses
- Taking the wrong dose
- Stopping a medication without the physician's advice
- Taking a medication incorrectly
- Taking a medication at the wrong time
- Taking someone else's medication

Noncompliance is a major problem. Some form of noncompliance is associated with up to 93% of the 1.8 billion prescriptions filled annually in the United States.[3,4]

Causes and Consequences of Noncompliance

The results of noncompliance are substantial. Studies show that noncompliant patients are more likely to be hospitalized and to require more clinic visits than compliant patients. The National Council on Patient Information and Education estimates that noncompliance is a cause of 10% of all hospital admissions and of 25% of admissions among the elderly. The annual cost to the economy has been estimated at more than $100 billion.[5] (The total amount spent for purchasing prescription drugs, in contrast, was $62 billion in 1993.[6])

Certain groups of patients are more likely to be noncompliant than others. These include persons who take more than one drug, who have a chronic condition, who take a drug more than once a day, or who have a condition that produces no overt symptoms or physical impairment.[4,7-9] Compliance decreases as the complexity of drug therapy increases. It is also related to the type of condition for which treatment is advised. Patients with chronic diseases are often noncompliant because of the complexity of their drug therapy, side effects, and social factors. Treatment for diseases that have few or no symptoms (for example, hypertension) is difficult, because the patient may feel that the side effects are worse than the disease itself.

Compliance often hinges on how important or desirable the outcome of treatment appears to the patient. Health providers must help the patient understand the consequences of treatment and nontreatment. For example, a man with hypertension is more likely to be compliant if he is told that the medication will reduce his risk of heart attack or stroke than if he is told only that it will reduce his blood pressure. A woman with glaucoma will probably be more compliant if she is told that using the prescribed eye drops will save her eyesight rather than if she is told that it will reduce her intraocular pressure.

Noncompliance may be unintentional. One cause of unintentional noncompliance is visual impairment. Unintentional noncompliance also may occur if patients do not understand instructions for taking their medication. For example, a patient taking Sinemet CR® 50/200 told the pharmacist that he had trouble swallowing the tablets. The pharmacist jokingly suggested that the patient coat them with petroleum jelly. The patient followed the pharmacist's advice and, within a few days, suffered a marked decline in function and became fatigued and lost coordination. The patient called his pharmacist to report that the new drug was not working. Upon questioning, the pharmacist discovered that the patient had interpreted his advice on coating the tablets literally. The coating was impairing the drug's absorption.[10]

Reasons for Noncompliance

Reasons for noncompliance may be divided into three categories: knowledge deficits, practical barriers, and attitudinal barriers.

Knowledge deficits are a key cause of unintentional noncompliance. They occur when a patient receives incomplete or faulty information about a disease or treatment. Knowledge deficits may be overcome by providing more information or by providing the information in a more understandable form. Health providers should tailor the way in which they present information to the patient's level of education and understanding. Dispelling myths about treatment and disease may be part of this process.

Practical barriers to compliance include poor eyesight, illiteracy, poverty, adverse drug reactions, confusing dosing schedules, containers that are hard to open, and cognitive impairment. These barriers are not always immediately discernible. For example, the National Institute for Literacy estimates that 90 million Americans have limited reading skills.[11] Many of these individuals have jobs and function quite well. They hide their inability to read, in some cases so well that members of their own families are unaware of their deficit. These individuals rely on memory, association, color, shape, and other cues. If such a patient must take several medications, errors are inevitable unless a system is designed that can compensate for illiteracy. This might entail, for example, color coding the bottles.

Another barrier to medication compliance is side effects. Some of these, such as urinary incontinence, are not only very disturbing to the patient but also difficult to admit to the health provider.

Attitudinal barriers may be hardest to overcome because they are rooted in the patient's health belief system, which is formed by his or her culture, family, personal values, and previous experience with the health care system. Patients with such barriers may deny their condition or express frustration with treatment. Some may exhibit a lack of trust for the health care establishment and seek alternative treatments such as homeopathy or herbal remedies.

Some patients, by contrast, seek professional advice for every ache and pain. Although they, too, present a challenge to the health provider, they are usually compliant with medication regimens.

Compliance is based on the patient's understanding of the disease and medication and the belief that treatment is necessary and beneficial. Health professionals can help patients minimize physical and practical barriers, but tackling attitudes is more challenging.

Specific Patient Populations

Most of the advice in this chapter applies to persons receiving medications in any setting. However, special considerations arise with respect to the use of medications in certain patient populations.

Hospitalized Patients

During a hospital stay, a patient is placed in a dependent role. All responsibilities that he or she normally bears, including that of safe drug use, are transferred to professionals. It is understandable that patients are reluctant to ask questions. They do not want to be labeled "troublesome." As a result, they hesitate to question anything, even if they believe that something is wrong. Such a climate increases the likelihood of medication errors.

Hospitalized patients need to play active roles in their treatment. They should take their medicine record and medications with them to the hospital. Medications should be in their original containers. After the physician, nurse, or pharmacist has seen the medications, a family member should take them home. Most hospitals do not allow patients to take their own medications while they are hospitalized. One reason for this is to prevent the patient from receiving a double dose—one from the nurse and one that is self-administered. Another reason is that the patient's drug regimen often changes during a hospital stay.

Hospitalized patients should query the health care professional about the name and purpose of their medications. Because the patient may not be well enough to do this, a family member or friend should be fully aware of the

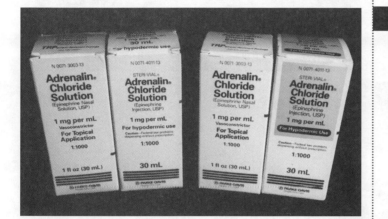

Figure 13-2

Confusion existed when the packaging of Adrenalin® Chloride Solution for topical application and for hypodermic use appeared similar (left); redesigned packaging (right) helped to distinguish the two products.

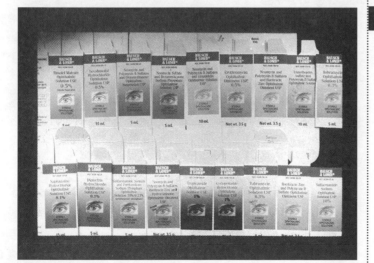

Figure 13-5

Color coding can actually increase the potential for error, as illustrated by the similar packaging of these ophthalmic products.

Figure 13-6

Effective use of color is shown by the red warnings printed on these bottles of sodium chloride injection.

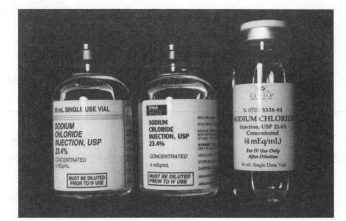

Figure 13-7

Improvements to the package labeling of Mivacron® included adding labels to the back of the foil miniwrap (left); the old packaging (right) was difficult to identify without labeling on the back.

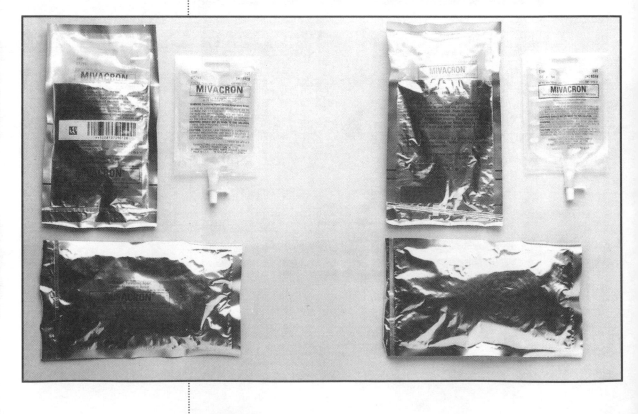

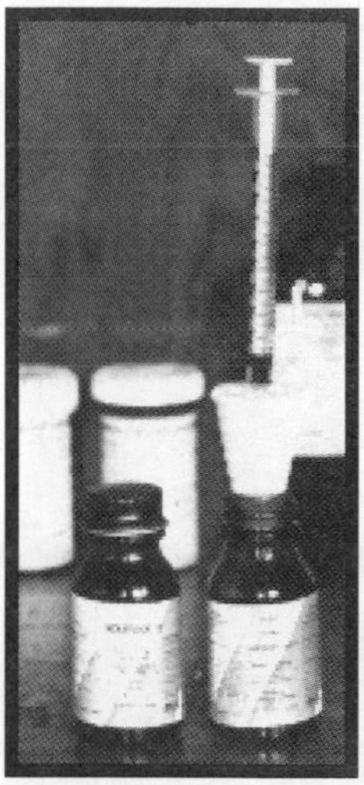

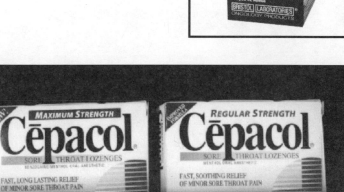

Figure 13-14

Epinephrine and vitamin E packaged in vials that are nearly indistinguishable.

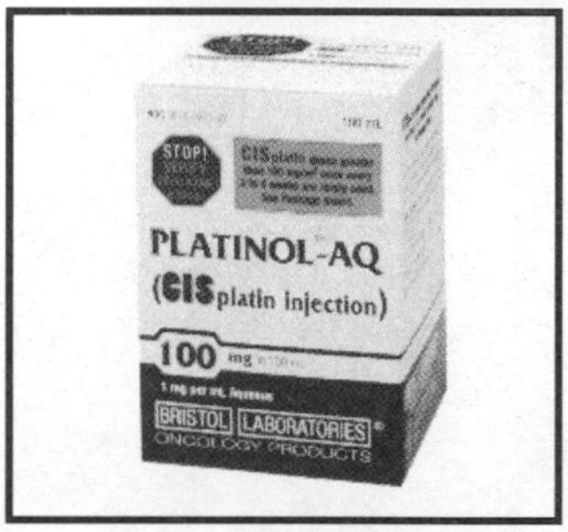

Figure 13-25

Changes to the package labeling of Platinol® (cisplatin) were made to avoid its confusion with Paraplatin® (carboplatin).

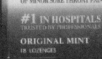

Figure 14-1

These packages look nearly identical, but only one of the products contains benzocaine.

patient's medication regimen and be prepared to ask questions on the patient's behalf. The literature contains many examples in which a family member intervened to prevent a medication error. For example, the mother of a leukemic child who was to receive a daily injection of interferon noticed that the solution in the syringe that the nurse was about to use was brown instead of its usual color. The mother questioned it and learned that the syringe actually contained Imferon (iron dextran).[12]

Before a patient is discharged, a health care provider should talk with him or her about any new prescriptions and about changes in the prescriptions that the patient had been taking prior to hospitalization. If the patient has brought a medication list to the hospital, it should be updated. If no list was brought, this is the time to create one.

The importance of patient education at the time of each hospital discharge is underscored by the following example.[13] A child with leukemia was discharged from the hospital with a nasogastric tube in place for intermittent enteral feeding. He was readmitted for chemotherapy. During this admission, he developed an infection, and a peripherally inserted central catheter (PICC) line was placed for administration of IV antibiotics. The patient improved and was discharged to home care with the PICC still in place. Shortly thereafter, the PICC line clotted. The child's mother called the home care nurse. When the nurse arrived, she found that the mother had drawn up ginger ale into a syringe and was about to inject it into the PICC line. Having been taught to clear the child's nasogastric tube with ginger ale, the mother assumed that all tubes could be cleared by the same technique. Had the home care nurse not intervened, the child would have been exposed to a possible infection and a carbon dioxide-induced (air) embolism. Predischarge counseling would have greatly reduced the potential for this error.

Older Patients

One-third of all older patients take three or more prescription medications, and 10% take five or more.[14] Special care should be taken in counseling older patients, who not only are often taking more than one medication but who may also have mental impairment. Older patients should be approached with sensitivity; advice should not be confused with nagging. If possible, a family member or friend should be engaged in the counseling process.

A medication schedule can be especially helpful for these patients. This schedule can be hand drawn or produced by a computer. Table 14–3 shows a sample chart for an elderly patient taking diltiazem, warfarin, and aspirin. The medications should be listed by time of day they are taken so that the patient can check off each time a dose is taken. Patients who use charts are less likely to take a double dose because they can easily refer to the list when in doubt. It is vital to update the chart when changes in drug therapy are made.

Older patients may want to use medication organizers, which allow them to prepackage up to a week's worth of medicine. The organizers are divided by time of day and provide space for multiple daily doses. Some are available in Braille. Patients using these organizers must be able to identify their medications by sight, in case the contents spill or the dosage is changed while the organizer is full. If a medication organizer is not used, the patient must be instructed to keep all medications in their original containers. Medications should never be mixed in a single bottle.

Older patients may have trouble swallowing medications. Cutting or crushing a tablet or capsule may not be safe[15] and may impair the action of some products. Patients should be instructed to ask the pharmacist if it is okay to break the tablet or to request a liquid form.

Pediatric Patients

Causes of noncompliance among children are similar to and different from those among older persons. First, children may be reluctant to take medications because they do not understand the difference between drugs that help people and those that hurt people. Children with chronic illnesses may feel hopeless about their disease and may be noncompliant for this reason.[16] Children often feel that they lack control over many aspects of their lives. Compliance with drug therapy is one thing they can control.[17] In addition, children harbor myths about drug therapy; they may believe, for example, that a higher dose will lead to a faster cure[18] or that taking someone else's medicine will give them that person's disease.[19] Despite these differences, rates of compliance for children and adults are virtually the same.[17]

Accidental poisonings are a separate but related concern with respect to children and safe medication use. If a medicine tastes too good, children may consume the entire bottle; this is quite common with cough syrups, chewable analgesics, vitamins, and antibiotics. Children may also consume cleaning substances and personal care products such as toothpaste and shampoo if they are left in an accessible location.[20]

Table 14-3

Example of medication schedule kept by patient

Time	Medication	Date		
		10/11	10/12	10/13
8:00 AM	Diltiazem 60-mg capsule			
	Aspirin 81-mg tablet			
12 noon	Diltiazem 60-mg capsule			
6:00 PM	Diltiazem 60-mg capsule			
10:00 PM	Warfarin 2-mg tablet			
	Diltiazem 60-mg capsule			

Child-resistant packaging has decreased the number of poisonings of children, but it has not eliminated the risk. Often this is because containers are not properly closed.[21,22] To meet the requirements of the Poison Prevention Act of 1970, 85% of children less than 5 years of age must be unable to open the package within 5 minutes, and 80% must be unable to open it even after being shown how to do so.[23] Nonetheless, the problem remains. One study performed in an emergency department showed that properly closed, child-resistant packaging failed to deter children under the age of 5 in 20% of cases; in another 12.5% of the cases, the container had been improperly closed.[24]

Adults can play an important role in encouraging medication safety. Medications should be stored with caps securely fastened, on a high shelf or in a locked box. Adults should never take medications in the presence of children, because a positive or negative reaction on the part of the adult may influence the child's perception of medications. When visiting with their children, parents should ask their hosts whether they have placed their medications in a place where they are not accessible to children.

Because accidental childhood poisonings do occur, even with the best precautions, parents should keep a bottle of syrup of ipecac on hand to induce vomiting. Some substances should not be vomited; for this reason, parents should always call the local poison control center before administering syrup of ipecac. They should take measures to determine how much the child has ingested. This may be done by marking the bottle each time it is appropriately used.

Unit dose packaging of oral solids makes it more difficult for children to ingest drugs. Many new over-the-counter drugs, as well as some prescription products, are packaged this way. The FDA now requires that iron tablets be individually packaged.

Conclusion

Patients can play an important role in their medication therapy and error prevention by asking questions of health care providers. Patients also should provide information to their physicians, nurses, and pharmacists. They should maintain accurate, up-to-date medication records. Because informed patients have prevented medication errors many times and can serve as the final check on medication administration, health care providers should encourage patients to take an active role in this process.

References

1. McGuckin M, et al. *Handwashing Compliance: The Effect of a Patient Education Program*. Presented at Society for Healthcare Epidemiology in America annual meeting, St Louis, Mo, April 1997.

2. O'Keefe JH, Kwong EM, Tancredi RG. Transgingival nitrate syncope. *N Engl J Med*. 1986; 315: 1030.

3. Berg JS, Dischler J, Wagner DJ, et al. Medication compliance: a health care problem. *Ann Pharmacother*. 1993; 27: S5–S19.

4. Greenberg RN. Overview of patient compliance with medication dosing: a literature review. *Clin Ther*. 1984; 6: 592–98.

5. Task Force for Compliance. Noncompliance with medications: an economic tragedy with important implications for health care reform. Presented at meeting of the National Council on Patient Information and Education, Baltimore, Md, November 1993.

6. US Pharmaceutical Market Year-In-Review 1993. West Port, Conn: IMS International Inc; 1994.

7. Hulka BS, Kupper LL, Cassel JC, et al. Medication use and misuse: physician-patient discrepancies. *Journal of Chronic Disease*. 1975; 28: 7–21.

8. Eraker SA, Kirscht JP, Becker MH. Understanding and improving patient compliance. *Ann Intern Med*. 1984; 100: 258–68.

9. Col N, Fanale JE, Kronholm P. The role of medication noncompliance and adverse drug reactions in hospitalizations of the elderly. *Arch Intern Med*. 1990; 150: 841–45.

10. Cohen MR. Caution: what patients hear may be taken literally. *Hosp Pharm*. 1996; 31: 603–04.

11. Newsletter. National Institute for Literacy. Vol 3, No 2, May/June 1996.

12. Cohen MR. Do not confuse interferon with imferon. *Hosp Pharm*. 1992; 27: 784–85.

13. Patient teaching needed before home care patients leave the hospital. *ISMP Medication Safety Alert!* March 26, 1997; 2: 2.

14. Cartwright A. Medicine taken by people aged 65 or more. *Br Med Bull*. 1990; 46: 63–76.

15. Mitchell JF. Oral solid dosage forms that should not be crushed. 1998 update. *Hosp Pharm*. 1998; 33: 399–415.

16. Szefler S. Children's drug-information needs are explored at USP conference. *Am J Health Syst Pharm*. 1996; 53: 2782–83.

17. Bearison DJ. Children's drug-information needs are explored at USP conference. *Am J Health Syst Pharm*. 1996; 53: 2782–83.

18. Aramburuzabala P. Children's drug-information needs are explored at USP conference. *Am J Health Syst Pharm*. 1996; 53: 2782–83.

19. Bibace R. Children's drug-information needs are explored at USP conference. *Am J Health Syst Pharm*. 1996; 53: 2782–83.

20. Litovitz TL, Felberg L, White S, et al. 1995 Annual Report of the American Association of Poison Control Centers Toxic Exposure Surveillance System. *Am J Emerg Med*. 1996; 14: 487–94.

21. McIntire MS, Angle CR, Grush ML. How effective is safety packaging? *Clin Toxicol*. 1976; 9: 419–25.

22. Jacobson BJ, Rock AR, Cohn MS, et al. Accidental ingestions of oral prescription drugs: a multicenter survey. *Am J Public Health*. 1989; 79: 853–56.

23. Poison Prevention Packaging Act of 1970. Pub Law 91-601; December 30, 1970.

24. Lembersky RB, Nichols MH, King WD. Effectiveness of child-resistant packaging on toxin procurement in young poisoning victims. *Vet Hum Toxicol*. 1996; 38: 380–83.

Part IV:

Medication Errors in Relation to Specific Diseases and Conditions

15.
Preventing Medication Errors in Cancer Chemotherapy

Michael R. Cohen, MS, FASHP

Institute for Safe Medication Practices
Huntingdon Valley, Pa.

Roger W. Anderson, MS

Division of Pharmacy
University of Texas M.D. Anderson Cancer Center
Houston, Tex.

Richard M. Attilio, MS

Mercy Suburban Hospital
Norristown, Pa.

Laurence Green, PharmD, FASHP

Amgen Corporation
Thousand Oaks, Calif.

Raymond J. Muller, MS

Division of Pharmacy Services
Memorial Sloan-Kettering Cancer Center
New York, N.Y.

Jane M. Pruemer, PharmD

Department of Pharmacy
University of Cincinnati
Cincinnati, Ohio

Reprinted with permission from *American Journal of Health-System Pharmacy*, Volume 53, April 1, 1996, pages 737–46. Based in part on a meeting held during the annual meeting of the American Society of Hospital Pharmacists, Philadelphia, Pa., June 7, 1995.

The contributions of Rebecca S. Finley are acknowledged.

Medication errors during cancer chemotherapy continue to make national headlines. The consequences of errors involving anticancer drugs can be devastating because these drugs typically have narrow therapeutic ranges. In addition, chemotherapy regimens have become increasingly complex and intensive as supportive care (e.g., antiemetics, colony-stimulating factors, bone marrow transplantation) has improved. These newer chemotherapy regimens carry greater risks of injury.

An episode at a comprehensive cancer center in New England in 1994 may have been a turning point because of the unprecedented publicity.[1] Betsy Lehman, a 39-year-old health care reporter for the *Boston Globe*, died of a drug overdose during treatment of metastatic breast cancer. According to the investigational protocol, the cyclophosphamide dose was "4 g/sq m over four days." This ambiguous order was misinterpreted by a number of health professionals. What should have been ordered was a daily dose of 1 g/m^2 for 4 days in a row. Instead, the patient received cyclophosphamide 6.52 g per day for four consecutive days, for a total of 26.08 g instead of a total of 6.52 g. The error was not adequately detected by any health care provider. Death was attributed to cardiotoxicity.

The Lehman case, and other case reports, prompted one of the authors to review the literature on medication errors, summarize how measures to prevent errors may apply to cancer chemotherapy, and invite a panel of experts to discuss the resultant document at a meeting held by the Institute for Safe Medication Practices (ISMP) in conjunction with the 1995 American Society of Hospital Pharmacists (ASHP) annual meeting. Audience members also participated in the discussion. The session was tape recorded and later reviewed to incorporate salient comments by the panelists and audience into the original document. The authors reviewed the revised draft, added appropriate literature citations, and considered additional revisions on the basis of guidelines developed by the Royal College of Physicians and the Royal College of Radiologists.[2]

The drug manufacturer, regulatory agency, prescriber, unit clerk, nurse or other professional responsible for drug administration and documentation, pharmacist and other pharmacy personnel, and patient all play important roles in the safe use of medications. As for all medications, the goal of drug administration in cancer chemotherapy is to ensure delivery of the right drug to the right patient in the right dose and dosage form at the right time. Achieving this goal requires a comprehensive, systematic approach by multiple providers.

Many steps are required to prevent medication errors. This article address-es the following measures as they relate to cancer chemotherapy: educating health care providers, verifying the dose, establishing dosage limits, stan dardizing the prescribing vocabulary, working with drug manufacturers, educating patients, and improving communication. The need to increase pharmacist involvement throughout these steps is also discussed.

Educating Health Care Providers

The single most important reason why medication errors reach patients is that information about the patient and the medication is not available when it is needed.[3] Ideally, each institution should provide a computerized system that makes important patient-specific information available. However, few hospitals have institution-wide computer systems that make patient-specific and more general information available to practitioners at the time of pre-scribing, dispensing, or drug administration. Therefore, practitioners contin-ue to rely heavily on traditional educational methods to bring information to practitioners.

Educational Process

The educational process should be customized according to whether an individual will be involved in prescribing, dispensing, or administering anti-neoplastic drugs. Before these privileges are granted, all health care providers should undergo a specific orientation program and possibly test-ing about mechanisms involved in documented cases of serious medication errors; this should become a specific requirement of the Joint Commission on Accreditation of Healthcare Organizations (JCAHO). Certification may be necessary before pharmacists and pharmacy technicians are permitted to dispense antineoplastic drugs.[4] Education is also indicated when a new agent is added to the formulary or involved when the institution is in an investigational drug protocol. This could be achieved with a traditional newsletter, guidelines, or a checklist.[5] By signing off on this information, a staff member indicates that he or she understands the appropriate use of the new agent.

Pharmacy education should not be limited to clinical specialists or oncology hospitals. Despite efforts to restrict administration times to periods of optimal staffing, cancer chemotherapy may be required in the evenings or on week-ends. Therefore, all staff pharmacists must be involved in a program to ensure competent 24-hour coverage. Pharmacists who practice in commu-nity hospitals encounter unique problems because of lack of standardiza-tion. A patient may be admitted to an oncology hospital where specialists who are familiar with investigational regimens prescribe and administer the initial dose, but subsequent doses may be administered in the community. This practice was a factor in the inadvertent administration of doxorubicin by the intrathecal route.[6]

In addition, independent oncologists who do not participate in cooperative studies write orders differently. For example, a private oncologist may try a new regimen after reading a new article or may modify an existing protocol. Even if protocols are followed, different protocols may specify different administration methods. Another obstacle to standardization is the use of both body surface area and patient weight in dosage calculations.

Pharmacists should initiate and participate in educational sessions for other health care providers. Pharmacists are uniquely qualified to instruct new house staff and attending physicians about institutional policies on prescribing and administering antineoplastics.

Describing actual medication errors, especially the consequences of nonstandard prescribing practices that occurred within the institution or that have been published, can be highly effective. Having an automated clinical intervention program initiated by pharmacists allows for these errors to be presented and discussed by the institution's pharmacy and therapeutics committee in a nonthreatening, evaluative manner.[7] Likewise, it may be instructive to ask another institution to share preventive measures or information on prescribing practices standardized there.

Reference Materials

Reference materials should be developed and made readily available to all health care providers involved in the prescribing, dispensing, and administration of antineoplastic drugs. These resources should cover the appropriate use of these agents (FDA-approved labeling and investigational uses), precautions, adverse effects, dose-limiting effects, instructions on infusion methods, usual adult and pediatric doses, and doses for single and multiple courses of therapy. Excellent resources have been published,[8–10] but textbooks alone are not sufficient because they become rapidly outdated. Institution-specific resources, especially in cancer research centers, should also be developed. A medium that can be easily updated is preferred. Institution-specific summary sheets, notebooks, computerized databases, and combinations thereof work well. These reference materials should be placed in all pharmacy locations (including all satellites) and at strategic locations throughout the institution (e.g., nursing stations). In addition, complete copies of treatment protocols, along with the patient's informed-consent sheet, should be readily available in all pharmacies that dispense antineoplastic agents.

PDQ (Physician's Data Query), a computerized database provided by the National Library of Medicine, contains basic information on different cancer therapies, along with current information on some protocols. This database can be accessed online at little expense. CancerNet, run by the National Cancer Institute, provides access to portions of PDQ and the Cancerlit database as well. Micromedex (Boulder, Colo.), a computerized drug information service, provides information about specific agents and has charts giving dosing and other important drug information. Another source of information is the annual "Guide for the Administration and Use of Cancer Chemotherapeutic Agents."[11]

Verifying the Dose

Although computerized dose-verification systems are available, a straw poll of practitioners attending the ISMP session on chemotherapy medication error prevention at the 1995 ASHP Annual Meeting showed that only a handful had this capability built into their current hospital computer system. Therefore, each institution should develop a dose-verification process with as many *independent* manual checks as possible. The process should specify how the prescribing physician, unit clerk, nurse, dispensing pharmacist, clinical pharmacist, pharmacy technician, and staff responsible for drug administration will interact. A comprehensive, detailed checklist covering prescribing, transcribing, dispensing, and administration is needed. For example, do house staff physicians have independent prescribing privileges, or must orders be co-signed by an attending physician?

Because of the inherent risk of misinterpretation of oral drug orders, it is recommended that such orders not be acceptable for antineoplastic agents. Faxed orders may be acceptable under certain circumstances, but faxes should not be accepted unless all the information is clear. Also, these drugs should be ordered only during specified working hours so that adequately trained staff members are on hand to provide necessary clinical reviews.

All doses should be calculated independently by the physician who writes the order, the pharmacist who checks the order and dispenses the drug, and the nurse who administers it. This is especially important in cancer chemotherapy, because repeating doses within a cycle or during subsequent cycles multiplies any error in calculation. This implies that the prescription should specify both the dose according to body surface area or body weight and the calculated amount. Physicians should be encouraged to specify doses in this format when ordering chemotherapy to permit double-checking of dosage calculations (e.g., "25 mg/sq m [50 mg]" for a patient whose body surface area is 2 m²). In addition, dosage modifications may be made because of drug-induced bone marrow suppression or renal dysfunction. Pharmacists must become familiar with the necessary formulas and have access to laboratory data. Computer software should link appropriate laboratory test results (e.g., white blood cell counts, platelet counts, and serum creatinine levels) with dosage adjustment criteria so that necessary modifications in the dose can be determined automatically. Simple dosing tables for all regimens that list the dose for given body surface areas or body weights or both could serve as a ready reference against which to compare calculated doses. This would help ensure that those responsible for prescribing, dispensing, and administering a drug have properly interpreted the dosage requirements of the protocol.

The dose-verification policy should specify whether the prescriber must identify the protocol (e.g., by listing the protocol number, institutional review board number, or a published citation) on the order form. If the regimen is unfamiliar, the pharmacist should verify the dose by reviewing at least two independent literature sources. It is possible that erroneous information may appear in a published article. When a journal article inadvertently indicated that the dose of vincristine sulfate was 1.4 mg/m² on days 1–8 instead of days 1 *and* 8, an accidental overdose resulted, even though the pharmacist initially recognized a problem.[12,13] A uniform method for pharmacist checking of antineoplastic drug orders that is in use at the National Institutes of Health appears in the Appendix.

Establishing Dosage Limits for Antineoplastics

It is recommended that hospitals define situations in which pharmacists should not dispense selected antineoplastic agents without further expert review. Such would be the case, for example, when a prescribed dose exceeds a preset maximum single dose or cumulative dose. Pharmacists should work with physicians, nurses, and other health care providers to identify dosage limits and to establish the review process (involving individuals other than the prescriber and reviewing pharmacist) required before a drug that exceeds a preestablished limit is dispensed.

Serious toxicity or death has been attributed to overdoses for many antineoplastic drugs during monotherapy, including cisplatin,[14–16] melphalan,[17] mitoxantrone,[18] mechlorethamine,[19] vinblastine,[20] and vincristine,[21–23] as well as in patients receiving multiple agents.[24] In some cases, an excessive dose was recognized during the order-review process. However, communication breakdowns, failure of the prescriber to fully consider the clinical implications of the dose in question, and failure of pharmacists and nurses to stand their ground have sometimes led to patient harm. With preset limits and a review process for exceptions, the chance that an improper dose will be administered is greatly reduced. Each institution should form a committee comprising oncologists, pharmacists, and nurses to establish maximum doses for all FDA-approved antineoplastic agents. The dosage ceiling should be based on the literature[25] and on clinical studies at the specific institution. At least four types of dosage limits are necessary for antineoplastic agents: (1) the maximum amount for a single dose, (2) the maximum amount per 24 hours, (3) the maximum amount per course of therapy (definable for each drug), and (4) the maximum amount per patient lifetime. These limits should be described in terms of milligrams, units, milligrams or units per square meter of body surface area, or milligrams or units per kilogram of body weight.

Although establishing maximum doses may be challenging in community hospitals, each oncologist should be invited to agree in advance to limits beyond which no drug should be dispensed. It may not be feasible to establish strict limits for all antineoplastic agents because of the diversity of doses and treatment methods used for different malignancies. However, it is safer to establish a limit and a review process when the limit is exceeded.

Pharmacists should work with computer programmers or software vendors to develop electronic warnings and order-screening routines that will not permit processing of orders when the established dosage limit is exceeded. Although such an automated system can help identify doses that surpass established ceilings, a manual verification and tracking program must also be in place. For example, if the maximum single dose of carboplatin in a comprehensive cancer center is determined to be 1200 mg, a manual system can augment a pharmacist's judgment and not allow the dispensing of another dose for at least 3 weeks. If a dose is ordered sooner, the pharmacist must contact the prescriber to verify the dose and identify the treatment protocol before the dose can be dispensed. If the pharmacist does not agree with the prescriber's decision and the issue cannot be resolved to the ultimate satisfaction of the pharmacist and the prescriber, a preestablished peer-review committee would make a judgment.

Tailoring the labeling on drug containers can sometimes help reduce the likelihood of a medication error. Bristol-Myers Squibb Oncology now places a message stating the dosage limit for cisplatin directly on the Platinol® packaging.[26] Placing statements on the container may be appropriate for other drugs, especially vincristine. Pharmacists might want to add their own dosage warnings on certain drug containers.

Warnings about dosage limits should not be restricted to the packaging and labeling. Consideration should be given to including dosage limits in chemotherapy protocols and on preprinted order forms. Pharmacists should include maximum doses in summary sheets. The limits must be communicated during employee orientation and in-service programs, as well as placed in strategic locations where these drugs are prescribed, stored, dispensed, and administered.

Other types of limits related to administration should also be established, such as the minimum duration of infusion and the appropriate route. There have been many case reports of death after inadvertent intrathecal administration of vincristine;[27–34] survival is rare.[35–37] These case reports prompted the ISMP to ask the U.S. Pharmacopeia (USP) to issue an official dispensing standard.[38] When vincristine is dispensed in other than its original container, the drug must be packaged in an overwrap that bears the following statement: "Do not remove covering until moment of injection. Fatal if given intrathecally. For intravenous use only." Recently, the FDA asked manufacturers to provide overwrap and labeling to facilitate dispensing. Manufacturers are now also required to provide a label that can be affixed directly to an extemporaneously prepared syringe. Another drug that has caused major toxicity after intrathecal administration is doxorubicin.[6] In addition, drugs that are suitable for intrathecal administration can be highly toxic if the dose intended for systemic use is given intrathecally (e.g., cytarabine[39] and methotrexate[40]).

Once limits are identified and endorsed by other health care providers, pharmacists must not become complacent. Although electronic messages and labels are useful tools that augment the dose-verification process, they should not become substitutes for other checks.

Standardizing the Prescribing Vocabulary

Failure to control the prescribing vocabulary is a major cause of medication errors. Conversations among oncology experts are replete with abbreviations, acronyms, and coined names. Efforts to squeeze large amounts of information into abstracts presented at meetings help perpetuate this problem.

While these shortcuts may be convenient for oncology specialists, they are an obstacle to health care providers who are less familiar with cancer chemotherapy, and they can easily lead to misinterpretations. For example the abbreviation "MTX" has been misinterpreted as "Mustargen®" (mechlorethamine).[41] An order for the bone-resorption inhibitor Aredia® (pamidronate) was misread as "Adria," a popular nickname for the brand name of doxorubicin.[42] A vague order for "platinum" led to the substitution of cisplatin for carboplatin.[43] A computer entry for "BUS10" resulted in busulfan 10 mg being dispensed instead of the antianxiety agent BuSpar® (buspirone hydrochloride) 10 mg prescribed for a 5-year-old child.[44] Acronyms like "COPP" and "MOPP" are other examples of risky shortcuts. These case reports illustrate the importance of using only approved generic names (United States Adopted Names [USAN]).

An equally troublesome source of medication errors is confusion between the individual dose and the total dose over a course of therapy. For example, the order "cisplatin 100 mg/sq m continuous infusion days 1–4" is ambiguous. The prescriber intended that the patient receive a total of 100 mg/m^2 over the entire 4-day period, a dose well within the usual limit of 120 mg/m^2 per course, which usually is repeated every 4 weeks. The order was misinterpreted, and the drug was dispensed as 100 mg/m^2 daily for 4 days.[15] The patient died. The preferred method for writing the order is "cisplatin 25 mg/sq m/day (or "daily") as a 24-hour continuous i.v. infusion on 7/5/95, 7/6/95, 7/7/95, and 7/8/95."

A study protocol can be a source of a medication error if it is subject to misinterpretation. Practicing pharmacists and nurses must be involved in the early stages of protocol development to ensure that dosage regimens are easily understood—written properly and as simply as possible. A pharmacist should be a voting member of the institutional review board that approves the scientific and ethical treatment of all patients enrolled in a research protocol. For example, the Eastern Cooperative Oncology Group (ECOG) has a pharmacy committee to evaluate its protocols. This should be mandatory for all study groups. Once protocols are written, prescribing patterns should be reviewed routinely to ensure compliance. Noncompliance may indicate the need for clarification.

As with other drug classes, decimal points should be placed judiciously. Missing decimal points were responsible for three of five vincristine overdoses.[21] Whereas leading zeros are mandatory (e.g., vincristine sulfate 0.9 mg), trailing zeros should be eliminated because they may lead to an overdose (e.g., vincristine sulfate 1.0 mg could be read as 10 mg).

The need to indicate both the dose according to body surface area and the calculated dose was identified earlier. The method for calculating body surface area should be standardized within an institution. Different formulas can lead to clinically important dosing differences, especially in children. Likewise, formulas for modifying the dose because of drug-induced bone marrow suppression, renal dysfunction, hepatic failure, and other organ toxicity should be standardized.

Many of the recommendations made in this and previous sections can be adhered to by using preprinted chemotherapy order forms.[45] Each facility should create its own form and ensure that it goes through the appropriate approval process.[46] Pharmacists should contribute to the development of these forms to ensure ease of use and interpretation, completeness, adherence to ASHP's Guidelines on Preventing Medication Errors in Hospitals,[47] institutional compatibility, and instructional value to the house staff. Another advantage of the preprinted order form is the ability to physically separate orders for antineoplastics from orders for other medications. Color, shading, and other methods of enhancement may be used to further distinguish the form. These recommendations are also applicable to computerized physician order-entry systems.

The following summary of guidelines for writing antineoplastic drug orders is based on guidelines established by Memorial Sloan-Kettering Cancer Center:

- Always double-check the dose against the protocol.

- Use only the full generic name of the drug. Do not refer to drugs by brand names, nicknames, abbreviations, acronyms, or company names. Do not use common drug class names (e.g., does "platinum" mean cisplatin or carboplatin?).

- Prescribe all drug doses by metric weight (e.g., milligrams [mg] or grams [g]) or units. Include the dosage interval.

- Do not use dangerous abbreviations in specifying doses (e.g., "U" for units could be read as "0," and the patient could receive a 10-fold overdose).

- Use a leading zero when the dose is less than a whole unit (e.g., write "0.1 mg," not ".1 mg").

- Do not use a trailing zero (e.g., "10.0 mg" could be read as "100 mg").

- Express the dose in milligrams per meter squared (mg/m^2) or, when applicable, milligrams per kilogram (mg/kg). Give the daily dose times the number of days; do not list the total course dose (e.g., "cisplatin 25 mg/sq m [50 mg] daily x 4 days [6/1, 6/2, 6/3, and 6/4]").

- Round doses above 5 mg to the nearest whole number (e.g., 6 mg, not 5.8 mg).

- Date all orders with the month, day, and year.

- Specify the route of administration and the duration of infusion in hours for all injections.

• Record the patient's current body surface area or body weight on the drug order.

Working with Manufacturers

Nomenclature problems occur when names of different medications look or sound alike. Accidental substitution of vincristine for vinblastine led to a massive overdose and permanent peripheral paresthesia.[23] Substitution of cisplatin for carboplatin led to a massive overdose of cisplatin in the absence of intravenous hydration. The patient suffered severe myelosuppression, renal failure necessitating a kidney transplant, and permanent deafness.[14] Likewise, the names "mitoxantrone," "mitomycin," and "Mithracin®" (plicamycin) are easily confused.[41] Although the USAN Council and the FDA are reluctant to change established names, this has been done (e.g., "mithramycin" was changed to "plicamycin" because of confusion with "mitomycin"). These organizations are also receptive to testing names on panels of practitioners before nomenclature is finalized.[48]

Pharmacists need to work with manufacturers and the FDA to eliminate ambiguous dosing information from official resources. The following wording appears in the cyclophosphamide package insert,[49] as well as in many textbooks:

> Although a few instances of cardiac dysfunction have been reported following use of recommended doses of cyclophosphamide, no causal relationship has been established. Cardiotoxicity has been observed in some patients receiving high doses of cyclophosphamide ranging from 120 to 270 mg/kg administered over a period of a few days, usually as a portion of an intensive antineoplastic multidrug regimen or in conjunction with transplantation procedures.

It is not clear whether 270 mg/kg was given daily for several days or in divided doses over several days. The former alternative is obviously a massive overdose. Many would argue that the latter is also an overdose. In reality, cyclophosphamide 270 mg/kg given over a period of a few days was the upper limit tested in a dose-ranging study, not the upper limit of a regimen that remains in clinical use.

Three vinorelbine overdoses can also be attributed to ambiguity.[50] When the drug was investigational, the computer-generated label indicated that the vial contained vinorelbine (as the tartrate) 10 mg/mL, but the total volume was on a portion of the label far removed from the drug name and concentration. Nurses assumed that the vial contained only 10 mg of drug, instead of recognizing that the 5-mL vial contained 50 mg.

These and other problems come under the auspices of manufacturers and regulatory agencies. In cooperation with the USP Medication Errors Reporting Program, ISMP works to bring such information to the attention of authorities as well as practitioners. Practitioners can effect change by participating in the USP–ISMP program (to report an error, telephone 1-800-23-ERROR).

Educating Patients

Pharmacists have a responsibility to educate patients about their drug therapy. Transient pancytopenia has occurred when patients did not understand complex treatment regimens and failed to stop taking chlorambucil,[51] lomustine,[52] or procarbazine.[53] The death of Betsy Lehman demonstrates that even the best-informed consumers are at risk.[1]

A patient should be informed of the proprietary and generic names of each antineoplastic agent he or she is to receive, the indication, the usual and actual dosages, expected and possible adverse effects, and methods of preventing or managing adverse effects.[54] A patient may be interested in other therapeutic options, including unapproved or alternative therapies. Pharmacists should make educational materials available to patients and direct them to the National Cancer Institute, libraries, or bookstores for more extensive information.

Pharmacists should become patient advocates and offer advice on how patients can protect themselves from medication errors. For example, an inpatient should observe that his or her wristband is checked before each course of cancer chemotherapy; an outpatient should repeat his or her name to the provider. The importance of double-checking the details of chemotherapy cannot be overstated. Patients or a family member should be invited to become part of the care team so they can help check doses and request recalculation if body weight or (in children) height changes.

Consent forms should be designed for readability and completeness.[55] Patients should be informed of their right to ask questions and seek satisfactory answers. After the therapeutic plan is described to the patient or family, the patient must be given sufficient time to gain a complete understanding of the treatment and what should be expected. Patients should consider enlisting the support of family members or friends who understand the language of medicine. Alternatively, the practice site should have a formal method for providing assistance to the patient or patient advocate as necessary.

Caregivers should always take time to listen carefully when patients have questions about their therapy or when they call attention to any situation they deem to be of concern. Alert and knowledgeable patients may serve as the last line of defense in preventing a medication error. In some cases, patient concerns that have gone unheeded could have warned hospital staff of a pending crisis.[56]

The pharmacist's responsibility does not end with the provision of traditional drug information. Pharmacists should become public relations agents and explain their role to their patients. Without a clear understanding of the benefits of comprehensive pharmaceutical services, a patient may opt for the convenience of a small physician's office that lacks pharmacist involvement.

Improving Communication

Miscommunication or lack of communication among physicians, pharmacists, and nurses can lead to medication errors. Other health care providers should be invited to identify potential problems and solutions. Multidisciplinary discussions can occur spontaneously, after a medication error, or routinely (e.g., annually) as part of the quality improvement process. If other health care providers do not offer specific suggestions, pharmacists can direct the discussion. What should the pharmacist do in the event of a disagreement with the prescriber? What are the most effective techniques for making this type of inquiry? If the discrepancy cannot be resolved, should the pharmacist refuse to dispense the drug? Policies should be developed on the basis of these multidisciplinary discussions. Pharmacists and others should be trained, through role playing, to handle these situations.

Pharmacist Involvement

An implied or overt theme throughout this discussion has been the need for greater pharmacist involvement in cancer chemotherapy. A pharmacist should be involved at all sites where antineoplastic agents are dispensed. Pharmacists can help to establish sound policies for drug administration, provide indispensable safety checks, and perform other services consistent with pharmaceutical care. A pharmacist was absent when vincristine overdoses contributed to the deaths of three of five children[21] and, more recently, when vinorelbine overdoses caused two deaths and one serious injury.[50]

Increasingly, cancer chemotherapy is being provided in outpatient settings because of greater convenience and lower cost. Some ambulatory care clinics and most private oncologist offices lack extensive pharmacist involvement. Each organization should establish a minimum acceptable level of pharmacist involvement in its outpatient settings, such as in prospective order review, screening of laboratory test results, provision of drug information, patient counseling, and reviews of drug storage. Investigational protocols should be initiated only at sites where comprehensive pharmaceutical services are available.

Pharmacist involvement in cancer chemotherapy remains less than ideal even in some hospitals. In some institutions there is a growing practice of having pharmacy technicians or nurses prepare doses that are not checked by a pharmacist. There is a danger that this trend will increase as financial pressures cause staffing reductions.

Need for Multidisciplinary Guidelines

This article has summarized available guidelines and incorporated suggestions by pharmacists who have extensive experience with cancer chemotherapy. The authors encourage pharmacy organizations to use this article as a starting point for developing guidelines on improving the quality of cancer chemotherapy. A draft of such a document should be distributed to other health care providers for their review and comment. The American Society of Clinical Oncologists (ASCO), the Oncology Nursing Society (ONS), and the American Cancer Society (ACS) are logical targets for cooperative efforts. In fact, ONS members have expressed concern about preparing doses of antineoplastic agents and have shown a willingness to work with pharmacists. After multidisciplinary endorsement of such guidelines is obtained, the next step is to present them to an accreditation agency like JCAHO and organizations that accredit cancer research centers, such as the National Cancer Institute. In the meantime, this article serves to provide preliminary recommendations to pharmacists for preventing medication errors.

Conclusion

Although even the most seasoned health care provider can make a mistake, it is possible to keep most medication errors from reaching patients if caregivers work together. All medication errors should be reported so that we can learn from them. Each error should be reviewed by a multidisciplinary team to search for ways to improve the system. Institutions should establish dosage limits for antineoplastic agents, set up dose-verification procedures that stress multiple independent checks, and work to standardize the prescribing vocabulary. Patients and health care providers must be educated about cancer chemotherapy.

Recent tragic accidents involving antineoplastic drugs generated widespread publicity and concern. Because of their training and experience, pharmacists should take the lead in implementing policies that will minimize the risk of future errors.

• • • •
References

1. Knox RA. Response is slow to deadly mixups. Too little done to avert cancer drug errors. *Boston Globe.* June 26, 1995: 29, 33.

2. United Kingdom Joint Council for Clinical Oncology. *Quality Control in Cancer Chemotherapy. Managerial and Procedural Aspects.* Oxford, England: Royal College of Physicians of London; 1994.

3. Leape LL, Bates DW, Cullen DJ, et al. Systems analysis of adverse drug events. *JAMA.* 1995; 274: 35–43.

4. Peters BG, Wilson AL, Lunik MC, et al. Certification program in antineoplastic drug preparation for pharmacy technicians and pharmacists. *Am J Hosp Pharm.* 1994; 51: 1902–06.

5. Melamed AJ, Nacov CG, Muller RJ. Antineoplastic agents: some preparation and handling considerations. *Pharm Pract News.* 1986; 13: 18–19.

6. Aricó M, Nespoli L, Porta F, et al. Severe acute encephalopathy following inadvertent intrathecal doxorubicin administration. *Med Pediatr Oncol.* 1990; 18: 261–63.

7. Wang Chin JM, Muller RJ, Lucarelli CD. A pharmacy intervention program: recognizing pharmacy's contribution to improving patient care. *Hosp Pharm.* 1995; 30: 120, 123–26, 129–30.

8. Finley RS, Balmer CM, Dozier N, et al. *Concepts in Oncology Therapeutics. A Self-Instructional Course.* Bethesda, Md: American Society of Hospital Pharmacists; 1991.

9. Dorr RT, Von Hoff DD. *Cancer Chemotherapy Handbook.* Middleton, Conn: Appleton & Lange; 1994.

10. Perry MC, ed. *The Chemotherapy Sourcebook.* Baltimore, Md: Williams & Wilkins; 1992.

11. Flannelly BP, Gregory RE, Kim Y, et al. Guide for the administration and use of cancer chemotherapeutic agents. *Pharm Pract News.* 1995; 22 (8): 47–51.

12. Lopez TM, Hagemeister FB, McLaughlin P, et al. Small noncleaved cell lymphoma in adults: superior results for stages I–III disease. *J Clin Oncol.* 1990; 8: 615–22.

13. Cohen MR. Misprint in journal article leads to vincristine overdose. *Hosp Pharm.* 1994; 29: 294, 302.

14. Chu G, Mantin R, Shen Y-M, et al. Massive cisplatin overdose by accidental substitution for carboplatin. *Cancer.* 1993; 73: 3707–14.

15. Pike IM, Arbus MH. Cisplatin overdosage (letter). *Am J Hosp Pharm.* 1992; 49: 1668.

16. Schiller JH, Rozental J, Tutsch KD, et al. Inadvertent administration of 480 mg/m^2 of cisplatin (letter). *Am J Med.* 1989; 86: 624–25.

17. Jost LM. Overdose with melphalan (Alkeran): symptoms and treatment. A review. *Onkologie.* 1990; 13: 96–101.

18. Hachimi-Idrissi S, Schots R, DeWolf D, et al. Reversible cardiopathy after accidental overdose of mitoxantrone. *Pediatr Hematol Oncol.* 1993; 10: 35–40.

19. Zaniboni A, Simoncini E, Marpicati P, et al. Severe delayed neurotoxicity after accidental high-dose nitrogen mustard (letter). *Am J Hematol.* 1988; 27: 305.

20. Conter V, Rabbone ML, Jankovic M, et al. Overdose of vinblastine in a child with Langerhans' cell histiocytosis: toxicity and salvage therapy. *Pediatr Hematol Oncol.* 1991; 8: 165–69.

21. Kaufman IA, Kung FH, Koenig HM, et al. Overdosage with vincristine. *J Pediatr.* 1976; 89: 671–74.

22. Kosmidis HV, Bouhoutsou DO, Varvoutsi MC, et al. Vincristine overdose: experience with 3 patients. *Pediatr Hematol Oncol.* 1991; 8: 171–78.

23. Maeda K, Ueda M, Ohtaka H, et al. A massive dose of vincristine. *Jpn J Clin Oncol.* 1987; 17: 247–53.

24. Kim IS, Gratwohl A, Stebler C, et al. Accidental overdose of multiple chemotherapeutic agents. *Korean J Intern Med.* 1989; 4: 171–73.

25. DeVita V, Hellman S, Rosenberg M, eds. *Cancer. Principles and Practice of Oncology.* 4th ed. Philadelphia, Pa: Lippincott; 1993.

26. Cohen MR. Cisplatin vial seals to carry message on dose limits. *Hosp Pharm.* 1995; 30: 538–39.

27. Al Fawaz IM. Fatal myeloencephalopathy due to intrathecal vincristine administration. *Ann Trop Paediatr.* 1992; 12: 339–42.

28. Bain PG, Lantos PL, Djurovic V, et al. Intrathecal vincristine: a fatal chemotherapeutic error with devastating central nervous system effects. *J Neurol.* 1991; 238: 230–34.

29. Gaidys WG, Dickerman JD, Walters CL, et al. Intrathecal vincristine. Report of a fatal case despite CNS washout. *Cancer.* 1983; 52: 799–801.

30. Manelis J, Freudlich E, Ezekiel E, et al. Accidental intrathecal vincristine administration. Report of a case. *J Neurol.* 1982; 228: 209–13.

31. Schochet SS Jr, Lampert PW, Earle KM. Neuronal changes induced by intrathecal vincristine sulfate. *J Neuropathol Exp Neurol.* 1968; 27: 645–58.

32. Shepherd DA, Steuber CP, Starling KA, et al. Accidental intrathecal administration of vincristine. *Med Pediatr Oncol.* 1978; 5: 85–88.

33. Slyter H, Liwnicz B, Herrick MK, et al. Fatal myeloencephalopathy caused by intrathecal vincristine. *Neurology.* 1980; 30: 867–71.

34. Williams ME, Walker AN, Bracikowski JP, et al. Ascending myeloencephalopathy due to intrathecal vincristine sulfate. A fatal chemotherapeutic error. *Cancer.* 1983; 51: 2041–47.

35. Bleck TP, Jacobsen J. Prolonged survival following the inadvertent intrathecal administration of vincristine: clinical and electrophysiologic analyses. *Clin Neuropharmacol.* 1991; 14: 457–62.

36. Dyke RW. Treatment of inadvertent intrathecal injection of vincristine. *N Engl J Med.* 1989; 321: 1270–71.

37. Zaragoza MR, Ritchey ML, Walter A. Neurourologic consequences of accidental intrathecal vincristine: a case report. *Med Pediatr Oncol.* 1995; 24: 61–62.

38. Cohen MR. Warning: vincristine practice standard must be followed by pharmacists and others. *Hosp Pharm.* 1995; 30: 740–41.

39. Lafolie P, Liliemark J, Bjork O, et al. Exchange of cerebrospinal fluid in accidental intrathecal overdose of cytarabine. *Med Toxicol Adverse Drug Exp.* 1988; 3: 248–52.

40. Ettinger LJ. Pharmacokinetics and biochemical effects of a fatal intrathecal methotrexate overdose. *Cancer.* 1982; 50: 444–50.

41. Davis NM, Cohen MR, Teplitsky B. Look-alike and sound-alike drug names: the problem and the solution. *Hosp Pharm.* 1992; 27: 95–98, 102–05, 108–10.

42. Cohen MR. "Adria," a dangerous abbreviation for Adriamycin, looks like Aredia. *Hosp Pharm.* 1994; 9: 141, 158.

43. Cohen MR. Safety alert—overdoses of Platinol (cisplatin) and Paraplatin (carboplatin). *Hosp Pharm.* 1992; 27: 991–92.

44. Sullivan P, Heaney J. Hospital admits giving wrong drug to sick child. *Boston Herald.* April 6, 1995: 7.

45. Slimovitz R. Thoughts on a medical disaster (letter). *Am J Health Syst Pharm.* 1995; 52: 1464–65.

46. Cohen MR, Davis NM. Developing safe and effective preprinted physician's order forms. *Hosp Pharm.* 1992; 27: 508, 513, 528.

47. American Society of Hospital Pharmacists. Guidelines on preventing medication errors in hospitals. *Am J Hosp Pharm.* 1993; 50: 305–14.

48. DiDomizio G, Cohen MR. Medication errors: who's at fault and who's counting. *Med Malpract Law Strategy.* 1995; 12 (5): 1–4.

49. Cyclophosphamide package insert. Princeton, NJ: Bristol-Myers Squibb; 1995.

50. Cohen MR. Cancer chemotherapy needs improved quality assurance. *Hosp Pharm.* 1995; 30: 258–59.

51. Enck RE, Bennett JM. Inadvertent chlorambucil overdose in adult. *NY State J Med.* 1977; 9: 1480–81.

52. Hörnsten P, Sundman-Engberg B, Gahrton G, et al. CCNU toxicity after an overdose in a patient with Hodgkin's disease. *Scand J Haematol.* 1983; 31: 9–14.

53. Hadjiyanni M, Valianatou K, Tzilianos M, et al. Prolonged thrombocytopenia after procarbazine "overdose" (letter). *Eur J Cancer.* 1992; 28A: 1299.

54. Muller RJ, Agre P. Patient education: a multidisciplinary approach to influence patient compliance. *Top Hosp Pharm Manage.* 1991; 10 (4): 50–58.

55. Grossman SA, Piantodosi S, Cvahay C. Are informed consent forms that describe clinical oncology research protocols readable by most patients and their families? *J Clin Oncol.* 1994; 12: 2211–15.

56. Knox RA. Doctor's orders killed cancer patient. *Boston Globe.* March 23, 1995: 1, 16.

Recommendations for Preventing Cancer Chemotherapy Medication Errors

1. Educate health care providers

   a. The educational process should be customized according to whether the individual will be involved in prescribing, dispensing, or administering antineoplastic agents.

   b. Consider a certification process to validate knowledge before allowing practitioners to prescribe, dispense, or administer antineoplastics.

   c. The pharmacy department should provide informational guidelines or a checklist when a new drug is added to the formulary. The guidelines should include therapeutic indication, usual dosage range (for single and multiple courses), reconstitution instructions (if applicable), infusion guidelines, and a description of adverse effects. Information on solution incompatibilities is helpful.

   d. Pharmacists should participate in educational sessions with prescribers and with nurses who administer the drugs. Describing actual medication errors and the consequences of nonstandard prescribing methods can be highly effective. Each institution, especially clinical research centers, should develop specific educational resources.

2. Verify the dose

   a. Each institution should develop a dose verification process with as many independent manual checks as possible. A computer system to verify the dose and route would be ideal but is not present in most hospitals.

   b. All doses should be calculated independently (e.g., by the physician who writes the order, the pharmacist who prepares the dose, and the nurse who administers it).

   c. All health care providers should have ready access to resources for verifying a patient's laboratory test data and body surface area.

   d. Investigational doses must be verified by checking the institutional review board protocol number and/or two independent sources.

3. Establish dosage limits

   a. Maximum single and total-course doses should be established at each institution. The limits should be communicated during employee orientation programs and in-service education programs.

   b. Maximum dosage limits should be entered into pharmacy computer systems and listed on preprinted order forms.

   c. Limits should be established for minimum duration of infusion and appropriate route of administration.

   d. Manufacturers should help practitioners avoid medication errors by improving package labeling.

4. Standardize the prescribing vocabulary

   a. Use full generic name of drug. Brand names and abbreviations are not acceptable.

   b. Express all drug doses in milligrams or units.

   c. All orders should be dated with the month, day, and year.

d. Use a leading zero when the dose is less than a whole unit (e.g., write "0.1 mg," not ".1 mg").

e. Do not use a trailing zero when writing an order ("2.0 mg" looks like "20 mg" if the decimal point is overlooked).

f. Include the current body surface area with the order.

g. Do not refer to drugs in terms of common drug classes (e.g., does "platinum" mean cisplatin or carboplatin?).

h. The use of preprinted order forms should be encouraged.

5. Work with drug manufacturers

a. Errors should be reported to the Medication Errors Reporting Program operated by USP in cooperation with the Institute for Safe Medication Practices.

b. Pharmacists should work with manufacturers to eliminate ambiguous dosing information from educational resources (package inserts, textbooks, company-sponsored educational programs, etc.).

6. Educate patients

a. Patients should be informed of the name of the antineoplastic agent, therapeutic indication, usual and actual doses, expected and possible adverse effects, and methods for preventing or managing adverse effects.

b. Patients should be instructed on how they can protect themselves from medication errors. Patients should be informed of their right to ask questions and seek satisfactory answers.

c. Health professionals need to listen carefully to what patients are telling them.

7. Improve communication

a. An interdisciplinary team at each practice site should review medication errors and resolve the miscommunication that is a leading cause of problems.

Guidelines for Checking Antineoplastic Drug Orders at the National Institutes of Health Clinical Center

The following are verified by a pharmacist assigned to check protocol-related orders:

- The medical information system (MIS) order (the label printout) reflects the most current order entry.

- The order includes the protocol number (so the appropriate treatment and drug supply can be determined).

- All drugs that should be ordered have been. Ancillary medications (e.g., dexamethasone, filgrastim) that are part of the protocol should also be checked. Judgment should be used to ensure that other supportive care medications (e.g., antiemetics) are ordered when appropriate, even if they are not specifically outlined in the protocol.

- The timing of drug administration within the chemotherapy cycle is appropriate.

- The dose is consistent with the dose specified in the protocol.

- The height and weight recorded in the MIS are the most recent values.

- The reason for major deviations of the pharmacist-calculated dose from the ordered dose (10% or greater for adults; 5% or greater for pediatric patients) is determined.

- The latest laboratory test values are satisfactory according to the protocol.

- The patient's pharmacy chemotherapy record (work card) is checked for any comments related to prior dosage modifications, cumulative dosage limits (e.g., for doxorubicin), expected changes in treatment, or other information.

- The administration route, diluent, infusion time, and infusion device are consistent with protocol specifications.

- The proper number of doses or days of therapy is ordered. Any deviations from the protocol specifications that have not been previously approved should be confirmed by contacting the prescriber, attending or senior physician, research nurse, or principal investigator. Notes should be made on the work card to reflect any current or future changes in treatment.

Checklist for Preparing and Labeling Antineoplastic Drugs

For each order you check, verify that each element is correct with a check mark.

Patient ❑ Drug ❑ Date ❑

Label Check

Patient name is same as on front of work card ❑

Dose on label matches dose written on back of work card ❑

Diluent on label matches diluent written on back of work card ❑

Volume of diluent on label matches volume of diluent on back of work card ❑

Correct date to prepare ❑

Expiration date and time ❑

Correct time (expiration date not greater than administration time) ❑

For Each Drug/Additive

Drug used ❑

Drug concentration in each vial ❑

Additives, such as sodium bicarbonate solution, for which large stock bottles are used (which remain in hood) are visually checked, lot number is verified, and technician is asked to verify volume used ❑

Syringe plunger is pulled back to volume required for dose ❑

Drug lot number on each vial matches lot number written on work card ❑

Calculations are checked ❑

Drug has not expired ❑

For Each Diluent

Correct diluent ❑

Volume of diluent ❑

Diluent has not expired ❑

Special Instructions Followed

Tubing ❑

Diluent for reconstitution ❑

Correct container ❑

Final Miscellaneous Steps

Chemotherapy work card checklist is in card pocket ❑

Solution is inspected for impurities/floaters ❑

Label is initialed (on left-hand side of label just below last additive or drug) after being affixed to correct admixture ❑

Work card is initialed ❑

Pharmacist's initials ❑ Date ❑

Supervisor's initials ❑ Date ❑

Checklist for Initial Setup of Chemotherapy Work Card

This form should be completed by the pharmacist checking the work card. Place check mark (or N/A) in each space after each check is completed. Your check marks and initials at the bottom of this worksheet are your personal assurance that you checked all these items for accuracy in the setup and transcription of information onto the work card. Each drug requires a separate checklist.

Patient ❑ Drug ❑

Start date ❑

Administration time ❑

Stop date ❑

Duration ❑

Drug name ❑

Number of doses ❑

Dose ❑

Drug concentration ❑

Drug volume ❑

Diluent ❑

Volume of diluent ❑

Expiration time ❑

Special delivery devices (tubing, cassette, container, etc.) ❑

Correct route of administration ❑

Correct mixing instructions (special directions, e.g., "Do Not Filter") ❑

Auxiliary label information (e.g., "Do Not Refrigerate," "Use In-line Filter" "For Intrathecal Use Only") ❑

Correct total volume ❑

Pharmacist's initials ❑ Date ❑

16. Pediatric Medication Errors

Yvonne C. D'Antonio, PharmD

University of the Sciences of Philadelphia
Philadelphia, Pa.*

Michael R. Cohen, MS, FASHP

Institute for Safe Medication Practices
Huntingdon Valley, Pa.

Pediatrics ranks second only to internal medicine as the medical specialty that is most frequently involved in legal actions resulting from drug-related events.[1] Few published reports, however, provide specific information about drug errors in pediatric patients.[2,3] A review of those that do provide such information reveals that certain drug categories tend to be implicated in errant medication orders in pediatrics. These include antibiotics, theophylline, digoxin, fluids and electrolytes (including total parenteral nutrition solutions), analgesics, and chemotherapeutic agents.[4]

Drug treatment of the pediatric population has always been a challenge. Until the last 15 to 20 years, drug dosages for children were usually based on a ratio of an adult dose, according to the child's age, weight, or body surface area.[5] There was no regard for the differences in maturational changes in body fat composition, renal and hepatic function, and drug absorption among pediatric patients—variables that require individualization of drug dosing based on factors such as status of prematurity, age, and weight.[5-7] Pharmacokinetic and pharmacodynamic differences between adults and children are often overlooked when medications are prescribed unless the health care professional has received specialized training and experience in pediatrics.

*At the time that this chapter was written, Dr. D'Antonio was serving as the Marsam Fellow at the Institute for Safe Medication Practices and the Center for Proper Medication Use.

There is little published dosing and monitoring information for many drugs used in the treatment of pediatric patients. The results can be tragic. For example, five deaths from overdoses of chloral hydrate syrup have been reported in pediatric patients, and all have been associated with a lack of familiarity with the drug and with pediatric dosing guidelines. In two cases, overdoses were given by technical support personnel who were unauthorized to administer the medication. Because of a lack of training and experience, they did not recognize that the dose was incorrect. In the third case, a dentist ordered too much of the medication, prescribing 12 teaspoons of 500 mg/mL syrup (6 g; maximum dose is supposed to be 2 g per 24 hours) on the basis of a 13-year-old child's weight of 150 pounds (75 mg/kg x 70 kg = 5.25 g). In the last two cases, overdoses were administered to the children by their parents at home.

Confusion at the pharmacy led to these errors. One child received chloral hydrate syrup (500 mg/5 mL) instead of the prescribed concentration of 250 mg/5 mL. The dose was prescribed by volume and the concentration was not noted, which made detection of the error impossible. The other child received 120 mL, instead of the intended 12 mL, of the chloral hydrate syrup. The pharmacy dispensed a 4-ounce bottle, even though only 12 mL was needed. The mother gave the child the entire bottle.

Drug products themselves may have deficiencies that can lead to problems in young patients. These include lack of suitable formulations and dosage forms, lack of desirable concentrations and strengths, and the presence of unlabeled or undesirable ingredients. In 1990, a Pennsylvania hospital reported that three premature neonates died after receiving erroneous injections of potassium chloride. This error originated in the sterile-products area of the pharmacy and involved a mix-up between look-alike vials of potassium chloride and an extemporaneously prepared dilute heparin solution. The pharmacy was preparing the heparin because of a lack of commercially available formulations for use in flushing intravenous lines of infants.

Many of today's drug products also lack pediatric indications and dosage guidelines.[6,8,9] The absence of one or more of these factors increases the risk of medication errors. The thalidomide disaster of the early 1960s, the "gray-baby" syndrome associated with chloramphenicol, and the deposition of tetracycline in the teeth and bones of children can all be traced to a lack of information about the effect of these drugs in the pediatric population at the time of the marketing of these drugs.

Pediatric pharmacology and drug dosing have evolved as a result of problems that have been reported when drugs have been used in children and infants without regard to the pharmacokinetic and pharmacodynamic differences between pediatric patients and adults and among pediatric patients. The U.S. government has taken measures to support this trend. For example, the Kefauver-Harris Act of 1962 mandated that approval of a drug by the Food and Drug Administration (FDA) for use in children must be contingent on evidence that the drug is safe and effective in the pediatric population.

Nonetheless, progress has not been as rapid as some might hope. In 1968, the noted pharmacist-pediatrician Harry Shirkey emphasized the limited amount of data available to support individualized dosing in children.[6,10] He noted that "by an odd and unfortunate twist of fate, infants and children are becoming therapeutic or pharmaceutical orphans."[10]

In 1994, the FDA strengthened its position on pediatric-specific drug recommendations by enacting regulations requiring that the pharmaceutical industry provide more pediatric dosage information and prescribing guidelines on product labels and package inserts. As former FDA Commissioner David Kessler, a pediatrician, has noted, "Children are not miniature adults; you cannot simply calculate a pediatric dose based on the dose that is safe and effective in an adult."[11]

Medication errors—those in which a patient is given an inappropriate drug or a drug at the wrong dose or frequency or via an incorrect route—have also contributed to adverse events in children and infants.[8,9,12] The errors most frequently recognized in association with pediatric drug therapy include computation errors of dosage and dosing interval, errors in drug orders (including written instructions and interpretation), and errors in drug preparation or conflicts with prescribed dosages.[8] Dosing and administration errors may occur because an appropriate drug concentration for the pediatric population is not commercially available or because medications are incorrectly measured. Infants and most children depend on an adult caregiver to administer medications; this individual may or may not be familiar with how to properly administer the medication.[6,12]

Pediatric Formulations, Dosage Forms, and Concentrations

Health care professionals are often unable to prepare and administer the appropriate dose of a medication needed for a pediatric dosage from a commercially available formulation.[3,8] For example, the inability of small children to swallow tablets or capsules may render some commercial preparations unusable.

Consequently, doses for pediatric patients are often altered. Tablets may be crushed, capsules may be opened and their contents added to food (e.g., applesauce or ice cream) or beverages (e.g., juices, formula, or soda). These situations increase the potential for solubility and bioavailability problems.[2,3,8] Unfortunately, many dosage forms, such as tablets, capsules, patches, and sustained-release products, cannot be reformulated into dosage forms that are suitable for infants and children. Even if reformulation were possible, problems might arise from the lack of information about product stability, sterility, and bioavailability, not to mention the lack of prescribing guidelines for children.

Much of the reason for the lack of pediatric formulations and dosing guidelines stems from economic considerations. If the anticipated market for a drug or dosage form used in the pediatric population is limited, the industry has little incentive to develop the product.[8] This is unfortunate, because the new formulations would decrease the potential for errors associated with cutting or diluting an adult dose in order to administer it to a child or infant.

Even when manufacturers produce both adult and pediatric concentrations (e.g., Tylenol® and Lanoxin®), there is still potential for errors. The pediatric and adult products are commonly stored next to each other in pharmacies or on shelves. If the pharmacist or customer does not read the package label, he or she may choose the wrong concentration of the drug.

Many of the drugs available as liquids for oral use or parenteral administration lack concentrations that are suitable for the small volumes required for pediatric patients. Volumes that are too small to measure accurately (even in a 1-mL tuberculin syringe) must be diluted before they are administered. Unless an appropriate dilution technique is used, serious errors may occur.[8] Pharmacists often use a technique requiring a premeasured amount of concentrated drug to be transferred to a mixing vial or container, where the appropriate diluent is added. The resulting drug concentration is then used to administer the prescribed drug dose accurately.

Inactive Ingredients

Inactive ingredients, such as benzyl alcohol, phenol, ethanol, sucrose, dyes, and surfactants, may affect the stability, sterility, palatability, and even the appearance, of a drug product. These additives have been associated with adverse effects such as intraventricular hemorrhage, arrhythmias, and seizures. Benzyl alcohol has been associated with "gasping syndrome" in neonates. Prolonged use of products containing phenol can cause accumulation of toxic metabolites.

Ethanol can accumulate in pediatric patients to the level of intoxication. This drug can also produce a disulfiram-like reaction when it is taken in combination with metronidazole. The American Academy of Pediatrics recommends that the ethanol content of nonprescription drugs be no greater than 5% by volume. A prescribed dose should not produce a blood alcohol level of greater than 25 mg/dL. An appropriate dosing interval should be selected to prevent alcohol accumulation.[13]

Measuring Devices

Parents of sick children are often anxious and sleep deprived. Children are sick and irritable; they may also be apprehensive and unwilling to take their medication.[14] The lack of convenient measuring devices, as well as of dosage forms, may complicate the already difficult situation of safely administering medication to a child.

Droppers, cylindrical spoons, oral dosing syringes, medication cups, and small-volume dosers with attachable nipples can be used to administer medications to children, provided that caregivers are familiar with the function of these devices and understand the differences in their calibration.[14] Nonetheless, errors are reported with the use of these devices because of an adult's unfamiliarity with the calibrations and volume equivalents. For example, a mother inadvertently gave her child a fivefold overdose of children's acetaminophen elixir (640 mg instead of 120 mg) because she thought that the cup included with the product held one dose.[15]

When using oral dosage syringes, parents should be cautioned to remove the syringe caps before drawing fluid into the syringe or forcing fluid into the child's mouth. Caps have popped off into the child's throat, causing asphyxiation.

Oral liquids are generally prescribed as a fraction of a teaspoon; however, measuring devices may express calibrations in terms of milliliters (mL), cubic centimeters (cc), fractions of teaspoons, and, in some cases, combinations of all three. Increments of calibration vary from one measuring device to another. For example, a 1-mL oral syringe is calibrated in increments of 0.1 mL, whereas the calibration of a 5-mL syringe is in 0.2-mL increments.

Houseware manufacturers do not intend for their equipment to be used for medication dosing, but the occurrence is commonplace and has led to dosing errors in infants and children.[16] The volume of a standard household teaspoon, for example, ranges from 3 mL to 6 mL. Measuring spoons are likewise unsatisfactory. For example, EKCO Housewares, Inc. (Franklin

Park, Ill.), manufactures measuring-spoon sets sold in supermarkets and variety stores. The stainless-steel spoon set (no. 00412) has a one-quarter-teaspoon size that is also marked 1 mL. If 5 mL is considered one teaspoon, a child who is supposed to take one-quarter teaspoon of a liquid medication would receive a 20% underdose if the 1 ml marking is correct. However, if that spoon indeed contained one-quarter teaspoon, a 25% overdose would result if the prescriber intended the child to receive 1 mL. EKCO also manufactures a plastic measuring spoon set (no. 00400). The one-quarter teaspoon is marked "1.2 mL." In both cases, if the spoon is filled to the point of meniscus stability, it will contain even more liquid than intended. Although it is difficult to transfer the entire amount without spilling, a child could still receive a significant overdose.

Calculations

All health care professionals who work with children are aware of the risks posed by dose miscalculations. Because of the nature of drugs used in pediatric patients, even simple computation errors may have harmful effects.

Dosages of medications for infants and children may be calculated on the basis of age, status of prematurity, weight, and body surface area (height and weight). Unlike adults, dosage calculations for children are a standard of practice for the pediatric population (defined as children aged ≤12 years and weighing ≤40 kg). To reduce the potential for error, prescribers should indicate the actual patient weight and the calculated dose, as well as the dose per weight or body surface area, on the medication order. For example, a dose of amoxicillin for a 15-kg pediatric patient should be written as amoxicillin "250 mg (50 mg/kg/day) orally every 8 hours." Pediatric patients should be weighed at least every other day to ensure the accuracy of the drug dose.

Perlstein et al.[17] reported that 1 of every 12 dosages calculated by 95 registered nurses in a neonatal intensive care unit contained errors that would result in the administration of doses 10 times larger or smaller than the prescribed dose. Eleven pediatricians made errors at the rate of 1 of every 26 computations attempted. Five pharmacists demonstrated far better computational skills than either the nurses or the physicians.[8,17]

Koren et al.[18,19] described several situations involving major dosage calculation errors. They reported up to 10-fold errors in the administration of drug doses to pediatric patients, including neonates. The drugs included phenobarbital, pancuronium, digoxin, aminophylline, atropine, and gentamicin. The consequences of these errors included coma, respiratory failure, cardiac arrest and tachycardia, and transient renal failure.[17] The most frequent computational error was a misplaced decimal point. The second most frequent set of errors was associated with careless and unclear writing that led to misinterpretation of the order. This risk may be minimized with the use of peer-reviewed, preprinted order sheets and standardized dosing for medication ordering. Communication between physicians, nurses, and pharmacists will also benefit from the use of these order sheets.

Another type of computation error may occur during the preparation of a nonstandard strength or concentration of a medication.[17] Usually the pharmacy prepares a dilution from the adult medication to a concentration that can be accurately measured for administration to a pediatric patient. If the weight or volume of the portion of adult medication is not appropriately calculated, the resulting concentration may lead to an overdose or underdose.

Problems with drug calculations exist partly because of an inability of health care professionals to accurately calculate the amount needed to initiate a drug order or a failure to question the appropriateness of an order. One solution would be to require certification of the computational capabilities of all health care personnel who dispense or administer the drugs. Another would be to implement a system of independent checks (pharmacists, physicians, and nurses) for all pediatric dosages.[8,17,18] Whenever possible, an institution should also standardize all pediatric drug dosages.

Preventing Pediatric Medication Errors

The most effective means of reducing errors is prevention. Only those health care personnel who have been educated in pediatric medicine and who are familiar with pediatric dosages should order, dispense, and administer these products. All dosages and routes of administration should be double-checked by two health care professionals. Attention should be focused on the possibility of calculation error, decimal error, and concentration error of solutions for oral or parenteral use in pediatric patients.

Doses of medications intended for children should be calculated on the basis of the patient's weight. The age, birth date (if less than 1 year), weight, height, and body surface area of an infant or child should be documented on the patient's profile and admission record. Up-to-date references such as the *Pediatric Dosage Handbook* and the *Harriet Lane Handbook* should be used by all health care personnel involved with infants and children. Finally, caregivers and older pediatric patients should be educated about their medications and taught how to use pediatric measuring devices and how to interpret their calibrations. The Institute for Safe Medication Practices and the Pediatric Pharmacy Administrative Group have published guidelines for preventing medication errors in pediatric patients.[5]

•••• *References*

1. Mill DH (ed). *Report on the Medical Insurance Feasibility Study*. San Francisco, Calif: Sutter Publications; 1977.

2. Nahata MC. Paediatric drug therapy II: drug administration errors. *J Clin Pharm Ther*. 1988; 13: 399–402.

3. Rosati JR, Nahata MC. Drug administration errors in pediatric patients. *Quarterly Review of Biology*. 1983; 9: 212–13.

4. Folli HL, Poole RL, Benitz WE, et al. Medication error prevention by clinical pharmacists in two children's hospitals. *Pediatrics*. 1987; 79: 718–22.

5. Cohen MR, Blanchard N, Federico F, et al. Draft guidelines for preventing medication errors in pediatrics. *J Pediatr Pharm Pract*. 1998; 3: 189–202.

6. Skaer TL. Dosing considerations in the pediatric patient. *Clin Ther*. 1991; 13: 526–44.

7. Nykamp D. Nonprescription medications in the pediatric population. *American Pharmacy*. 1995; NS35: 11–27.

8. Leff RD, Roberts RJ. Problems in drug therapy for pediatric patients. *Am J Hosp Pharm*. 1987; 44: 865–70.

9. Galinsky RE, Nickman NA. Pharmacists and the mandate of pharmaceutical care. *Drug Intelligence and Clinical Pharmacy*. 1991; 21: 431–34.

10. Shirkey HC. Therapeutic orphans (editorial). *J Pediatr*. 1968; 72: 119–20.

11. Conlan MF. FDA lays down new rules on pediatric dosing. *Drug Topics*. 1995; 139: 68.

12. Jonville APE, Autret E, Bavoux F, et al. Characteristics of medication errors in pediatrics. *Drug Intelligence and Clinical Pharmacy*. 1991; 25: 1113–16.

13. American Academy of Pediatrics, Committee on Drugs. Ethanol in liquid preparations intended for children. *Pediatrics*. 1984; 73: 405–07.

14. Chater RW. Pediatric dosing: tips for tots. *American Pharmacy*. 1993; NS33(5): 55–56.

15. Institute for Safe Medication Practices. Safety briefs. *ISMP Medication Safety Alert!* April 9, 1997; 2: 1.

16. Institute for Safe Medication Practices. Safety briefs. *ISMP Medication Safety Alert!* February 26, 1997; 2: 1.

17. Perlstein PH, Callison C, White M, et al. Errors in drug computations during newborn intensive care. *Am J Dis Child*. 1979; 133: 376–77.

18. Koren G, Barzilay Z, Greenwald M. Tenfold errors in administration of drug doses: a neglected iatrogenic disease in pediatrics. *Pediatrics*. 1986; 77: 848–49.

19. Koren G, Barzilay Z, Modan M. Errors in computing drug doses. *Can Med Assoc J*. 1983; 129: 721–24.

17.

Recognizing and Preventing Errors Involving Immunologic Drugs

John D. Grabenstein, PhD, FASHP

U.S. Army Medical Department
University of North Carolina
Chapel Hill, N.C.

Michael R. Cohen, MS, FASHP
Susan M. Proulx, PharmD

Institute for Safe Medication Practices
Huntingdon Valley, Pa.

Vaccines, antibodies, and other immunologic drugs are no more or less likely to be involved in medication errors than are other drugs. Nonetheless, it is instructive to consider this subset of medications and to illustrate how errors can be anticipated and prevented. It is also important to consider the unique consequences of errors with immunologic medications.

Categories of Medication Errors

Medication errors are systemic in nature and can thus be categorized on this basis. This review of errors with immunologic products is based on the system categories summarized in Table 17–1 and discussed in greater detail in Chapter 20. A single error can involve the failure of multiple features of the drug delivery system, as illustrated in the examples that follow.

This chapter was modified, with permission, from Grabenstein JD, Proulx SM, Cohen MR. Recognizing and preventing errors involving immunologic drugs. *Hospital Pharmacy.* 1996; 31: 791–94, 799, 803–04.

The opinions or assertions contained herein are the private views of the authors and are not to be construed as official or reflecting the views of the U.S. Department of the Army or the Department of Defense.

Table 17-1

Categories of Medication Error

Type of Error	Examples
Manufacturer drug labeling, packaging, nomenclature, and advertising	Misinterpretation, incorrect product selection
Communication dynamics	Misinterpreted abbreviation, poor handwriting, misunderstood verbal (spoken) order
Lack of complete patient information	———
Drug preparation, compounding, or manufacturing	Incorrect measurement or product selection
Drug stock and storage	Misfilled machine, incorrect product selection, inadequate checks and balances
Staffing and environmental stressors	Inadequate staff, personnel turnover, stress, poor lighting, interruptions and distractions
Drug administration	Patient misidentification, wrong route of administration
Competency validation and staff education and knowledge	Inadequate training
Automated order processing	Failure to double-check order before dispensing, ambiguous mnemonics, inability of computer to signal excessive doses
Formulary	Lack of protocols for new formulary items
Quality assurance	Failure to encourage exchange of ideas about patient safety, failure to correct system problems known to occur at one's own site or elsewhere
Patient education	Misunderstanding of drug name, purpose, dose, regimen, or injection technique

Manufacturer Drug Labeling, Packaging, Nomenclature, and Advertising

On several occasions, pediatric-strength diphtheria–tetanus toxoid (DT) has been confused with adult-strength tetanus–diphtheria toxoid (Td). Td contains a lower dose of diphtheria toxoid than does DT. The upper- and lowercase D's in the acronyms are intended to reflect the relative dose, even though the doses are inversely proportional to age. (Adults receive a lower dose of diphtheria toxoid to avoid reactions at the injection site.) These mix-ups occur because the names of the products are similar and because the wording and type styles on the labels do not clearly distinguish the two products.

Another source of error (i.e., a knowledge system error) may occur when a health care worker does not realize that two different products are available. The consequences of this error are a painful arm for the adult given a DT injection or inadequate protection for the child given Td.[1]

In a related error, Td was inappropriately injected intradermally by a nurse who mistook the Td vial for purified protein derivative (PPD) of tuberculin for skin testing. The patients developed indurations ranging from 30 mm to 60 mm in diameter. Eventually, they were prescribed isoniazid. The diagnosis of tuberculosis was questioned, and tuberculin tests were reapplied. Results were negative. Inquiry revealed that the office stored Td and PPD on the same shelf in the refrigerator and that the packages were quite similar in appearance.

The wrong vaccines have also been given when health care workers have confused the vaccine against measles with that against German measles because of similarity between the two names. Alternative terms for these diseases (rubeola and rubella, respectively) are also quite similar. One solution is to encourage the use of the official titles of these two vaccines (i.e., measles and rubella). The consequence of this error is vulnerability to the disease against which one is not vaccinated.

Examples of other hazards posed by similar names include the series of hyperimmune globulins distributed by Bayer Corporation (Bayer Pharmaceutical Division, Biological Products, West Haven, Conn.) (i.e., BayHep B™, BayRab™, BayRho-D™, and BayTet™).[2,3]

Tripedia® diphtheria–tetanus–acellular pertussis vaccine (Pasteur Mérieux Connaught, Swiftwater, Pa.) can be used as the diluent for the powdered ActHIB® brand of *Haemophilus influenzae* type b (Hib) vaccine for patients of certain ages. The combination of Tripedia® and ActHIB® is marketed under the trade name TriHIBit®. TriHIBit® may be confused with ProHIBiT®,

a different brand of Hib vaccine, even though the combination of Tripedia®
and ActHIB® has nothing to do with ProHIBiT.

Communication Dynamics

Vaccines have been developed for a number of viruses that have sound-
alike and look-alike names: varicella and vaccinia, hepatitis A and hepatitis B, Hib and viral influenza, and Hib and hepatitis B. These names can be
confused in verbal (i.e., spoken) as well as in written communications.
Vaccinating someone who is already immune is generally harmless,
although local side effects at the injection site can occur in immune persons
given certain vaccines, such as those for tetanus and pneumococcus.[2,4]

Merck & Co. (West Point, Pa.) now distributes Comvax®, a combination vaccine against Hib and hepatitis B virus. Under no circumstances should this
vaccine be informally called the "H & H" vaccine, because when the
Twinrix™ form of hepatitis A–hepatitis B vaccine (SmithKline Beecham
Pharmaceuticals, Philadelphia, Pa.) is approved, it, too, could be referred to
as an "H & H" vaccine. Similarly, once Twinrix™ is licensed, one should
resist the temptation of calling it the "A & B" vaccine, because it may then
be confused with the influenza vaccine whose label reads "Influenza Virus
Vaccine, Trivalent, Types A & B."

Suffixes are a special source of confusion when a product is being dispensed. For example, an error occurred when a supply system inadvertently sent Imovax Rabies I.D. Vaccine® (a pre-exposure rabies vaccine) instead
of Imovax Rabies Vaccine® (a pre- and post-exposure vaccine). The error
was not caught until the patient received pre-exposure–only vaccine for two
of the five doses. Luckily, the patient suffered no ill effects. Early proprietary
names for some monoclonal antibodies varied only in their suffixes, even
though the products had drastically different uses.[2]

The brand-name suffixes -mune and -gam have traditionally referred only
to vaccines and hyperimmune antibodies, respectively, manufactured by
Lederle Laboratories (Philadelphia, Pa.). Two new, recently named products
may cause confusion, however: Viramune® is Roxane Laboratories'
(Columbus, Ohio) brand of nevirapine, a reverse transcriptase inhibitor
used in the treatment of human immunodeficiency (HIV) disease; and
Zagam® is Rhône-Poulenc Rorer's (Collegeville, Pa.) brand of sparfloxacin,
a quinolone antibiotic.

Abbreviations are also a major source of medication errors.[5,6] Because so
many vaccines are identified by their abbreviations, the potential for error
when mnemonics are used for their names is great. DTP is commonly understood to refer to diphtheria–tetanus–pertussis vaccine, but in some practice

sites it is used as shorthand for a sedative cocktail of Demerol®, Thorazine®, and Phenergan®. Several children for whom the sedative mixture was prescribed have been vaccinated instead. "MR" is another ambiguous abbreviation. To some, it means measles–rubella vaccine (as in Merck's M-R-VAX IIV®); to others, it means mumps–rubella vaccine (as in Merck's Biavax II®). It is the prescriber's responsibility to make his or her intention clear.

In France and French-speaking parts of Canada, the abbreviation "DTP" refers to *vaccin diphtérique-tétanique-poliomyélitique*, or diphtheria-tetanus-poliomyelitis vaccine, whereas in English-speaking areas this abbreviation refers to diphtheria-tetanus-pertussis vaccine. In Francophone areas, "diphtheria-tetanus-pertussis vaccine" is abbreviated "DCT" (*diphtérique-coqueluceux-tétanique*). In German-speaking countries, "typhus vaccine" refers to a vaccine against *Salmonella typhi*, the cause of typhoid fever, not to one against *Rickettsia prowazekii*, the cause of epidemic typhus.

Table 17–2 lists look-alike and sound-alike proprietary names. Some of these names have been trademarked in anticipation of approval by the Food and Drug Administration (FDA).

Other sources of error stem from poor handwriting. Using abbreviations such as "U" for units has led to overdoses when the U was mistaken for the numeral zero (0) or four (4). The word "units" should never be abbreviated. Trailing zeroes after a decimal point have led to 10-fold overdoses. To prevent this error, one should write "4 mg," not "4.0 mg"; in this way, there is less possibility that the number will be misinterpreted as "40." On the other hand, a zero should always precede a decimal point for amounts less than one (e.g., write "0.2 mL," not ".2 mL").

Verbal (i.e., spoken) orders should be discouraged. If such an order must be taken, it should always be repeated for clarification. Numbers in the teens (e.g., 16) should be repeated as "one-six" to avoid confusion with the number 60, and so forth. Another technique is to imitate the technique used to confirm orders by ship captains: One person says, "Set heading 123," and the other responds, "Heading set 123, aye."

Patient Information

Nearly all children need immunization with the DTP vaccine. A few children who have had a serious side effect to DTP vaccine, however, should not receive the pertussis vaccine component but instead should be immunized with pediatric-strength DT. It is altogether possible that some children have received DTP rather than DT vaccine because the person giving the vaccine was uninformed of a prior adverse event. Failure to communicate can occur when pediatricians refer patients to local health departments for immuniza-

Table 17-2
Sound-alike and look-alike vaccines and other drugs
Acel-Imune®, Acelluvax™[a], Actacel™, Actimmune[b]
ActHIB®, ActHIB®–DTP
Alferon N®, Alkeran®, Imferon[b], interferon
Candin, Cantil®[b], Vantin®[b]
Combivax™, Recombivax HB®
Engerix-B®, Infanrix™, Twinrix™
Flu-Imune, Pnu-Imune®
Imogam®, Imovax®, Imovax® Rabies I.D.®
Ipol®, Opol™, Optipol™, Pediopol™, Poliovax[b]
Leukeran®, Leukine®, Prokine, Proleukin®[b]
Neupogen®, Pnu-Imune®
Pentacel™, Pentasure™
Tetracel™, Tetramune
Tine Test PPD®, T.R.U.E. Test®[b]
Tri-Immunol, Tripedia®
Varicella immune globulin, varicella-zoster immune globulin

[a] TM = trademarked, but not licensed, in the United States as of January 1998.
[b] Product vastly different from others listed.

tion, when charts are not marked adequately, when patients and parents are not queried about previous adverse reactions, or when clinicians do not make efforts to identify valid adverse events after immunization.

Drug Preparation, Compounding, and Manufacturing

The most commonly reported errors with immunologic drugs are probably those involving dose measurements, compounding, and manufacturing procedures. Although overdoses are most common, underdoses have also occurred.

The agent most often associated with error may be hepatitis B vaccine, for which a wide variety of doses are recommended, depending on the patient's age and the brand of vaccine to be administered. Two products are available, and both are equally safe and effective when administered according to product labeling, even though the doses are different.[2] When the wrong vaccine was inadvertently administered at one hospital, some 1400 newborns were left vulnerable to hepatitis B over a 2-year period because they received an amount that was correct for one of the products but only half of the amount that should have been given for the new product. Investigation revealed that one reason for the error was that the institution's preprinted order forms had not been updated to reflect the new volume after the hospital changed from one brand to the other. As a corrective measure, the pharmacy decided to dispense prefilled single-dose syringes. It also expanded its educational programs.[7]

Another potential error stems from use of informal terminology for different concentrations of PPD of tuberculin. The slang terms *first, intermediate,* and *second strength* have been used to describe the concentrations of 1, 5, and 250 tuberculin units (TU) per 0.1 mL, respectively. These imprecise terms can lead to a significant error. Too high a dose can lead to severe cutaneous reactions. Tuberculin products should always be described by numerical concentration. Few pharmacies need to routinely stock 1-TU and 250-TU PPD. These concentrations can be procured only when patients needing them have been identified by name.

The complexity of products and schedules for Hib vaccines also presents opportunities for error. Health care workers are often accustomed to obtaining most vaccines from a single manufacturer. Occasionally, prophylactically equivalent vaccines or immunoglobulins are available from a short list of manufacturers; these are accompanied by comparable instructions for their use.

The existence of four inequivalent Hib vaccines presents a different situation, namely, one disease for which there are four available but unique vaccines used on three different schedules. If an institution believes that confusion over the four vaccines poses possible harm to patients, it might decide to color code the labels and vial caps. A similar practice has been used to distinguish the different strengths of dopamine injection, and at one time, different colors were used for various concentrations of insulin. Relying on color is not, however, a panacea. Many errors occur even when the products have different-colored packaging.

An entry on an electronic bulletin board recounted an instance in which health professionals misinterpreted the package inserts for two forms of lyophilized Hib vaccine powder, OmniHIB™ (SmithKline Beecham) and ActHIB™ (Pasteur-Mérieux-Connaught). They misconstrued the following phrase:

> *Haemophilus b Conjugate Vaccine (Tetanus Toxoid Conjugate)–OmniHIB™ (distributed by SmithKline Beecham Pharmaceuticals) is identical to Haemophilus b Conjugate Vaccine (Tetanus Toxoid Conjugate)– ActHIB™....*[8]

The phrase was misinterpreted to mean that the complete packages were identical. In fact, OmniHIB™ powder is distributed with a saline-based diluent, whereas ActHIB™ powder is distributed with fluid DTP vaccine under the name "ActHIB™/DTP." When these professionals administered OmniHIB™, they thought they were protecting their patients against four diseases; in reality, they were giving only Hib vaccine. After this error was discovered, many children had to be recalled for additional immunizations.

Manufacturers of some biotechnology products have used different potency measurement systems at various times in the "life cycles" of these medications. For example, the current international standard of potency for interferon beta-1b (Betaseron®; Berlex Laboratories, Wayne, N.J.) supersedes a standard developed by the National Institutes of Health (NIH) for native interferon beta. Doses of 1.6 million international units (IU) and 8 million IU in the international system are equivalent to 9 million IU and 45 million IU, respectively, in the NIH system. For aldesleukin (Proleukin®; Chiron Therapeutics, Emeryville, Calif.), the labeling refers to IU, but two other potency systems have been used. One Roche unit is approximately equivalent to 3 IU; one Cetus unit is approximately equivalent to 6 IU. For botulinum toxin, several potency systems are in use.[9] Each of these distinctions poses an opportunity for a dosage error.

Two children with leukemia developed BCG (bacillus Calmette-Guérin)-associated meningitis, possibly as a result of a pharmacy compounding error. Neither child had been given BCG as therapy and neither had ever been vaccinated with BCG. One explanation is that BCG bacteria contaminated a container of methotrexate in the chemotherapy compounding area. When the methotrexate was administered intrathecally, the BCG may have been introduced across the blood-brain barrier. Extensive review of pharmacy techniques failed to identify any means by which contamination might have occurred, but genomic DNA from the vaccine strain matched BCG bacteria found in the patients' cerebrospinal fluid. The hospital in question now has designated one compounding area solely for the preparation of BCG.[10]

Allergen extracts and Hymenoptera venoms are initially administered at extremely low doses. Therapy continues with progressively higher doses. If a patient is challenged with too high a dose too soon, the results may be fatal. Double-check systems are essential at each step in the compounding process to minimize transcription errors, inaccurate calculations or measurements, and transposition of vials or labels.[2,11,12]

Vaccines have been adulterated when vials were contaminated or needles or syringes were reused. For example, DTP and measles vaccine vials have been contaminated with streptococci and staphylococci. Transmission of hepatitis B virus or HIV in this manner is also of concern.[13-15]

Meticulous technique is essential when conducting mass influenza vaccination programs. Health system vaccine practices should be closely regulated and inspected. In 1997, the medical director of Monroe, Conn., resigned after administering adulterated vaccines to 468 people. He used fresh needles when preparing doses of the vaccine from multiple-dose vials but did not always change syringes between patients. Therefore, blood was aspirated into a syringe with one of the patient's injections, and it may have contaminated a second patient. The doctor claimed that he was unaware that the method he used was improper.

This incident is one of several indicating a lack of awareness both of the risk of medication errors and of appropriate infection control procedures during vaccination programs. A 1993 report from the Centers for Disease Control and Prevention (CDC) described physicians in Washington, D.C., and Bucks County, Pa., who injected patients and drew up the next patient's dose with the same needle.[14] Although they changed the needle before injecting the next patient, the vial may have been contaminated.

Drug Stock and Storage

If adult-strength Td is prescribed but DTP is delivered, the error is in the drug distribution system. Was there no Td on hand? Were both products stored in the refrigerator but in the wrong locations? Did the person who took the DTP out of the proper bin in the refrigerator not understand the distinction between the products? A related case involved the administration of Hib vaccine that was inadvertently stored in the location designated for measles-mumps-rubella vaccine. The way to prevent errors of this sort lies in changing the purchasing, environment, or education process.

In another case, health care workers selected the neuromuscular blocker pancuronium instead of influenza vaccine from the refrigerator. This error was repeated dozens of times before being discovered. Fortunately, no harm came to the patients, who had been given the 0.5-mL dose of pancuronium. The facts that the labels were similar in color and the vials similar in shape contributed to this error. Several instances of using pancuronium or succinylcholine to reconstitute vaccine powders have been reported.[15]

In this phenomenon, called "confirmation bias," the practitioner relies on familiar evidence (e.g., the color or shape of the vial) and ignores contrary evidence (e.g., the name on the container). Health care professionals can reduce errors of this type by repeating to themselves the name of the drug as they prepare to select it ("I need 0.5 mL of adult Td") and then reading the container label ("I see 0.5 mL of adult-strength Td in my hand").[4,16,17]

Another way to avoid the pancuronium mistake is to restrict its availability. Neuromuscular blocking agents should not be easily accessible. They should be stored in a separate location, away from other medications. A clearly visible warning label (e.g., "Warning! Paralyzing agent!") may also be affixed to the package.

Several cases have been reported of inadvertent administration of veterinary vaccines to humans. A teenager ingested live Newcastle disease vaccine intended for immunization of chickens. After induced catharsis, the patient remained asymptomatic and did not seroconvert. In another instance, a woman was exposed to infectious bursal disease vaccine intended for chickens. Her exposure consisted of skin contact and inhalation of aerosolized vaccine. Her symptoms were treated and she recovered. Other cases have been reported; the common element in all of them was inappropriate handling of the vaccines.[18]

In Yemen, insulin was dispensed instead of BCG vaccine during a government-sponsored tuberculosis prevention campaign.[19] Twenty-one children died. Apparently, a medical worker sent insulin instead of vaccine to the site at which the vaccinations were administered. Quality assurance measures are an essential element of every step of mass vaccination programs, because a single error can affect many people.

Staffing and Environmental Stressors

A recent confidential report concerned two employees reporting to the occupational health clinic. One was to be vaccinated against hepatitis B virus, and the other was to be immunized with Td. Both received hepatitis B vaccine. No reason for the error was reported; however, this error could well have been caused by a telephone call or a visitor distracting the clinic nurse. Alternatively, it may have resulted from a lapse in attention, from stress, or from miscommunication.[20]

Intradermal injections are difficult to administer. Personnel turnover or inadequate staffing can place health care workers in a situation where they are called on to give injections they have not been adequately trained to give. Other environmental factors that contribute to medication errors include poor lighting, interruptions, distractions, and stress.

Drug Administration

Questions frequently arise about the consequences of inadvertently administering an intramuscular vaccine by the subcutaneous route. Subcutaneous injections are generally absorbed more slowly than an equivalent volume of intramuscular vaccine. This may result in reduced antibody titers.[2] Revaccination is usually not warranted.

A related case involves an intradermal injection that is actually delivered subcutaneously. Hepatitis B vaccine, for example, is effective intradermally at a lower dose than that of intramuscular administration.[21,22] CDC does not recommend its use in this way because of concerns about improper vaccination technique.

The U.S. Pharmacopeia (USP) Drug Product Quality Review Program reported a case in which oral attenuated poliovirus vaccine was injected intramuscularly. No harm came to the vaccinee, but the proper dose was delayed. In other cases, BCG vaccine intended for scarification was injected intradermally. Similar packaging and labeling may have contributed to these errors.[23,24]

Competency Validation and Staff Education

The various formulations of DTP, DT, and Td are discussed earlier in this chapter. Monovalent tetanus toxoid is also manufactured in two forms, fluid and adsorbed.[2] If a health care worker does not understand the differences between these drugs or is unaware even that two forms exist, he or she cannot prevent an error that originates in some other area of the drug delivery system.

At least seven pregnant women have been given varicella vaccine instead of varicella-zoster immune globulin.[25] Mistakes such as this are more likely when new drugs are first introduced, such as following the licensing of the varicella vaccine in 1995.[2]

Mumps skin test antigen (MSTA®; Pasteur-Mérieux-Connaught) and mumps vaccine (Mumpsvax®; Merck) have been repeatedly confused. MSTA® has been administered in a futile attempt at immunization, and mumps vaccine has been given in a fruitless effort to assess cell-mediated immunity. In many cases, these errors result from rapid staff turnover and lack of training. This particular error is abetted by system failures related to nomenclature and distribution.[10]

Automated Order Processing

Computers can help speed delivery of medications to patients and can provide a basis for information retrieval and storage; however, they can also contribute to medication errors. A computer system is only as good as the people who use it. Every order entered into the computer by pharmacists or technicians must be double-checked against the original order before the product is dispensed.

The potential for error is compounded by the use of mnemonics, which is particularly common with immunologic products. These so-called "short codes" can be interpreted in different ways by different people.

Formulary

Control over product selection can deter medication errors. For example, if fluid tetanus toxoid or 250 TU PPD is not kept in stock or is segregated from normal storage locations, errors can be averted. Prefilled syringes should be stocked only if the labels are distinctive. This will help avoid selection errors.

Patient Education

Many errors have been prevented by a well-informed patient or family member. Simply noting the color of an injectable medication (for example, the difference between Intron®, which is clear, and iron dextran [Imferon®], which is brown) may help a patient prevent a serious error at the bedside.

Quality Assurance

Any quality assurance system needs a means of evaluating medication errors and taking action to prevent their recurrence. One important method of ensuring safety—namely, discussing reports of medication errors experienced outside one's own practice site—is often overlooked. The

Institute for Safe Medication Practices, FDA, and USP publish accounts of errors in professional journals and newsletters. A review of external errors should be a routine quality assurance measure at all institutions.

The importance of error reporting cannot be overemphasized. Silent errors pose a serious threat to patient welfare. If they remain undetected, they may affect hundreds of patients. All involved in the medication use process must acknowledge that even the most experienced health care professionals do make errors.[17] Hospitals and other institutions need to create open, guilt-free systems in which preventing errors takes precedence over blaming and punishing employees for errors that have already occurred. Employees must have an opportunity to communicate their error prevention ideas. Regular feedback to staff on errors that have been reported is essential because it maintains the two-way flow of information needed to support risk management efforts.

Implications for Health Care Practitioners

Vaccines are expected to perform minor miracles: to confer immunity for a decade or more. By the same token, the consequences of an error, such as vulnerability to a preventable infection, may also be felt for a long time and, in addition, may be fatal.

Flynn and Barker note in Chapter 6 that at least one medication error occurs for every patient hospitalized on every day. Health professionals who want to avoid medication errors with immunologic agents should be involved in the selection of immunologic agents used at their practice site. They should consider the potential for mix-ups when storing immunologic products, keep up-to-date reference materials for each agent, and educate their colleagues about proper use. Double-checking and independent checking can eliminate many errors.

Maximum use of unit-dose packaging helps reduce errors. The added cost of packaging is far outweighed by increased patient safety. Preprinted forms or computer order sets can help ensure patient safety, but only if they are routinely revised as conditions warrant. The fact that children are more vulnerable to the effects of medication errors than adults must always be borne in mind. Finally, patient counseling is essential in the prevention of errors with immunologic and other drug products.

References

1. Smith G, Norman A, Banks J. Management of school leavers given a diphtheria and tetanus vaccine intended for children instead of the intended low dose preparation. *Commun Dis Rep Rev.* 1997; 7: R67–68.

2. Grabenstein JD. *ImmunoFacts: Vaccines & Immunologic Drugs.* St. Louis, Mo: Facts & Comparisons; 1997.

3. Cohen MR. "Bay" this and "Bay" that. *Hosp Pharm.* 1997; 32: 836.

4. Davis NM, Cohen MR, Teplitsky B. Look-alike and sound-alike drug names: the problem and the solution. *Hosp Pharm.* 1992; 27: 95–98, 102–05, 108–10.

5. Cohen MR. Play it safe. Don't use these abbreviations. *Nursing 87.* July 1987; 17: 46–47.

6. Davis NM. *Medical Abbreviations: 12,000 Conveniences at the Expense of Communications & Safety.* 8th ed. Huntingdon Valley, Pa: Davis Associates; 1997.

7. Cohen MR. Insufficient dose of hepatitis B vaccine given to 1400 newborns; formalin accidents. *Hosp Pharm.* 1995; 30: 938–39.

8. *1998 Physicians' Desk Reference.* Montvale, NJ: Medical Economics; 1998: 2848.

9. Pearce LB, First ER, Borodic GE. Botulinum toxin potency: a mystery resolved by the median paralysis unit. *J R Soc Med.* 1994; 87: 571–72.

10. Stone MM, Vannier AM, Storch SK, et al. Meningitis due to iatrogenic BCG infection in two immunocompromised children. *N Engl J Med.* 1995; 333: 561–63.

11. Grabenstein JD. Allergen-extract compounding by pharmacists. *Hosp Pharm.* 1992; 27: 145, 149–53, 165.

12. Grabenstein JD. Immunotherapy for Hymenoptera insects: bees, wasps, hornets, and fire ants. *Hosp Pharm.* 1992; 27: 883, 887–90, 905.

13. Stetler HC, Garbe PL, Dwyer DM, et al. Outbreaks of group A streptococcal abscesses following diphtheria-tetanus toxoid-pertussis vaccination. *Pediatrics.* 1985; 75: 299–303.

14. Centers for Disease Control and Prevention. Improper infection-control practices during employee vaccination programs—District of Columbia and Pennsylvania, 1993. *MMWR Morb Mortal Wkly Rep.* 1993; 42: 969–71.

15. World Health Organization. Vaccine supply and quality: surveillance of adverse events following immunization. *Wkly Epidemiol Rec.* 1996; 71: 237–42.

16. Cohen MR. Drug product characteristics that foster drug-use-system errors. *Am J Health Syst Pharm.* 1995; 52: 395–99.

17. Cohen MR. To prevent mix-ups, learn to talk to yourself. *Hosp Pharm.* 1996; 31: 184, 187–88.

18. Crosby AD, Geller RJ. Human effects of veterinary biological products. *Vet Hum Toxicol.* 1986; 28: 552–53, 569; 1987; 29: 24.

19. Institute for Safe Medication Practices. *ISMP Medication Safety Alert!* June 4, 1997; Vol 2, No 11.

20. Davis NM, Cohen MR. Sterile cockpit. *American Pharmacy.* 1995; 35 (12): 11.

21. King JW, Taylor EM, Crow SD, et al. Comparison of the immunogenicity of hepatitis B vaccine administered intradermally and intramuscularly. *Rev Infect Dis.* 1990; 12: 1035.

22. Woodruff BA, Moyer LA, Bryan JP, et al. Intradermal vaccination for hepatitis B. *Clin Infect Dis.* 1992; 15: 1063–66.

23. Miles MM, Shaw RJ. Effect of inadvertent intradermal administration of high-dose percutaneous BCG vaccine (letter). *Br Med J.* 1996; 312: 1205.

24. Puliyel JM, Hughes A, Chiswick ML, et al. Adverse local reactions from accidental BCG overdose in infants. *Br Med J.* 1996; 313: 528–29.

25. Centers for Disease Control and Prevention. Unintentional administration of varicella virus vaccine—United States, 1996. *MMWR Morb Mortal Wkly Rep.* 1996; 45: 1017–18.

Part V:

Medication Errors and Risk Management

Medication Error Reporting Systems

Diane DeMichele Cousins, RPh

Vice President for Practitioner Reporting Programs
United States Pharmacopeial Convention, Inc.
Rockville, Md.

Rita Calnan, RPh

Coordinator, Human Drug Programs
United States Pharmacopeial Convention, Inc.
Rockville, Md.

Human beings, by their nature, learn from the experiences of others. Teaching others by our experiences, however, requires us to be willing to share our mistakes as well as our successes. Today, health professionals have shown themselves to be willing to do so. As a result, the national medication errors database created by the U.S. Pharmacopeia (USP) enables thousands of health care practitioners to learn from the experiences, and indeed sometimes the tragedies, of their colleagues.

Not long ago, many health professionals felt embarrassed or ashamed about divulging a medication error. Individuals and facilities became so fearful of legal exposure that there was an unwritten, unspoken, but clearly understood rule: Silence is golden.

Times are changing. We have begun to realize that the admission and open discussion of errors can allow us to better analyze a situation, more appropriately predict behavior, and more safely and reliably design systems and processes. In fact, the North Carolina Board of Pharmacy views reporting as a mitigating factor in its disciplinary hearings (Rule 21 NCAC.2502[m]). In other words, the liability lies in *not* reporting.

The health care community—practitioners and administrators alike—must recognize that both people and systems contribute to medication errors. Reducing the incidence of errors requires changing the way we think. Neither committing nor reporting an error should become the basis for disciplinary or punitive action by an employer. Rather, the focus should be on identifying the error-prone aspects of the medication use continuum—prescribing, ordering, dispensing, administering, and monitoring—with the goal of improving system safety and reliability through remedial action.

Developing internal systems for reporting and tracking errors is a first step toward identifying problems. However, we must not stop there. Contributing to national reporting systems facilitates large-scale tracking and trend analysis that can help office staff in hospitals, nursing homes, pharmacies, and physicians' offices to learn from the experiences of others. National reporting systems can also have a strong impact on the development of practice guidelines, standards for product packaging and labeling, standardized procedures, and fail-safe systems. Ultimately, medication error reporting can also save unnecessary health care expenditures. By preventing the incidence of such errors, reports to a national system can help substantially reduce related medical and hospitalization costs.

National Medication Error Reporting Programs

In the United States today, two national programs collect experiences and observations relative to medication errors: the USP Medication Errors Reporting Program (MERP) and MedWatch, which is operated by the Food and Drug Administration (FDA). The two programs have a common goal: to identify the circumstances in which errors occur and to educate the health professional so that the chances of recurring errors are lessened.

Although USP MERP began only in 1991, the USP has actually administered reporting programs for health professionals since 1971. In addition to USP MERP, current USP programs in this area include the Drug Product Problem Reporting Program, the Drug Product Problem Reporting for Radiopharmaceuticals (operated in cooperation with the Society of Nuclear Medicine), and the Veterinary Practitioners' Reporting Program (operated in cooperation with the American Veterinary Medical Association). These programs are known collectively as the USP Practitioners' Reporting Network.

USP MERP was created in response to requests by Michael Cohen and Neil Davis, who approached USP to help coordinate a MERP that had developed out of monthly features on preventing medication errors that Cohen was publishing in national health care journals. Cohen would later become president of the Institute for Safe Medication Practices (ISMP), currently a cooperating organization in USP MERP.

USP's experience with national programs, its established processing and database operations (including toll-free telephone reporting), and its mechanisms to share information with product manufacturers and the FDA were acknowledged assets for further development of the USP MERP on a national level. USP agreed to coordinate the program.

Through the program, USP hoped to learn of those instances in which a product's design or characteristics may be contributing to an error. This information in turn would enable USP to modify standards and requirements as necessary to help eliminate the potential for such errors. USP also hoped to gain insight about the safer use of medications for inclusion in its USP Drug Information (DI) database.

An early sign of the acceptance of USP MERP by the health care community occurred in 1992, when USP created a new program designed to enable state boards of pharmacy to convey errors filed with the boards. The database of the Board of Pharmacy MERP provides additional insight into problems occurring nationwide.

As the program grew, the need for specialization of roles became evident. USP acquired the program and its database from ISMP in September 1994. In its present role as a cooperating organization of MedWatch as well as USP MERP, ISMP receives copies of all USP reports. It reviews reports submitted to both programs and uses the information to make recommendations, discuss reports with manufacturers, and educate health care providers. ISMP also interacts with the FDA as the occasion warrants.

Although the FDA does not usually assert jurisdiction over practice issues or systems failures, which are often involved in medication errors, it is concerned with issues relating to product nomenclature labeling and packaging. For this reason, USP shares reported information with the FDA, and the USP MERP is a partner in MedWatch.

FDA's Center for Drug Evaluation and Research, Committee on Medication Errors, holds responsibility for evaluating medication error reports. FDA recommendations to companies may include, among other things, avoiding trademarks and packaging that are misleading or confusing, as well as guidance on avoiding look-alike packaging and sound-alike drug names.

USP shares reports of errors in reference books and computer software, as well as errors concerning drugs and medical devices, with the product manufacturer so that appropriate corrections and improvements can be made. All information on medication errors that is received at USP MERP is computerized. In 1998, the USP announced MedMARx, a national database of medication errors for use by hospitals. Reports are submitted anonymously, and the USP has established standardized reporting elements and facility profiles that will make possible comparative analyses and, eventually, the benchmarking of medication errors by participating facilities.

Information from the USP MERP Database

Between 1991 and 1997, 2467 reports were submitted to USP. Of these, 1481 were shown to be actual errors. The remainder were potential errors, which are also regarded as important because of the possibility that they may lead to actual errors.[1] Pharmacists and nurses were most likely to have initiated the reported errors (475 and 332 errors, respectively); physicians were reported to have initiated errors in 267 reports. Pharmacists were more likely than nurses to have intercepted errors (187 and 108, respectively); physicians intercepted 14 errors. These reports underscore an important outcome of reporting: Health professionals who handle the medication order at the earliest point in the process are in a position to benefit from the safety checks of other professionals who follow them in the chain. Physicians are often protected from committing an error that reaches the patient because nurses and pharmacists can intercept it.[2] The information in a national database is important to determine trends. It can indicate a need for additional training, limiting responsibilities of support staff, or designing safety nets or system redundancies into particular areas.

Tracking Trends in Medication Errors

As a result of its data collection and analysis, USP MERP has identified certain medications that are prone to misuse and are the most common causes of errors (see Tables 18–1 through 18–4).

Errors by Drug

Heparin, lidocaine, morphine sulfate, digoxin, and potassium chloride have made the "top 10" list of drug errors nearly every year (Table 18–1). For heparin, two common causes of error were the use of "U" for units (a cause of 10-fold dosing errors) and confusion of the drug with others that have similar packaging and labeling.

Of all reported errors that reached the patient in 1998, 3.6% resulted in fatalities. Lidocaine, potassium chloride, and morphine sulfate are among the most frequently reported drugs to cause fatalities (Table 18–2).

Table 18–3 lists examples of circumstances leading to fatal errors.

Reporting a Medication Error to USP

To report an actual or potential medication error, health care providers or consumers can phone or send a fax to USP (1-800-23-ERROR) or FDA (1-800-FDA-1088) at any time of day.

Electronic access to USP and FDA reporting forms is available through the Internet (www.usp.org/prn and www.fda.gov/medwatch) or on free diskette (Microsoft Word or Novell WordPerfect, both for Windows 6.0/6.1). USP staff are available to assist callers between 9 AM and 4:30 PM Eastern Time, Monday through Friday. Each report is treated confidentially. The identity of the reporter is protected by the FDA under federal statute, and USP offers an option for anonymous reporting.

Callers should be prepared to provide the following information:

- Describe the error, including the sequence of events, the personnel involved, and the work environment in which it occurred (e.g., during a code, a change of shift, or when the pharmacy was closed).

- Was the medication administered to or used by the patient?

- What was the patient outcome (e.g., death, injury or impairment, adverse reaction)?

- When and how was the error discovered, and by whom (e.g., nurse, physician, pharmacist, technician)?

- Where did the error occur (e.g., hospital, nursing home, outpatient or retail pharmacy, patient's home)?

- What level of staff (e.g., pharmacist, nurse, technician) made the initial error?

- Was the error unwittingly perpetuated by another practitioner?

- Had the patient received counseling on proper use of the medication?

- What product was involved (if applicable)? Who is the manufacturer?

- What was the dosage form, strength, concentration, and type and size of container (if applicable)?

Types of Errors

Table 18–4 lists the types and causes of medication errors most frequently reported to USP between 1991 and May 1998. Those most likely to be associated with fatal outcomes were overdoses, selection of the wrong drug, and deficits in practitioner knowledge. Selecting the wrong drug most commonly occurs because of similarities in labeling or packaging; it can also result from mix-ups between drugs with similar names.

Table 18-1	Period	Drug
Drugs most frequently involved in error reports to USP MERP, 1991–1998	August 1991 to April 30, 1993	Epinephrine
		Heparin
		Lidocaine
		Potassium chloride
		Cefazolin
		Ampicillin
		Morphine sulfate
		Phenytoin
		Doxorubicin
		Digoxin
	May 1, 1993, to May 31, 1994	Norvasc® (amlodipine)
		Navane® (thiothixene)
		Digoxin
		Morphine sulfate
		Potassium chloride
		Lidocaine
		Levoxine
		Sodium chloride
		Heparin
	June 1, 1994, to May 31, 1995	Heparin
		Digoxin
		Morphine sulfate
		Insulin
		Warfarin
		Lidocaine
		Nitroglycerin
		Mesalamine
		Ketorolac
		Potassium chloride
	June 1, 1995, to May 31, 1996	Heparin
		Morphine
		Lidocaine
		Potassium chloride
		Sodium chloride

Table 18-1 (continued)

	Digoxin
	Furosemide
	Gentamicin
	Ritonavir
	Zidovudine
	Hydroxyzine
	Omeprazole
	Midazolam
	Cefazolin
	Esmolol
	Insulin
	Erythromycin
	Phenytoin
	Haloperidol
	Metoprolol
	Warfarin
June 1, 1996, to May 31, 1997	Sodium chloride
	Morphine sulfate
	Glyburide
	Warfarin sodium
	Potassium chloride for injection concentrate
	Digoxin
	Heparin sodium
	Amlodipine besylate
	Lamotrigine
	Furosemide
June 1, 1997, to May 31, 1998	Morphine sulfate
	Meperidine hydrochloride
	Heparin sodium
	Hydroxyzine hydrochloride
	Sodium chloride
	Digoxin
	Cefazolin sodium
	Warfarin sodium
	Lorazepam
	Diltiazem hydrochloride

Table 18-2	Period	Drug
Drugs most frequently associated with fatalities as reported to USP MERP, 1991–1998	August 1991 to April 15, 1993	Lidocaine hydrochloride (also confused with heparin sodium; sodium chloride) Potassium chloride (also confused with furosemide) Chloral hydrate Carboplatin Cisplatin (confused with carboplatin) Colchicine Digoxin Doxorubicin Heparin Hydromorphone hydrochloride (confused with morphine sulfate) Insulin
	April 16, 1993, to June 15, 1994	Mivacurium chloride (also confused with metronidazole; ranitidine) Potassium chloride (confused with furosemide; heparin; sodium chloride) Morphine sulfate (also confused with hydromorphone) Lidocaine hydrochloride (also confused with dextrose) Cisplatin Dobutamine hydrochloride (confused with acetazolamide sodium) Insulin (confused with heparin) Oxytocin (confused with vasopressin) Phenytoin Warfarin sodium
	June 16, 1994, to May 31, 1995	Vinorelbine tartrate Cisplatin Potassium chloride (confused with furosemide) Morphine sulfate (confused with meperidine hydrochloride) Hydromorphone hydrochloride (confused with meperidine hydrochloride) Dextrose (confused with sterile water) Aprotinin Cyclophosphamide Lidocaine hydrochloride (confused with hetastarch, sodium chloride) Salmeterol xinafoate

Table 18-2 (continued)

June 1, 1995, to May 31, 1996	Esmolol hydrochloride Potassium chloride (confused with furosemide) Morphine sulfate Atenolol (confused with digoxin) Bupivacaine hydrochloride (confused with vancomycin) Chloral hydrate Cisplatin Fluorouracil Lidocaine hydrochloride with epinephrine (confused with epinephrine) Diatrizoate meglumine, diatrizoate sodium
June 1, 1996, to May 31, 1997	Potassium chloride for injection concentrate (confused with furosemide, heparin, sodium chloride) Irinotecan hydrochloride Dactinomycin Dextrose Isophane insulin (confused with isophane insulin human) Liposomal doxorubicin (confused with doxorubicin hydrochloride) Methylphenidate hydrochloride (confused with metolazone) Morphine sulfate Penicillin Ticlopidine hydrochloride
June 1, 1997, to May 31, 1998	Prednisone Albumin Amphotericin B (confused with amphotericin B lipid complex) Amiodarone hydrochloride (confused with amrinone lactate) Amrinone lactate (confused with amiodarone hydrochloride) Cisplatin Colchicine Digoxin Fosphenytoin sodium Levothyroxine sodium Morphine sulfate Nitroprusside sodium Potassium chloride for injection concentrate Vincristine sulfate Esmolol hydrochloride Oxytocin (confused with vasopressin)

Table 18-3

Circumstances leading to fatal medication errors reported to USP MERP, June 1995 to May 1996

Potassium chloride/furosemide

- A registered nurse gave a patient potassium intravenous push instead of furosemide.
- A nurse chose the wrong vial from the medication supply closet and put potassium chloride instead of Lasix® into the intravenous drip bag of an 82-year-old female hospital patient.

Esmolol hydrochloride

- A patient was supposed to receive 2.5 mg of esmolol hydrochloride; instead, 1.25 g of esmolol hydrochloride intravenous was administered via intravenous push.
- A patient received a 3.5-g intravenous bolus because a physician made an error when converting the dosage from micrograms to grams.

Cisplatin

A doctor mixed up the dosages, and the patient received four times the correct dose every day for 5 days.

Diatrizoate meglumine/diatrizoate sodium

The technician chose a dye that was not intended for use in the spinal cavity.

Automix/Micro mix

A total parenteral nutrition solution for a 600-g infant was incorrectly prepared.

Fluorouracil

A patient being treated for cervical cancer received a fourfold overdose.

Epinephrine/lidocaine hydrochloride with epinephrine

A patient received an overly strong concentration in a subcutaneous injection.

Strong iodine solution

A 5-day-old infant was given an overdose of Lugol's solution.

Morphine sulfate

A terminally ill cancer patient was receiving MS Contin® 60 mg every 12 hours. A nurse received a physician's order to increase the dosage to 10 mg every 15 minutes as needed; however, she transcribed the order as morphine 60 mg every 15 min as needed. This dose was administered.

Fatal Medication Errors (continued)

Diltiazem hydrochloride

> An 83-year-old patient chewed her Cardizem CD® capsules because they were too large for her to swallow. She became dizzy, weak, and lethargic every afternoon after taking the capsule. On learning of these symptoms, the physician changed the prescription to an immediate-release product. The patient did well and experienced no further side effects. At a check-up a few months later, the physician switched her back to Cardizem CD. She again chewed the capsule and 3 weeks later died suddenly.

Bupivacaine hydrochloride/vancomycin hydrochloride

> Instead of a scheduled dose of vancomycin, a patient received an infusion of bupivacaine that was intended for epidural use and that had been prepared and labeled for another patient.

Oxygen supply tubing 7'/back check extension set 30"

> An extension tube from the wall oxygen supply was connected to an intravenous port. Efforts to resuscitate the patient failed.

Digoxin/atenolol

> An order written for Lanoxin® was mistakenly filled with Tenormin®.

Midazolam hydrochloride

> A 41-year-old man was hospitalized for the treatment of congestive heart failure and asthma. He was not properly restrained and self-extubated. An intern administered an overdose of Versed® and tried to reintubate the patient. Efforts were not initiated in time. The patient went into a coma from which he never recovered.

Chloral hydrate

> A 6-year-old boy was scheduled to undergo computerized tomography at a health maintenance organization. A prescription for chloral hydrate was written so that the boy could be presedated at home. The prescription was written for 12 mL, but the community pharmacy dispensed 120 mL. The mother called the facility to check whether she was supposed to give the child the whole amount, and the person answering the phone replied "yes." She administered a 10-fold overdose.

Table 18-4	Period	Error Type/Cause	% Errors [a]
Types and causes of medication errors most frequently reported to USP MERP, 1991–1998	August 1991 to April 30, 1993 (N = 573)	Wrong drug	32
		Similar labeling and packaging	30
		Overdose	18
		Similar names	15
		Knowledge deficit	10
		Similar products	9
		System failure/floor stock	8
		Poor label design	7
		Transcription error	7
		Confusing/incomplete spoken/written order	6
	May 1, 1993, to May 31, 1994 (N = 348)	Wrong drug	49
		Similar labeling and packaging	29
		Similar names	23
		System failure/floor stock	17
		Knowledge deficit	16
		Overdose	16
		Poor label design	13
		Similar products	10
		Inaccurate order/label information	10
		Illegible order	10
		Look-alike drugs	9
		Transcription error	9
		Confusing/incomplete spoken/written order	9
		Confusing label information	6
	June 1, 1994, to May 31, 1995 (N = 552)	Wrong drug	34
		Similar labeling and packaging	18
		Overdose	18
		Similar products	13
		Similar names	12
		Illegible order	9
		Knowledge deficit	7
		Poor label design	7
		Missed dose	6
		System failure/floor stock	5

[a] Percentages do not add to 100 because error categories are not exclusive of one another.

Period	Error Type/Cause	% Errors [a]	**Table 18-4 (continued)**
June 1, 1995, to May 31, 1996 (*N* = 484)	Wrong drug	37	
	Similar labeling and packaging	35	
	Similar name	23	
	Overdose	20	
	Knowledge deficit	11	
	Faulty drug distribution system	10	
	Illegible order	10	
	Practitioner error	10	
	Wrong drug strength	8	
	Transcription error	7	
June 1, 1996, to May 31, 1997 (*N* = 564)	Similar names	39	
	Wrong drug	30	
	Similar labeling/packaging	24	
	Wrong dose	18	
	Illegible order	15	
	Knowledge deficit	12	
	Faulty drug distribution system	12	
	Right drug, wrong strength	7	
	Poor label design	5	
	Confusing or incomplete spoken or written order	4	
June 1, 1997, to May 31, 1998 (*N* = 1014)	Wrong drug	24	
	Similar names	23	
	Wrong dose	13	
	Similar labeling/packaging	13	
	Transcription error	11	
	Omission error	10	
	Inadequate safeguards	10	
	Right drug, wrong strength	9	
	Faulty drug distribution system	9	
	Established procedure/protocol not followed	7	

Impact of USP MERP

The impact of the USP MERP can be seen in changes to USP's standards and drug information database and educational outreach programs.

Drug Standards and Requirements

Two important changes have been made as a result of reports filed with USP MERP. Reports of accidental direct injection of undiluted, concentrated potassium chloride triggered changes in the nomenclature, labeling, and packaging requirements for that drug. The official name of the product was changed to "Potassium Chloride for Injection Concentrate." The container's cap, the overseal, or both now must be black and bear the words "Must be diluted." The product label must bear the following boxed warning immediately following the name: "Concentrate—Must Be Diluted Before Use" (see Chapter 13, Figure 13–16). No other injectable products may have black caps.

Because of reports of accidental intrathecal injection of vincristine, USP now requires that vincristine labels bear the following statement: "Fatal if given intrathecally. For intravenous use only." Further, the individually prepared dose must be placed by the dispenser in an overwrap bearing the words "Do not remove covering until the moment of injection. Fatal if given intrathecally. For intravenous use only."

Another important area of improvement instigated by the USP MERP resulted from reports concerning the confusion and inconvenience caused by the apothecary system of measurement. Errors were reported in the interpretation of product labeling and prescriptions, in calculations and conversions, and in the appropriate use of devices marked in apothecary units. Because of such errors, the Table of Metric–Apothecary Dose Equivalents and the Equivalents of Weights and Measures Table were deleted from the *United States Pharmacopeia XXIII/National Formulary XVIII* (*USP XXIII/NF XVIII*). The table of reference was the conversion of apothecary measures, which had commonly been used in pharmacy, to metric measures. It was published in the *United States Pharmacopeia/National Formulary* (*USP/NF*), which is the combined book of the USP and the National Formulary. By eliminating the table, *USP/NF* officially ceased to recognize the apothecary system and thereby discouraged its further use in medicine.

Unless otherwise specified in a USP monograph, the strength of a drug must now be expressed on the container label only in metric units. Unless otherwise indicated in an individual monograph, USP also requires that prescriptions for compendial articles state the quantity or strength desired in metric units. If an amount is prescribed by any other system of measurement, only an amount that is the metric equivalent of the prescribed amount may be dispensed.

DI Database

Reports of the unsafe use of certain drugs sparked a review of those monographs in the USP DI. Information on medication errors, when available, is now included under the subheading "Caution" in the "Dosage Forms" section of USP DI monographs. This action creates a specific area for such information to be located and a searchable, tagged field for identification of the information in the USP DI database. Information on the following four drugs has been added.

Colchicine. Reports of the deaths of hospitalized patients resulting from accidental overdoses of colchicine led to the inclusion of a warning about the toxicity and narrow margin of safety for therapeutic doses of colchicine, especially when used intravenously for acute attacks of gout.

Cisplatin and Carboplatin. The antineoplastic drugs cisplatin and carboplatin have similar brand names (Platinol® and Paraplatin®, respectively) and generic names. Following two reports of accidental deaths resulting from a mix-up of these products, a cautionary statement was added to the monograph. It warned of the similarity of both the brand and generic names and cautioned that a sixfold overdose of cisplatin could occur if cisplatin is administered in place of carboplatin.

Chloral Hydrate. USP reports conveyed that the use of chloral hydrate for sedation prior to diagnostic or therapeutic procedures in pediatric patients had resulted in three fatal overdoses. The "Precautions to Consider" section of this monograph now warns about the need to calculate proper doses and recommends administration of the drug only at facilities where appropriate monitoring can be instituted.

Esmolol. Confusion caused by two substantially different concentrations of esmolol hydrochloride resulted in several tragic incidents. Both concentrations are available in 10-mL containers. The more concentrated form, intended to be diluted for intravenous infusion, is packaged in 10-mL, break-open, 2500-mg ampuls. The less concentrated, ready-to-use form is intended for direct bolus injection and is packaged in 10-mL vials containing 100 mg. The monograph now provides specific information on the proper use of each package size and a warning regarding the appropriate handling of the more concentrated product.

Educational Programs

The USP has developed educational resources designed for consumers, health care practitioners, and students of the health professions.

The "Just Ask!...About Your Medicines" campaign focused its first program on the consumer's role and responsibility for his or her medication therapy and for helping to prevent medication errors. Experiences of consumers, reported through USP MERP, were the basis for the common errors described.

The curricular resource "Understanding and Preventing Medication Errors" is available in most U.S. colleges of pharmacy. It takes a multidisciplinary approach to teaching students about the causes of medication errors and how to prevent them. USP conducted a Faculty Training Institute with 10 professors in pharmacy schools nationwide to introduce the resource. State boards of pharmacy have expressed interest in using the curriculum for remediation programs. The overwhelming interest in the pharmacy curricular resource resulted in its adaptation for use in colleges of nursing. The curriculum has also been adapted for use as an educational resource for continuing education and in-service programs for practitioners.

Multidisciplinary Approaches to Error Reduction

National Coordinating Council for Medication Error Reporting and Prevention

In 1995, a multidisciplinary group of national organizations formed the National Coordinating Council for Medication Error Reporting and Prevention. The council comprises 17 organizations and agencies representing the health professions and the general public, licensing boards and accrediting bodies, the pharmaceutical industry, health care facilities, and standards-setters and regulators. Members are the following:

- American Association of Retired Persons
- American Health Care Association
- American Hospital Association
- American Medical Association
- American Nurses Association
- American Pharmaceutical Association
- American Society of Consultant Pharmacists
- American Society for Health Care Risk Management
- American Society of Health-System Pharmacists

- Food and Drug Administration
- Generic Pharmaceutical Industry Association
- Institute for Safe Medication Practices
- Joint Commission on Accreditation of Healthcare Organizations
- National Association of Boards of Pharmacy
- National Council of State Boards of Nursing, Inc.
- Pharmaceutical Research and Manufacturers of America
- USP Advisory Panel on Medication Errors, Chairperson (ex officio)
- U.S. Pharmacopeia (Member and Secretariat)

The council has the authority, mechanisms, and resources to find workable solutions, despite the complexity and seriousness of medication errors. By examining the prescribing, dispensing, administration, and use of drugs by health professionals and patients alike, the council has set forth on its mission "to promote the reporting, understanding, and prevention of medication errors." Its goals are as follows:

- To examine and evaluate the causes of medication errors;

- To increase awareness of medication errors and methods of prevention throughout the health care system, including health care organizations and facilities, delivery systems, practitioners, manufacturers, regulators, and consumers;

- To recommend strategies relative to system modifications, practice standards and guidelines, and changes in packaging, labeling, and product identity;

- To stimulate the development and use of medication error reporting and evaluation systems in individual health care organizations;

- To stimulate reporting to a national system for review, analysis, and development of recommendations to reduce and prevent medication errors.

Among the first activities of the council was to develop a consensus on the definition of medication error. This definition follows:

> *A medication error is any preventable event that may cause or lead to inappropriate medication use or patient harm, while the medication is in the control of the health-care professional, patient, or consumer. Such events may be related to professional practice, health-care products, procedures, and systems including: prescribing; order communication; product labeling, packaging, and nomenclature; compounding; dispensing; distribution; administration; education; monitoring; and use.*

Table 18-5

Index for categorizing medication errors

Type of Error/Category	Results
No error A	Circumstances or events that have the capacity to cause error.
Error, no harm[a] B	An error occurred, but the medication did not reach the patient.
C	An error occurred that reached the patient but did not cause patient harm.
D	An error occurred that resulted in the need for increased patient monitoring but no patient harm.
Error, harm E	An error occurred that resulted in the need for treatment or intervention and caused temporary patient harm.
F	An error occurred that resulted in initial or prolonged hospitalization and caused temporary patient harm.
G	An error occurred that resulted in permanent patient harm.
H	An error occurred that resulted in a near-death event (e.g., anaphylaxis, cardiac arrest).
Error, death I	An error occurred that resulted in patient death.

[a] The National Coordinating Council for Medication Error Reporting and Prevention defines harm as death or temporary or permanent impairment of body function and/or structure requiring intervention. Intervention may include monitoring the patient's condition, a change in therapy, or active medical or surgical treatment.

Source: Adapted from Hartwig SC, Denger SD, Schneider PJ. A severity-indexed, incident report-based medication error-reporting program. *Am J Hosp Pharm.* 1991; 48: 2611–16.

The council has urged researchers to adopt this definition as a first step toward standardizing medication error classification and analysis. Health care facilities can also implement this definition into the design of internal reporting mechanisms.

To further assist researchers, practitioners, and others in standardizing errors recorded, in July 1996 the council adopted a severity grading system to categorize errors by level of harm to the patient (Table 18–5).[2] In that

Avoiding Errors in Prescriptions	Table 18-6

National Coordinating Council for Medication Error Reporting and Prevention recommendations to correct error-prone aspects of prescription writing

1. All prescription documents must be legible. Prescribers should switch to a direct, computerized, order entry system.

2. Prescribers should avoid abbreviations, including those for drug names (e.g., HCTZ) and Latin directions for use.

3. Prescription orders should include a brief notation of purpose (e.g., "for cough") unless the prescriber believes this is inappropriate. This notation can help ensure that the proper medication is dispensed. Certain medications and disease states may, however, warrant confidentiality.

4. All prescription orders should be written in the metric system except for those that use standard units (e.g., insulin, vitamins). Units should be spelled out; the abbreviation "U" should not be used.

5. Prescribers should include the patient's age and, when appropriate, weight, on the prescription or order. The most common errors in dosage occur in pediatric and geriatric populations in whom low body weight is common. Providing patient age and weight can be an important double check.

6. Prescribers should not use vague directions such as "Take as needed" or "Take as directed." Clear directions help the dispenser verify the proper dosage and provide appropriate counseling.

7. The medication order should include drug name, exact metric weight or concentration, and dosage form.

8. A leading zero should precede a decimal expression of less than one. A terminal or trailing zero should never be placed after a decimal.

same month, after reviewing errors submitted to the USP MERP, the council developed eight strategies (Table 18–6) to address errors in the earliest stage of the medication use process and prescription writing. The council encourages implementation of these recommendations by prescribers and inculcation of these concepts into staff education and orientation programs in hospitals and long-term care facilities.

USP Advisory Panel on Medication Errors

The USP has long relied on the expertise and commitment of experts to provide it with unbiased and state-of-the-art counsel. More than 1000 scientists, academicians, clinicians, regulators, and members of the general public serve on the USP Committee of Revision, its subcommittees, and advisory panels.

In keeping with this traditional structure, USP in 1996 appointed its first Advisory Panel on Medication Errors to review all reports submitted to the USP MERP. Panel members are nurses, pharmacists, and physicians in active practice who have first-hand experience in the handling of drugs and the systems in which they are prescribed, dispensed, and administered. Their function is to make recommendations for enhancing the USP MERP, revising or devising USP standards, and incorporating warnings or cautions into the USP DI database. It also submits recommendations for consideration by the National Coordinating Council for Medication Error Reporting and Prevention. The panel chair holds an ex officio, nonvoting seat on the National Coordinating Council for Medication Error Reporting and Prevention. The panel is expected to make recommendations relating to areas such as systems improvements, product standards, practice standards and guidelines, and product design and nomenclature. ISMP has a permanent seat on this panel.

Summary

Professionals who contribute information to a national reporting system can have a vast impact on improving health care products, practices, and systems. Identification of standardized information elements to capture medication errors is crucial to analysis and national benchmarking. As local reporting and tracking systems are developed, the systems approach to error reduction at the national level should help to revolutionize the way in which medication errors are perceived and acted on by health care systems.

• • • •

References

1. Edgar TA, Lee DS, Cousins DD. Experience with a national medication error reporting program. *Am J Health Syst Pharm.* 1994; 51: 1335–38.

2. Leape LL, Bates DW, Cullen DJ, et al. Systems analysis of adverse drug events. *JAMA.* 1995; 274: 35–43.

19.

The Role of Risk Management in Medication Error Prevention

Judy L. Smetzer, RN, BSN
Michael R. Cohen, MS, FASHP

Institute for Safe Medication Practices
Huntingdon Valley, Pa.

Charles J. Milazzo, CSP, ARM, ALCM

PHICO Insurance Company
Mechanicsburg, Pa.

Risk management has been defined as "the process of making and carrying out decisions that will minimize the adverse effects of accidental losses upon an organization."[1] In health care settings, the principles of risk management are applied to protect the safety and welfare of patients, visitors, and staff. To prevent or minimize the effects of loss, risks are identified, analyzed, treated, and evaluated.

The cornerstone of risk identification is an effective event reporting system. Because of the sensitive nature of adverse events, informal and formal channels of communication are of equal importance. Risk analysis involves ranking events in order according to their potential to produce adverse effects. This is accomplished by assessing the severity of loss, the probability that a loss will occur, and the probability that a similar loss may recur if the system is not modified.

Risk treatment strategies are based on the seriousness of the threat of loss to patients, visitors, staff, and the organization as a whole. If the probability of loss is minimal, the risk may be accepted and little or no change may be made in the system. If risk cannot be accepted or reduced, a decision may be made to avoid the service that gives rise to it or to transfer the potential financial loss to outside entities (e.g., through the purchase of additional insurance).

Risk Management and Quality Assurance

Risk management techniques and quality assurance (or quality improvement) activities frequently overlap. Improving staff performance through process and system changes, a primary goal of quality improvement, is also a means of achieving a major goal of risk management—namely, the safety of patients, visitors, and staff.

If there is no link between risk management and quality assurance, the goals of both are compromised. Quality assurance systems need the data obtained through risk identification and analysis to aid in identifying priority opportunities for improvement. Risk management needs the processes and tools of quality assurance analysis to help identify causes of problems and to make systemic changes that will eliminate or reduce risk.

Because these two activities are interdependent, most health care organizations combine or coordinate them. Such an arrangement minimizes redundancy, maximizes resources, and provides a means for collaborating to develop effective solutions.

Risk Management and Medication Errors

Medication use is a complex process, and the possibility for risk is substantial. Although many errors result in no harm to the patient, the potential for serious injury with certain medication types, classes, and routes of administration is substantial. In a study of closed claims, drug-related injuries were responsible for the highest expenditures for claims related to procedures.[2] Given the injuries and cost associated with preventable adverse drug events and the growing concern about medication errors by consumers,[3] health care organizations have an obligation to invest time and effort to reduce and prevent them. In this chapter, we explore the various aspects of reporting an adverse event, an activity that lies at the heart of risk management in health care systems.

Event Reporting

Purpose

Event reporting is the primary means through which adverse drug events and other risks are identified. The purposes of event reporting are to

- improve the management of an individual patient,
- identify and correct systems failures,
- prevent recurrent events,

- aid in creating a database for risk management and quality improvement purposes,
- assist in providing a safe environment for patient care,
- provide a record of the event, and
- obtain immediate medical advice and legal counsel.

Need for Consistent Terminology

To report an event clearly, consistent terminology is needed. Health facilities refer to adverse drug events as "unusual occurrences," "variances," "medication errors," "incidents," and a variety of other names. The word *incident* has come to mean "crisis" in many people's minds; for this reason, many organizations prefer the word *event*.

The American Hospital Association and other organizations define an event as "any happening which is not consistent with the routine operation of the hospital (or health care organization) or the routine care of a particular patient."[4] This definition is purposely broad in order to accommodate all potentially compensable events.

Many organizations recommend developing lists of specific reportable events. The American College of Surgeons estimates that 40% to 60% of all adverse occurrences can be identified through a reporting system that identifies the specific events to be reported.[5]

The National Coordinating Council for Medication Error Reporting and Prevention (NCC MERP) defines a medication error as[6]

> *...any preventable event that may cause or lead to inappropriate medication use or patient harm while the medication is in the control of the health care professional, patient, or consumer. Such event may be related to professional practice, health care products, procedures, and systems, including prescribing; order communication; product labeling, packaging, and nomenclature; compounding; dispensing; distribution; administration; education; monitoring; and use.*

The products included in a definition of medication error must be recognized. They may include oral, parenteral, and topical medications; anesthetic agents and gases; radiopharmaceuticals and radiopaque contrast media; blood-fraction medications; intravenous fluids; dialysis fluids; respiratory therapy agents; investigational medications; medication samples; medications brought into the facility by patients; and other chemical or biological substances.

The definition of an adverse drug event should include not only all situations that have the potential to lead to errors but also actual errors that never reach the patient. An organization that reports potential errors ("near-misses") is taking a proactive role in identifying system failures. This approach will ultimately produce cost savings as well as benefits in terms of patient care. Risk managers should not be concerned, moreover, that reporting near-misses will inflate their error statistics. For the purposes of tracking error rates, severity-leveling systems such as that developed by NCC MERP can help separate actual errors from potential errors.[6] The more potential errors reported (and appropriately addressed), the better. Additional information on national reporting systems appears in Chapter 18.

Event Reporting Mechanisms

Event reporting mechanisms should be flexible. Reporters should be able to file oral as well as written reports, and anonymity should be guaranteed. The importance of promoting and maintaining informal lines of communication cannot be overemphasized.

Today's integrated health care delivery systems may include several acute care facilities, each with its own specialty, as well as physician group practices, ambulatory clinics, home health services, assisted living centers, nursing homes, and other health care businesses. The staff of each of these entities needs to understand the system's overall event reporting system as well as alternative reporting systems. For example, an acute care hospital may use a telephone hot line and have a reporting form that is different from that used by a mental health facility. Physician practices and chain pharmacies may use still another means of reporting; for example, many prefer making oral reports to risk management. The corporate risk manager needs to be aware of all these alternative reporting systems and track their relative use and effectiveness.

Many liability insurers provide event reporting forms to their clients. Some accept facility-specific forms for internal reporting, providing that they meet specific criteria. Any external reporting requirements to the insurer, such as notification of potentially compensable events, can be met in standard fashion, regardless of the event reporting forms being used in the hospital.

Information on the Report Form

A report form should request all information necessary to describe the event accurately and completely. It should serve as a factual description of what happened. Minimal information to be included on this form is summarized in Table 19–1.

Table 19-1

Required Reporting Information

Patient:

Name, age, room number, attending physician, diagnosis, procedure

Volunteer or visitor:

Name, address, telephone number, reason for presence in facility

Event information:

- Date, time, and location
- Names and addresses of witnesses
  (e.g., roommate, visitor, staff member)
- Type of event (e.g., adverse drug event, fall, medical device event, surgical event, patient leaving against medical advice, customer complaint, destruction of property)
- Facts surrounding event
- Effect of event on patient, volunteer, or visitor
- Individuals advised of event and date of notification
- Individual completing the report (printed name and signature)
- Date of report

The report should never contain personal or professional conclusions, opinions, accusations, criticisms, or admissions. Information regarding why the event happened, as well as prevention strategies, should be documented separately as part of the organization's quality improvement processes. This information, which is related to the root causes of the event and underlying system failures, is gathered during peer review of the event.

Responsibility for Reporting

The best person to report an event is the individual who discovered or witnessed it. A person who learns of an adverse drug event second-hand may be included in the reporting process by documenting the information received.

Nursing departments are the most common source of event reports; however, they should not be the only source. Medication use is a multidisciplinary process that involves physicians, dentists, podiatrists, physician assistants, pharmacists, pharmacy technicians, nurses, secretaries, medics and paramedics, clinical laboratory technicians, medical and paramedical students, respiratory therapists, pharmaceutical companies, and patients. Individuals from any of these groups should report an adverse drug event or potentially dangerous situation involving medication use.

It is not advisable to allow pharmaceutical company representatives or patients to document an event on internal reporting forms. Information gathered from these individuals should be documented by persons who are employed by the organization.

When and to Whom to Report

Most organizations require that all adverse drug events that may cause serious harm or threaten the life of a patient be immediately reported to supervisors, physicians, and risk management staff. The pharmacy and medical director should also be notified immediately of all serious adverse events. For less severe events, reporting policies vary. The best approach is to immediately report every incident to at least the supervisor, no matter how insignificant it seems.

Immediate reporting has two advantages. First, adverse drug events that initially do not appear to be serious may in fact be so. By reporting the event immediately, the individual is not relying on independent judgment to determine its potential severity. Additional resources, such as the pharmacist or physician, may be secured. Second, immediate reporting gives the supervisor an opportunity to ask questions while the event is fresh in the reporter's mind.

Organizational policies concerning the time frame for submitting written reports to risk management staff vary, ranging from 24 hours to 1 week. Although it is important to notify risk management in a timely fashion, written reports that are hastily prepared because of unrealistic time frames are often incomplete and do not contain important information needed to identify system failures. A better approach is to require immediate oral reporting of serious or potentially serious events. Written reports can then be forwarded to risk management after all necessary information has been gathered. Such submissions should be made no later than 1 week after the event.

Shortcomings of Traditional Reporting Systems

In the early days of risk management, reporting was erratic and inconsistent; as a result, liability claims frequently came as a surprise. In 1985, the American College of Surgeons estimated that event reporting systems identified only 5% to 30% of adverse patient occurrences in hospitals.[5] Barker and McConnell found that errors were detected through observation 1422 times more frequently than through event reporting.[7] Shannon and DeMuth found that the observation method detected a mean error rate of 9.6%, whereas event reporting revealed a rate of only 0.2%.[8]

Reasons for underreporting include the following:

- Concern for personal liability,
- Limited participation in reporting (i.e., perceiving it as a nursing function),

- Reluctance to report incidents involving physicians,
- Lack of time,
- Perception that reporting has a low priority,
- Lack of knowledge about the advantages of an effective incident reporting system, and
- Fear of punishment.

When an Error Is Not Really an Error

The reasons why nurses report or do not report medication errors may be surprising. Some literature supports the idea that more experienced nurses make fewer errors, whereas other researchers believe that more experienced nurses report fewer errors. Recent research[9] identifies tacitly shared rules that nurses apply to clinical situations to determine whether a "real" medication error occurred. The rules frequently involve reading between the lines of medication orders or modifying organizational regulations. Even though this research involved nurses, physicians and pharmacists may have their own rules as well.

If it's not my fault, it is not an error. If the nurse cannot avoid the error, it is not an error. Examples include late drug administration or omission when the patient is off the unit or when the prescribed drug is not available on the unit.

If everyone knows, it is not an error. When everyone is aware that actual practice differs from policy and procedure, it is not an error. Applying transdermal patch medications at 0600 instead of the prescribed time of 0800 is an example. Since 0800 is not a routine time for medication administration, and the patch would likely be applied later than the prescribed time because of busy schedules, the nurses change the time of patch application. The physicians know and approve of this practice.

If you can make it right, it is not an error. More experienced nurses become innovative about making things right when an error has occurred. If a dose is omitted, the nurse may change the subsequent drug administration schedule to "get back on track." This mind set may also include documentation. When a discrepancy is noted, the nurse involved may be asked later to document a procedure that may or may not have actually been carried out.

If a patient's needs are more urgent than accurate medication administration, it is not an error. If, in the nurse's clinical judgment, other patient needs take priority, any irregularity in drug administration is not considered an error. Examples include dealing with emergencies, which often delay or otherwise alter drug administration.

A clerical error is not an error. Nurses frequently assume that there is no "real" error when faced with an apparent error in documentation. When a nurse on a previous shift fails to document drug administration or documents a dose in the wrong section of a medication administration record, often no one investigates because the nurse may already be at home sleeping or would not remember.

If it prevents something worse, it is not an error. If a nurse knows that she will be busy later due to planned admissions, discharges, and procedures, she may administer medications early rather than risk omitting doses. Technically, early administration is an error, but it is preferable to omission.

Medication errors should be reported regardless of the circumstances surrounding them. Institutions may have official organizational policies and procedures on medication administration and error reporting, but this study shows that, when faced with real clinical situations, nurses develop alternative tactics. Some of these tactics evolved because many managers look for individuals to blame instead of fixing the systems that failed. Fearful of punishment, nurses try to protect their colleagues and independently change practices when they feel it is in their patients' best interests. As a result, much important information about errors is lost. With this in mind, it is important to promote an atmosphere that encourages honest inquiry and stimulates discussion about the organization's medication use problems and possible solutions. One rule we hope is never used is: It was a blessing in disguise, so it's not an error.

The role of a punitive environment in inhibiting error reporting cannot be overemphasized. Some organizations do use event reporting to punish practitioners. A punitive reporting system is reactive. Reactive systems focus on the weaknesses of individuals, resulting in accusatory attitudes, rationalization and other self-deceiving behavior, and a sense of victimization.[10] At times, individuals may even use a reporting system in a punitive way to inappropriately "wage a war" with another individual (see Chapter 7).

Fear of punishment may be reinforced by the use of tracking systems that are tied to disciplinary consequences (e.g., written or verbal warnings, suspension, transfer, demotion, or termination). The El Dorado Medication Error Tool, for example, is used to evaluate errors and determine disciplinary action. It assigns points to individuals based on the type of error, route of administration, drug classification, and timeliness of reporting.[11]

Stephen Covey[10] notes that

> It is not what others do, or even our own mistakes, that hurt us the

most; it is our response to those things. Our first response to a mistake affects the quality of the next moment. It is important to [be able to] immediately admit our mistakes so they have no power over the next moment.

Failure to report errors creates a false sense of security. Those responsible for medication use do not receive the information and tools they need to correct system failures. A proactive approach to error reporting, by contrast, creates a true sense of security, provided that the incident is used to identify system problems and prevent them from recurring.

Promoting a nonpunitive reporting system is difficult. Managers may believe that punishment is indicated, especially if they are under pressure from consumers. Managers may also feel that they need a tracking system as a competency assessment tool. Medication errors, however, rarely assess individual competence, because they are the consequence of the system in which the individual works.[12–15] Errors do not measure individual performance but the combined effects of the system and an individual's effort.[16] The causes of most mistakes are outside the power of the individual. Patient safety is best served by a reporting system that places higher value on identifying and resolving systemic problems than on punishing individuals.[17]

Nonpunitive reporting systems and handling employees who make multiple or catastrophic errors are frequent topics raised by health care managers and practitioners who contact us. We always stress the need for leadership understanding and a solid commitment to a nonpunitive approach to errors. Employees are blamed for errors when administrative leadership is unaware of the significant influence of the system on individual performance. A nonpunitive approach is not possible unless there is support from top leaders—all the way up the leadership chain—who truly understand that errors are just symptoms of a "diseased" system and that error prevention efforts must be directed at the weaknesses in the system, not at individuals.

Several techniques are suggested for creating a nonpunitive environment that supports increased error reporting. A confidential reporting system in which everyone understands that errors will not be linked to performance appraisals is critical. It should be easy to report errors; doing so should be rewarded and timely feedback provided to show what is being done to address problems. A nonpunitive approach to errors should be consistently applied. If even one person is disciplined for an error, mistakes will be hidden. Alternative ways should be found to evaluate employees, based not on errors or lack of making mistakes but on positive measures that evaluate an employee's overall contribution to the organization.

A nonpunitive environment is truly tested when an organization is confronted with an employee who makes multiple errors or is involved in a catastrophic error. People often find it easier and in their nature to blame individuals and resort to familiar solutions such as counseling, disciplinary action, enforcing rules, or developing new rules. There is little or no remedial value in doing so, however, and this easy way out often leads back to problems that persist or worsen. In fact, when the only action is punishing individuals for errors, this can actually be dangerous to an organization. It leads to the ever-increasing need for more of the same familiar remedies—the philosophy of "what we need here is a bigger hammer." The root causes of problems are not identified, and the system is weakened even further.

Organizations face considerable pressure from the public and the legal system to discipline individuals for mistakes. Nevertheless, there is little advantage to terminating even those employees involved in multiple or catastrophic errors. This inadvertently sends the message that the organization has hired a defective employee and has not exercised good judgment in allowing the employee to provide care in the organization. Rather, it is more important to determine why errors are happening and to take action to effectively prevent these errors or minimize their consequences. The goal of patient safety is best served with a nonpunitive environment that places more value on reporting problems so that they can be remedied, rather than pursuing the largely unprofitable path of disciplining employees for errors.[a]

Traditional reporting systems have additional shortcomings. If the form is inappropriately designed, it will yield little or no useful data about the root causes of the event. Without such data, systems problems cannot be identified and corrected. Aggregate data needed for identifying patterns are of little value when they identify only types of errors and proximal causes. Attempts to capture data needed retrospectively are often fruitless because the information has been forgotten or is no longer available.

Another pitfall of reporting systems is the failure to include pharmacists in the initial review of adverse drug events. The pharmacy is a pivotal link in the medication use process, and pharmacists are in a unique position to recognize the root causes of errors that other disciplines may overlook. Pharmacists are also particularly well qualified to recommend and implement prevention strategies.[18]

[a] An excellent videotape on this subject is available at no charge through Bridge Medical, 120 South Sierra, Solana Beach, CA 92075-1811; 619-350-0100; www.mederrors.com. This is a California health care company that is focused on reducing the risks of serious medication errors through technology development. The tape is a documentary film on how medication errors affect all involved, practitioners and patients alike. The film features case histories of a pharmacist, a nurse, and a physician, each of whom has been involved in a fatal medication error.

Some organizations claim that they do not share information with the pharmacy because of fear of legal ramifications regarding the discoverability of event reports. However, failure to take action on problems brought to the attention of the organization may have even more serious consequences.

Event Reports and Discovery

Discovery is the legal process by which one party can obtain information from another party. Discovering an event report and using it as evidence are two different matters. The document discovered by a plaintiff's counsel can sometimes be protected from entry into evidence.

Event reports are discoverable in some locations if they are considered to be the only routine means of documentation of an organization. Depending on state law and the role of event reporting in an individual institution's quality assurance efforts, the report and other documents may be protected through attorney–client privilege or peer review statutes.[19] Practitioners should seek the advice of legal counsel in their jurisdictions to determine the extent of discoverability of documentation of adverse events. Considerations relating to protecting the information surrounding an adverse drug event from being admitted as evidence during litigation are summarized in Table 19–2.[19]

Because of liability concerns, many health care facilities believe that a serious adverse event should not be recorded on a form. This position is untenable. Adequate, legible, timely, and accurate records are the first line of defense against a medical liability claim. If litigation results from such an event, information that facilities do not have in writing may cause more harm than the information contained on an appropriately designed and completed adverse event form. If the event report is filled out objectively and accurately, it should be no problem if it is discovered and used in litigation.

Managing Publicity Surrounding a Serious Medical Event

Health care personnel are experienced in disaster management. Plans are devised, practiced, and evaluated for community accidents with mass casualties, loss of critical services such as electricity, and coping with a natural disaster.

All organizations should likewise have a plan for responding to serious medical events. Individuals who should be involved in the planning include the chief executive officer, chief of the medical staff, a risk management professional, director of pharmacy, director of nursing, public relations director, and an attorney. Key issues to be covered in the plan are discussed in the following paragraphs.[20]

Table 19-2

Safeguarding Adverse Drug Event Reports from Discovery

- The event report is not part of the medical record. It should not remain with the patient's chart unless state law dictates otherwise.

- The event report should not be photocopied.

- The fact that an event report has been completed should not be documented in the patient's medical record or chart.

- The report should include only a factual description of the event; it should not include opinions, conclusions, accusations, or admissions.

- The event report should be shared only through a peer review process involving those who participate in or are responsible for the medication use process.

- The purpose and appropriate use of the event report should be defined in the policies and procedures dealing with event reporting, as well as in the quality assurance and risk management plans that describe operational linkages between the two functions.

- All forms should contain a guarantee of confidentiality. Separate forms, which state their intended use for quality assurance purposes, should be used to document follow-up investigation, conclusions, and prevention strategies.

- Events that have a direct medical effect on the patient should be recorded in the medical record. Only the facts should be recorded, including a description of the patient's response to the event for at least 24 to 48 hours following the event.

Who will be responsible for the immediate investigation of the event? How will the review be carried out? Legal advice should be sought to determine the best way to proceed with the investigation. Risk management professionals are usually best suited to perform an investigation when there is a high probability that litigation will ensue.

How will the event and the information obtained from the investigation be documented? Legal advice should be sought on how to protect from discoverability the information gathered concerning the event, either through attorney–client privilege or state peer review statutes.

What is the internal and external notification process (coroner, professional staff, administration, state department of health, Food and Drug Administration, MedWatch and medical device reporting, manufacturer, U.S. Pharmacopeia Medication Errors Reporting Program)? It is important to identify mandatory and voluntary reporting requirements and to assign individuals the responsibility to carry out the required functions. All reports should be reviewed by a risk management professional before they are released.

What will be done to safeguard applicable documents and equipment? A copy of the medical record should be made immediately following a serious event. The original should be secured in a locked file in the medical records department. All containers, wrappings, equipment, or other items related to the event (e.g., defective equipment) should be sequestered by risk management for possible use in the event of litigation.

What communication and interaction should occur between the health care providers and the patient and family involved in the event? It is important to present the facts surrounding the adverse event; however, no opinions, accusations, or admissions should be offered. This interchange should be performed in a timely fashion by a professional who has been providing care to the patient and after consultation with risk management. The professional chosen to talk to the patient and family should explain what the institution is doing to investigate the event and to prevent its recurrence. Staff should continue to interact with the patient and family in a compassionate manner. Avoiding the patient and family is a common initial reaction, because staff may feel uncomfortable. A sincere expression of concern and continuing contact, however, help the patient and family feel that they have not been abandoned in a time of need.

When physicians err, they should put aside all concern about the potential negative consequences to themselves and disclose the errors to the patients, particularly when such disclosure would benefit patients' health. Wu and colleagues[21] believe that, in most cases, "...the fiduciary character of the doctor-patient relationship indicates that a physician has the ethical duty to disclose error to a patient when disclosure furthers the patient's health, respects the patient's autonomy, or enables the patient to be compensated for serious, irreparable harm." Damage-minimizing tips include disclosing promptly and openly, making apologies, and foregoing charges for associated care. When a mistake has a major adverse impact on the patient, an offer should also be made to cancel charges for subsequent care needed to remedy the consequences of the mistake and to provide any necessary supportive services.

If the event attracts media attention, how will the organization respond? Health care organizations have an ethical and a legal obligation to keep medical information confidential. Facilities should develop a policy on handling the media and make sure that all employees are aware of it. The patient and family should be consulted regarding their wishes for release of information. It is important to be specific rather than general. Family consent should be obtained in writing. Additional permission is needed for photographs, videotapes, or interviews with patients, families, and others.

The institution's public relations team must choose a spokesperson and a backup to gather the available facts related to the event. The team should decide what will be said and should have a plan to screen new information before its release. The goal should be to control the news going out, rather than to react to any particular aspect of the case being pursued by the news media. The spokesperson should emphasize what is being done or should let the press know that it is a confidential issue. The spokesperson should not make excuses or reply with "no comment."

Internal public relations is important. Administration should ensure that staff are kept up to date with the investigation of the event and proposed prevention strategies. Details of the peer review process, however, should not be shared with the entire staff.

What processes will be used to promote immediate and long-term remedial action? Immediate action may be indicated to prevent a similar event until the circumstances surrounding the event are explored. An in-depth analysis of the event should then be undertaken to identify systems failures. Following this analysis, long-range prevention strategies should be implemented.

How will visits from accreditation bodies, regulatory agencies, and other investigative agencies be accommodated? For example, after verifying the facts, the Joint Commission on Accreditation of Healthcare Organizations may send a surveyor to determine whether the organization would benefit from an in-depth analysis of the event. If so, the surveyor will provide education and materials on performing a root cause analysis and place the organization on Accreditation Watch.[22] Regulatory bodies such as the state department of health or the FDA may visit unannounced. The organization should designate a team of people who will respond to these visits and develop a procedure to follow for appropriate responses to requests for information.

What sort of counseling and other support will be available for persons involved in the event? The plan may include psychological counseling, social services intervention, and support through an employee assistance program. Coworkers should support involved staff.

Conclusion

To improve their reporting systems, organizations should focus on five important staff needs:

1. *Protection.* The promise of immunity from punitive consequences
2. *Purification.* The opportunity to admit mistakes
3. *Prevention.* The assurance that corrective action will be taken at the system level
4. *Philanthropy.* The knowledge that one's decision to report will help educate other practitioners and patients
5. *Process.* The use of brief, uncomplicated reporting methods

Administrators should remove barriers to reporting by promoting a nonpunitive reporting system. They should explore ways to recognize and reward reporting. They should make reporting as simple as possible. Reporters and other staff should receive timely feedback concerning any actions taken in response to the report. Finally, the institution should have a written plan for responding to serious errors that gain public attention.

References

1. Head GL, Horn S. *Essentials of the Risk Management Process.* Vol 1. 2nd ed. Malvern, Pa: Insurance Institute of America; 1987.

2. Bates DW, Spell N, Cullen DJ, et al. The cost of adverse drug events in hospitalized patients. *JAMA.* 1997; 277: 307–11.

3. Golodner L. How the public perceives patient safety. *National Patient Safety Foundation Newsletter.* Winter 1997.

4. ECRI. Event reporting. *Continuing Care Risk Management.* May 1996: 1–10.

5. US General Accounting Office. Health care initiatives in hospital risk management. Report to the Honorable Ron Wyden, US House of Representatives. Washington, DC: July 1989.

6. The United States Pharmacopeial Convention, Inc. National Council focuses on coordinating error reduction efforts. *Qual Rev.* 1997; 57.

7. Barker KM, McConnell WE. The problem of detecting medication errors in hospital. *Am J Hosp Pharm.* 1962; 19: 361.

8. Shannon RC, DeMuth JE. Comparison of medication error detection methods in the long term care facility. *Consultant Pharmacist.* 1987; 2: 148–151.

9. Baker H. Rules outside the rules for administration of medication: a study in New South Wales, Australia. *Journal of Nursing Scholarship.* 1997; 29 (2): 155–58.

10. Covey, SR. *The Seven Habits of Highly Effective People: Restoring the Character Ethic.* New York: Simon & Schuster; 1989: 66–94.

11. Cobb MD. Dealing fairly with medication errors. *Nursing 90.* March 1990: 42–43.

12. Cohen MR, Senders J, Davis NM. Failure mode and effects analysis: a novel approach to avoiding dangerous medication errors and accidents. *Hosp Pharm.* 1994; 29: 319–30.

13. Williams E, Talley T. The use of failure mode effect and criticality analysis in a medication error subcommittee. *Hosp Pharm.* 1994; 29: 331–38.

14. Leape LL. Error in medicine. *JAMA.* 1994; 272: 1851–57.

15. Leape LL, Bates DW, Cullen DJ, et al. Systems analysis of adverse drug events. *JAMA.* 1995; 274: 35–43.

16. Stevens T. Dr. Deming: management today does not know what its job is. *Industry Week.* January 1994; 17: 21.

17. Davis NM. Nonpunitive medication error reporting systems: tough to accept but safest for patients. *Hosp Pharm.* 1996; 31: 1036.

18. ECRI. Medication errors. *Continuing Care Risk Management.* May 1995: 1–25.

19. ECRI. Identifying and managing risks. *Continuing Care Risk Management.* November 1994: 1–14.

20. Cohen MR. Responding to a serious medication error. *Hosp Pharm.* 1991; 26: 1024–25.

21. Wu AW, Cavanaugh TA, McPhee SJ, et al. To tell the truth: ethical and practical issues in disclosing medication mistakes to patients. *J Gen Intern Med.* 1997; 12: 770–75.

22. ECRI. A look at accreditation watch. *Risk Management Reporter.* 1997; 16 (2): 1, 3.

Risk Analysis and Treatment

20.

Michael R. Cohen, MS, FASHP
Judy L. Smetzer, RN, BSN

Institute for Safe Medication Practices
Huntingdon Valley, Pa.

Once an adverse drug event has been reported, a risk assessment must be performed. Ideally, a medication safety committee should review each reported adverse event. When this is not possible, a reporting system that tracks errors by severity, such as that of the National Coordinating Council (NCC) for Medication Error Reporting and Prevention (MERP), may be helpful.[1] Each event should be evaluated to determine the severity of actual or potential harm to the patient, the probability that harm will occur, and the probability that the event will happen or recur.

Priority should be given to events that have a high potential to cause harm and a high likelihood of occurring or recurring. All adverse drug events of high priority should be then assessed to determine the root causes and systems failures. "Near misses" (i.e., events that did not actually cause harm to a patient but that well could have) should rank near the top of a priority list if the potential for harm is sufficient.

JCAHO's Sentinel Event Policy

The Board of Commissioners of the Joint Commission on Accreditation of Healthcare Organizations (JCAHO) has established a Sentinel Event Policy. In support of its mission to improve the quality of health care provided to the public, JCAHO includes a review of organizations' activities in response to sentinel events in its accreditation process, including all triennial and random unannounced surveys. A sentinel event is defined as an unexpected occurrence involving death or serious physical or psychological injury, or the risk thereof. Serious injury specifically includes loss of limb or function. The phrase "or the risk thereof" includes any variation in process for which a recurrence would carry a significant chance of a serious adverse outcome. Reportable events are those that result in an unanticipated death or major permanent loss of function that is not related to the natural course of the patient's illness or underlying condition. A reportable event may also be one that meets the following criteria, even if the outcome was not death or permanent loss of function:

- Suicide of a patient in a setting where the patient receives around-the-clock care,
- Infant abduction or discharge to the wrong family,
- Rape,
- Surgery on the wrong patient or the wrong body part,
- Hemolytic transfusion reaction.[2]

Organizations are not required to report sentinel events; however, voluntary disclosure is encouraged through the promise of less severe ramifications. If an organization reports a sentinel event to JCAHO, the organization will not automatically be placed on "Accreditation Watch." Rather, the organization will be given the opportunity to perform a "root cause analysis" within 45 days and submit it to JCAHO for approval. If a routine inquiry is made to JCAHO, the organization's accreditation status will be reported without making reference to the sentinel event. If JCAHO learns of a sentinel event that was not self-reported, such as through the media or during scheduled surveys, it will automatically place the organization on Accreditation Watch and require a root cause analysis of the event. Not only is an on-site visit from JCAHO probable, the organization's Accreditation Watch status will be publicly disclosed. There is a risk of loss of accreditation if it declines to share information arising from the root cause analysis with JCAHO.

The required root cause analysis focuses primarily on systems and processes—on why an event occurred. An acceptable analysis must be thorough, progressing from identification of special causes to common causes. Once the root of the problem is identified, an action plan and measurement strategy must be implemented. In order for the analysis to be credible, it must include the individuals who are closest to the process being reviewed, organizational leaders, and an evaluation of relevant literature. JCAHO strongly encourages organizations to use its suggested format, "Framework for Root Cause Analysis."

Only those sentinel events that affect recipients of care are included in this analysis. After review and approval at a future board meeting, JCAHO plans to provide organizations with specific examples of sentinel events that are and are not subject to their review.

Medication errors are the most prevalent type of sentinel event reported to JCAHO, and we support the principles of root cause analysis for these errors. Rather than blaming individuals, evaluating and improving the larger organizational systems that support the efforts of individuals is at the heart of preventing medication errors. The Institute for Safe Medication Practices (ISMP) has been assisting the U.S. Pharmacopeia (USP) and the NCC MERP in the development of an effective mechanism for providing JCAHO with critical and timely error prevention information (see Chapter 18). We can successfully predict where significant risks with medication use lie. By sharing this information with JCAHO, surveyors can probe for these risks and recommend prevention strategies during the survey process. The position of ISMP is that this would be a much more comprehensive and proactive process, rather than just retrospective awareness of a single random sentinel event that can potentially lead to the sanctions of Accreditation Watch.

Analysis of risk requires systems thinking. In this chapter, we discuss risk analysis from this perspective. We present 12 key elements that affect medication use and discuss the considerations that health professionals should take into account in dealing with them.

Systems Thinking and Medication Use

Most medication errors are more closely associated with faulty drug distribution systems, miscommunication, poor packaging and labeling, and other systems failures than with the competence of a single health care professional.[3–6] Consequently, the goal of a risk management program should be to predict how and where systems might fail and to intervene to prevent them. Health professionals and risk managers must also learn from failures that have already occurred and take action to ensure that problems associated with these events are corrected.

Senge[7,8] defines a system as "a perceived whole whose elements 'hang together' because they continually affect each other over time and operate toward a common purpose." Systems thinking entails seeing wholes rather than parts. It provides a framework for seeing the changing patterns and structures that underlie complex situations. It involves detecting the subtle influences and connections that give systems their character.[7,8]

Because of the complexity of the medication use process, systems thinking is essential. Systems thinking enables people to realize that the problems with complex processes such as medication use are in direct proportion to their inability to see the organization as a whole.[7,8]

Three principles lie at the heart of systems thinking.[7,8] The first is that structure influences behavior.[7] Regardless of how different they are, people tend to produce the same results when they are in a system. When problems arise, an organization with a linear view tries to assign responsibility for those problems to someone or something. In contrast, an organization with a systems perspective looks beyond individuals and events to the underlying structures that shape individual behavior and create the conditions under which events occur.

Senge's second principle is that structure in human systems is subtle.[7] For Senge, structure is defined by the pattern of interrelationships among the components of a system, not by the individuals who make it up. When an organization focuses on people, this underlying structure is often hidden.

The third principle is that leverage often comes from new ways of thinking.[7] Systems thinking can reveal a variety of potential solutions. Some of these actions have higher leverage than others. The action with the most potential to contribute to enduring improvements is not always immediately obvious (see Note).

Applying Systems Thinking to Key Elements of Medication Use

Medication use is a complex process that comprises the subprocesses of drug prescribing, order processing, dispensing, administration, and effects monitoring. The 12 key elements that most often affect the medication use process, and the common failures and medication errors associated with them, are presented in Table 20–1. The interrelationships among these 12 elements form the structure within which medications are used. In the following discussion, we outline the nature of errors that arise within these key elements and the questions that staff members should consider in devising a plan to reduce or eliminate them.

Patient Information

Many errors result from health professionals' lack of information about their patients. This missing information may include clinical data or background on social factors in the patient's life. In some cases, the needed information is not available or easily accessible; in others, it is available but not used.

For example, did the pharmacy dispense an oral medication to a patient who was not supposed to receive anything by mouth because staff had failed to check the patient's chart? Was a dosage for a cancer patient not

Principles That Govern Systems Thinking

Today's problems are yesterday's solutions. Systems are always changing, and solutions must change as well. The harder you push, the harder the system pushes back. Well-intentioned actions bring responses that may offset the positive benefits of the action. For example, an individual who quits smoking may gain weight and decide to resume smoking.

Behavior grows better before it grows worse. Low-leverage actions may work in the short term; however, long-term improvements cannot be realized if the solution cures only the symptoms and overlooks the underlying problem.

The easy way out usually leads back in. The fastest and easiest solutions are not usually the most effective.

The cure can be worse than the disease. Easy solutions can be dangerous. The consequence of nonsystemic solutions is an ever-increasing need for more solutions. Short-term improvements lead to dependence and may leave the system weaker than before.

Faster is slower. When improvement efforts are excessive, the system will compensate by slowing down. Action must be undertaken at a realistic pace.

The relation between cause and effect is not always apparent. The consequences or effects of a problem may not be closely related in time and space with the cause. The root cause of a problem with drug distribution, for example, may not reside in the pharmacy.

Small, well-focused actions can produce significant improvements. There are no simple rules for identifying high-leverage actions, but learning to use systems thinking helps increase the probability of success.

You can have your cake and eat it, too, but not at once. Lowering costs and increasing quality may both be possible, provided that one is willing to wait for one while focusing on the other.

Dividing an elephant in half does not produce two small elephants. The integrity of the system is compromised when it is divided. Systems thinking is not effective when it is practiced only by individuals, because optimum results depend on the interaction of major functions with diverse perspectives.

There is no blame. You and the cause of your problem are part of the system, and the problem will be remedied only when the system affecting your relationship is resolved.

Source: Adapted from Senge PM, Kleiner A, Roberts C, et al. *The Fifth Discipline Fieldbook: Strategies and Tools for Building a Learning Organization.* New York: Currency Doubleday; 1994: 87–112.

properly modified because laboratory data on the patient's renal function were not available to the prescriber? Is a patient "noncompliant" because she cannot afford to pay for her medications?

A multidisciplinary committee should explore how to prevent such incidents. How is the pharmacy notified of a patient who is pregnant, or of one who has

Key Elements	Common Failures	Examples of Resulting Errors
Patient information	• Lack of basic demographic, clinical, and social data • Lack of patient monitoring information	• Prescribing a medication to which the patient is allergic • Diagnostic reporting error resulting in inappropriate medication order • Lack of dose modification because laboratory data are not available or checked
Drug information	• Lack of computer screening for allergies, duplication of therapy, maximum dose limits, food and drug interactions • Lack of up-to-date, accessible, and easy-to-use drug references, protocols, and standardized dosing tables • Lack of pharmacists, physicians, and nurses for reference • Lack of accurate, up-to-date, and accessible medication administration records	• Wrong route ordered and administered because of lack of information • Overdose ordered, dispensed, and administered when the computer program failed to screen for maximum doses • Wrong dose of chemotherapeutic agent ordered due to an error in print reference • Extra dose administered because prior dose not documented
Communication dynamics	• Lack of clear, accurate, and timely written and oral communication related to the drug regimen • Lack of interactions that are free of fear of intimidation, punishment, and embarrassment	• Error in dosing or frequency because of the use of dangerous abbreviations, misplaced decimal points, or illegible handwriting • Delay in therapy because of inability to reach a physician for clarification • Wrong drug dispensed and administered as the result of failure to clarify an ambiguous order because of fear of intimidation
Labeling, packaging, nomenclature, and advertising	• Lack of clear drug labeling and packaging • Lack of distinctive drug and drug class names • Lack of accurate advertising	• Wrong drug dispensed and administered when drug names look alike • Error in route of administration when warning labels are not prominent • Dose error when container does not clearly state total dose in vial

Table 20-1 (continued)

Key Elements	Common Failures	Examples of Resulting Errors
Drug device acquisition and monitoring	• Lack of safety assessment and interventions for devices prior to purchase and use • Lack of effective preventive maintenance of devices	• Dosing error resulting from equipment failure because of lack of regular safety checks • Dosing error because of purchase and use of pumps not protected from free flow • Inadvertent administration of enteral fluid intravenously because of confusion with multiple unlabeled lines
Drug stock and storage	• Lack of safe drug storage and stocking practices • Lack of standardization of stock drug concentrations • Lack of standardized storage locations	• Drug interaction with the use of sample drugs • Dosing error because of availability of multiple drug concentrations • Wrong drug administered because of availability of dangerous drugs on nursing units • Incorrect base solution used in compounding because of availability of dangerous chemicals in compounding area
Stressors	• Lack of an environment that is free of stressors	• Errors related to frequent interruptions, poor lighting, or ambient distractions • Errors related to fatigue or personal stressors
Quality and risk management	• Lack of a culture that fosters exchange of ideas and proactive risk management efforts • Lack of a nonpunitive event-reporting system • Lack of feedback to staff regarding error prevention efforts • Lack of quality controls and safety nets • Lack of standards of practice and medication administration policies and procedures	• Dosing error with insulin when no system of double-checks in place • Dose concentration error with compounding when quality control checks on lines not completed • Dosing error resulting from miscalculation when not double-checked by another practitioner • Same error occurring on multiple units because of lack of feedback on internal errors and their prevention

Table 20-1 (continued)

Key Elements	Common Failures	Examples of Resulting Errors
Competency validation	• Lack of review of competency of new staff and with the introduction of new drug delivery systems or policies • Lack of orientation of staff to specific medication use policies, procedures, and protocols • Lack of credentialing and privileging of independent practitioners for use of targeted classes of drugs	• Overdose by practitioner not privileged to administer conscious sedation • Drug administered at the wrong time because of lack of knowledge of standardized times • Chemotherapy dose prescribing error when controls not in place to limit prescribing to credentialed physicians
Staff education	• Lack of ongoing staff education regarding unusual and new formulary drugs, new protocols, availability and use of drug references, targeted high-alert drugs and drug devices, drug calculations, and drugs with unusual or critical dosing considerations	• Error in route of administration stemming from unfamiliarity with drug not on formulary • Error in use of thrombolytic therapy because of lack of awareness of protocol • Same critical error occurring in multiple health care sites after error prevention strategies have been published in professional journals and newsletters
Staffing patterns	• Failure to match staff competency to patient and unit assignment • Failure to match staff with fluctuating patient census, acuity, and unit activity level • Lack of limits on number of hours or days worked in a row • Lack of appropriately placed supervisors for direction of experienced and inexperienced staff	• Dispensing and administration error because of inadequate supervision of inexperienced staff • Errors resulting from excessive workload • Errors caused by loss of concentration because of too many consecutive hours on duty
Patient education	• Lack of patient and family education by pharmacists, physicians, nurses, or other professionals concerning drug name (brand and generic); doses; directions for use; indications; side effects and adverse reactions; and proper storage, handling, and disposal	• Patient self-administration error resulting from lack of knowledge • Wrong drug dispensing undetected by patient because of lack of patient counseling • Patient noncompliance with medication regimen because of lack of knowledge • Errors related to patient or family use of devices because of inadequate education

liver disease, diabetes, or any other condition that may affect medication selection or dosage? Is there an adequate process for patient identification? What can be done to make patient information available to all who need it?

Drug Information

Lack of information about drugs and drug delivery systems contributes to medication errors. For example, a drug may be administered by the wrong route because drug reference texts are not accessible on the nursing units. A patient may receive an overdose if the hospital's computer system does not screen for maximum doses.

Are drug references and protocols accurate, up to date, and accessible? Do computer programs screen for food and drug interactions, allergies, dose limits, and duplication of therapy? If the system does have such capability, is it routinely used? Are pharmacists available for consultation? Are standardized dosing tables available for reference?

Communication

Obvious examples of communication breakdowns include misunderstood abbreviations, illegible handwriting, and inaudible verbal (i.e., oral) orders. Less obvious examples include confrontational behavior that leads to intimidation or embarrassment or punishment and failure to pass on information to the responsible party.

Solutions might include establishing a list of abbreviations that should never be used or requiring facsimile transmission to avoid oral orders. Another strategy is to develop a process to resolve conflicts over drug therapy. When a provider is concerned that a newly ordered medication might harm a patient, the matter should be pursued through an established process. Options should include refusing to dispense a drug until the matter undergoes peer review.

Drug Labeling, Packaging, Nomenclature, and Advertising

Many errors are caused by look-alike and sound-alike drug names, unclear labeling and packaging, and misleading advertising. Did an error occur because warning labels were not prominent? Was a wrong dose administered because the label did not clearly display the total dose in each container as well as the amount per milliliter? A unit clerk may misread a medication order because he or she is unfamiliar with a new drug whose name is similar to that of a well-established product.

Errors in this element may be hard to rectify because their cause is beyond the direct control of the institution. Actions can be taken, however, to minimize the possibility of drug mix-ups. The hospital may choose a new supplier or change its drug storage practices. In cases where internal action is insufficient, the ISMP, as well as the USP MERP, the FDA, and the manufacturer, should be notified and urged to advocate for changes.

Drug Device Acquisition and Monitoring

Is there an effective biomedical engineering program? Has there been an equipment failure, an automated compounder problem, a glucose monitor error, an infusion pump problem, or problems with pumps used for patient-controlled analgesia? Are devices standardized throughout the organization? Are safety measures (e.g., labeling lines for epidural analgesics and enteral feeding) in place to prevent mix-ups? The institution should take measures to ensure that all medical equipment is assessed for safety before it is purchased and used.

Drug Storage and Stocking

Are medications in storage protected from light and heat? Are expiration dates of medications in emergency carts regularly checked? Are drug samples controlled by the pharmacy? Is there a limit on the number of medications accessible from floor stock? Do nonpharmacists have access to the pharmacy after hours? Do nurses hoard medications or "borrow" medications from other patients?

Errors can also be attributed to lack of standardization of drug concentrations available in the pharmacy and as floor stock. A formulary ensures that the number and variety of drugs are controlled. Access to dangerous chemicals in pharmacy compounding areas or clinical areas must be restricted.

Stressors

The environment should be free of stressors that may cause staff to lose concentration. Common stressors include noise, frequent interruptions, poor lighting, extreme temperature and humidity, and fatigue. The level of unit activity and the acuity of patient care also may affect the accuracy of the medication use process.

Quality Control and Risk Management

Quality control checks must be incorporated throughout the medication use process, and special attention must be paid to areas that have proven particularly problematic. Do two nurses independently check insulin doses before giving them? Do pharmacists check on the dextrose concentration for all total parenteral nutrition solutions prepared in the pharmacy? Are proper sterility procedures used? Quality control checks should be built into the medication use process for high-risk tasks such as calculation of doses and preparation of intravenous admixtures.

Hospital management should create an environment in which problems can be aired and solutions discussed in a positive manner. Many nurses and pharmacists are initially full of ideas concerning quality improvement; however, they lose their enthusiasm if no one listens to them.

The way in which adverse drug event reporting is handled can stifle creative thinking. A nonpunitive reporting system and regular feedback to staff are essential. A pharmacy newsletter should communicate information about internal and external errors, discuss prevention methods, and describe corrective measures taken in response to identified errors.

Competency Validation

Is the competence of staff members assessed at the time they are hired and annually thereafter, as well as whenever new medication use devices, practices, and delivery systems are introduced? Are staff cross-trained before being assigned to specific patient care areas? Does the orientation include an explanation of medication use policies? Are procedures periodically reviewed? Must independent practitioners be credentialed before they are permitted to use targeted drugs or drug classes (e.g., anesthetic agents and chemotherapy agents)?

Staff Education

Lack of knowledge about a drug contributes to many adverse medication events. The challenge is to focus education on products with the highest leverage.

Is information on internal and external medication errors and techniques for their prevention shared with staff? Techniques include providing information on past medication errors during orientation sessions, writing newsletter articles, and lecturing on medication errors.

Are staff informed of educational resources and encouraged to use them? Is education provided on drugs or drug classes that have the particular potential to cause harm if used incorrectly? Are drugs with unusual or critical dosing considerations emphasized?

When drugs are added to the hospital formulary, adequate time must be provided for necessary protocols and educational programs to be developed. Computer systems can be enhanced to help workers recognize errors, and warning messages to nurses can be included in computer-generated medication administration records.

Staffing Patterns

Errors resulting from excessive workload, inadequate supervision, or loss of concentration from excessive days or hours on duty are included in the category of staffing patterns. Are staff adequately trained to work in the units to which they are assigned? Are staffing patterns matched to fluctuations in hospital census, unit activity, and patient acuity? Does the staffing plan consider the number of consecutive hours and days that staff can work without becoming fatigued? Are supervisors assigned strategically to meet the needs of experienced and inexperienced staff? Is student work properly supervised?

Patient Education

A well-informed patient is a safeguard against medication errors. Patients who know why they are taking a medication, understand its benefits and side effects, and know what the drug looks like and when it is to be taken have prevented many adverse drug events. Well-informed family members have also intervened to prevent medication errors.

The institution should emphasize to all staff the importance of patient education. Patients and families should receive as much information as possible from prescribers, nurses, and pharmacists. Providing information through the Internet and closed-circuit television in hospitals merits exploration.

Review of Internal Errors

Each site should have in place a structure for evaluating medication errors from a systems perspective. In large institutions, this function is often performed by a multidisciplinary medication safety team. At small practice sites, such as pharmacies or home intravenous-therapy companies, this role can be carried out by managers and staff. Pharmacists should take a lead role in all activities relating to safe medication use.

All high-priority medication errors should be examined to determine which key elements have failed. The committee must start as far back in the medication use process as possible and piece together the activities that should have occurred if the drug had been used properly. It can then determine at what point or points things went wrong. These failure points are referred to as "symptoms" of the adverse drug event.

As this analysis proceeds, the team must ask "why" questions repeatedly until the root causes of the problem are identified.[6] There is often more than one answer. The team should repeat this process for each answer. Gradually, it will uncover the root causes.

The team must focus this investigation on the system rather than on individuals. Even when an error can be directly traced to a specific individual (e.g., a pharmacist's improper dispensing), further probing might determine that poor order communication, dangerous storage practices, and look-alike labeling were root causes. In most cases, the error will be attributable not to a single cause but to failures in a number of key elements in the system.

Lesson from Denver: Look Beyond Blaming Individuals

In October 1996, a medication error occurred at a Denver area hospital that resulted in the tragic death of a newborn infant. The error involved the intravenous administration of a large dose of penicillin G benzathine, a medication that is insoluble and must not be injected intravenously. Since nurses are charged with the responsibility of knowing about the potential dangers of the drugs they administer, many who learned about the incident were quick to focus blame for the death solely on the nurses. The District Attorney of Adams County, Colo., brought this case before a grand jury. Three nurses who were involved in the infant's care were eventually indicted for criminally negligent homicide. In preparation for the trial that followed, a systems analysis was performed by ISMP on behalf of the defense team. The analysis revealed more than 50 latent failures in the system that contributed to the tragedy and allowed the accident to occur.

Latent failures are weaknesses in the structure of an organization, such as faulty information management or ineffective personnel training. These weaknesses are the result of both good and ill-conceived decisions made by upper management.[9] Even the best strategic decision in an organization carries with it both risks and benefits, as well as a certain degree of compromise. Individual winners and losers can be easily identified once a decision is made. However, the far-reaching effects of these decisions often go undetected. This is especially apparent when strategic decisions involve solutions that shift a problem from one part of a system to another and those solving the problem are different than those who ultimately inherit the new problem.[7]

Because it is not possible to immediately recognize all problems associated with management decisions, latent failures are inevitable in all organizations. They lie dormant in the system—hence the term *latent failures*. By themselves, they are often subtle and may cause no problems. Their consequences are hidden, becoming apparent only when they occur in proper sequence with each other and combine with the active failures of individuals to penetrate or bypass the system's safety nets.

Active failures are errors committed by individuals, such as physicians, nurses, or pharmacists, who are in direct contact with vulnerabilities and weaknesses in the structure of an organization. When individuals fall victim to these weaknesses, mistakes are made. Unfortunately, it is at these points of human fallibility that we often tend to focus our attention.[10] Although it may seem easier to concentrate on the human contribution to errors, the root causes of problems lie with latent failures in the system that are inherited by individuals in the work force, often without notice until an error occurs. Therefore, the only effective way to decrease the likelihood of medication errors is to strengthen the system's resistance to chance combinations of both latent failures and active failures.[10]

Many of the latent and active failures that were at the root of the medication error in Denver are identified in the brief description of the error that follows. A more detailed description has been published elsewhere.[11]

This case was riddled with both latent and active failures and thus provides a good exercise in identifying failures that may be present in an institution. If failures are found, it is recommended that they be brought up at a meeting of an institution's pharmacy and therapeutics committee for evaluation.

An infant was born to a mother with a history of syphilis. Despite a lack of complete patient information about the mother's past treatment for syphilis and the current status of both the mother and the child, a decision was made to treat the infant for congenital syphilis. (It was later learned that the mother had previously given birth to two healthy children after her disease was successfully treated and her laboratory tests were negative for syphilis.) After phone consultation with infectious-disease specialists and the health department, an order was written for one dose of "benzathine penicillin G 150,000 U IM."

The physicians, nurses, and pharmacists, unfamiliar with the treatment of congenital syphilis, also had limited knowledge about this nonformulary drug. The pharmacist consulted both the infant's progress notes and *Drug Facts and Comparisons* to determine the usual dose of penicillin G benzathine for an infant. However, she misread the dose in both sources as 500,000 units per kg—a typical adult dose, instead of 50,000 units per kg. Consequently, the pharmacist also incorrectly read and prepared the order as 1,500,000 units, a 10-fold overdose. Due to the lack of a consistent pharmacy procedure for independent double-checking, the error was not detected. Because a unit dose system was not used in the nursery, the pharmacy dispensed the 10-fold overdose in a plastic bag containing two full syringes of Permapen® 1.2 million units/2 mL each, with green stickers on the plungers to "note dosage strength." A pharmacy label on the bag indicated that 2.5 mL of medication was to be administered intramuscularly, to equal a dose of 1,500,000 units.

Figure 20-1

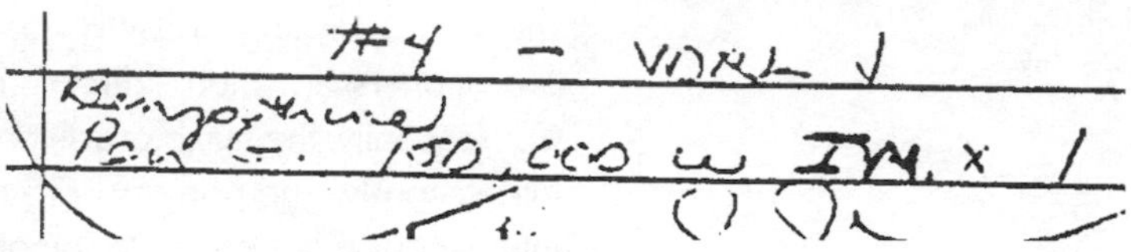

After glancing at the medication sent from the pharmacy, the infant's primary care nurse expressed concern to her colleagues about the number of injections required to give the infant the medication (since there is a maximum of 0.5 mL per intramuscular injection allowed in infants, the dose would require five injections). Anxious to prevent any unnecessary pain to the infant, two colleagues—an advanced-level staff nursery registered nurse and a neonatal nurse practitioner—decided to investigate the possibility of administering the medication intravenously instead of intramuscularly.

A misconception that "benzathine" was a brand name for penicillin G was reinforced by the physician's method of writing the drug order—with "Benzathine" capitalized and placed on a line above "penicillin G" rather than after it on the same line.

Neofax '95 was one of the medication resources relied upon by the two nurses to determine whether penicillin G benzathine could be administered intravenously. The *Neofax* monograph on penicillin G did not specifically mention penicillin G benzathine; instead, it noted the treatment for congenital syphilis with aqueous crystalline penicillin G intravenously slow push or penicillin G procaine intramuscularly. Nowhere in the two-page monograph was penicillin G benzathine mentioned, and no specific warnings regarding "intramuscular use only" for penicillin G procaine and penicillin G benzathine were present.

Unfamiliar with the various forms of penicillin G, the nurse practitioner believed that "benzathine" was a brand name for penicillin G. This misconception was reinforced by the physician's method of writing the drug order—with "Benzathine" capitalized and placed on a line above "penicillin G" rather than after it on the same line (Figure 20–1). In addition, many texts use ambiguous synonyms when referring to the various forms of penicillin. For example, penicillin G benzathine is frequently associated with the terms "crystalline penicillin" and "aqueous suspension" in texts. Believing that aqueous crystalline penicillin G and penicillin G benzathine were the same drug, the nurse practitioner concluded that the drug could be safely administered intravenously. The nurses knew that, although they were taught that only clear liquids can be injected intravenously, certain milky-white substances, such as intravenous lipids and other lipid-based drug products, can also be given intravenously. Therefore, they did not recognize the problem of giving penicillin G benzathine, a milky-white substance, by the intravenous route.

Hospital policies and practices did not clearly define the prescriptive authority of nonphysicians. However, the neonatal nurse practitioner assumed that she was operating under a national protocol that allows neonatal nurse practitioners to plan, direct, implement, and change drug therapy. Consequently, the nurse practitioner made a decision to administer the drug intravenously. The primary-care nurse, who was not certified to administer intravenous medications to infants, transferred the care of the infant to the advanced-level staff nursery registered nurse and the nurse practitioner.

While preparing for drug administration, neither nurse noticed the 10-fold overdose or that the syringe was labeled by the manufacturer "IM use only." The manufacturer's warning is very difficult to see because it is not prominently placed, and the syringe must be rotated 180 degrees away from the drug name to be visible (Figure 20–2). The nurses began to administer the first syringe of Permapen® via slow intravenous push. After about 1.8 mL was administered, the infant became unresponsive, and resuscitation efforts were unsuccessful.

It is important to recognize that, had even just one of these failures not occurred, either the accident would not have happened, or the error would have been detected and corrected before reaching the infant. Because most of what people do is governed by the system, the causes of errors belong to the system and, consequently, often lie outside the control of individuals, despite their best efforts. This case provides clear evidence that medication

Figure 20-2

Although this syringe is labeled "IM use only," the syringe must be rotated 180 degrees away from the drug name for the warning to be visible. Another problem is that the right-hand thumb can hide the warning.

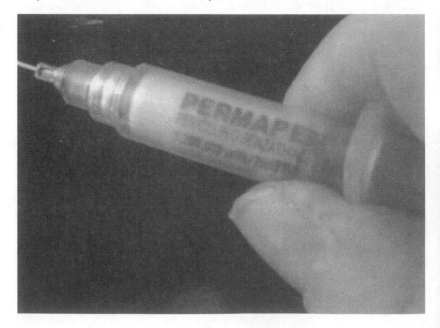

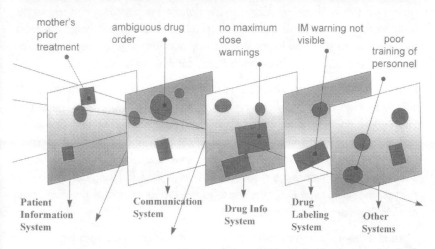

System Failures Leading to Denver Infant's Death

mother's prior treatment

ambiguous drug order

no maximum dose warnings

IM warning not visible

poor training of personnel

Patient Information System

Communication System

Drug Info System

Drug Labeling System

Other Systems

Figure 20-3

Medication errors are almost never caused by the failure of a single element, but rather are the result of the combined effects of latent failures in the system and active failures by individuals.

errors are almost never caused by the failure of a single element or the fault of a single practitioner. Rather, a catastrophic event such as this is the result of the combined effects of latent failures in the system and active failures by individuals (Figure 20–3).[9]

After being presented with the evidence during trial, the jury found the nurse "not guilty." By reaching this verdict, the jury also delivered an important message to health care providers: We must look beyond blaming individuals and focus on the multiple underlying systems failures that shape individual behavior and create the conditions under which medication errors occur.

Relieving "Stuck Thinking": Directed Creativity[a]

Directed creativity, a concept introduced by Paul Plsek,[12] is the purposeful production of creative ideas in a topic area, followed up by deliberate effort to implement some of those ideas. Many people incorrectly assume that creative thinking is a special gift, bestowed on only a few. Although it is true that we rarely see the extraordinary creativity of an Edison or an Einstein, modern research from the fields of the cognitive sciences indicates that the ability to generate innovative ideas for change in our work is a common gift that we all possess.

A Case of Late Meds. To illustrate what is meant by directed creativity, consider the following case of a hospital medication process quality improvement team. This team was a model of the scientific approach to

[a] Adapted from Plsek PE. *Creativity, Innovation, and Quality.* Milwaukee, Wis: ASQ Quality Press; © 1997 Paul E. Plsek. Used with permission. <www.DirectedCreativity.com>

quality improvement. Its members had gathered data on the problem, identified the key types of medication errors, constructed cause-and-effect diagrams and flow charts, collected more data, identified root causes, implemented remedial process changes, and measured improvement. The team members were successful with every medication error type they focused on except one: medications not administered on time, or so-called "late meds."

Interviews with the nurses indicated that the primary cause for late meds was simply that the nurses got busy and forgot to give medications at prescribed times. As a solution, the team had posted a log sheet as a reminder at the nurses' station, listing in chronological order all of the patients' medication times. As it turned out, however, the nurses were too busy to look at the log sheet. Unable to secure the resources to relieve the workload burden on the nurses, the team was frustrated and had decided to accept the remaining error rate as simply inevitable.

Here is a team stuck in its thinking. The team had gone down a logical path in its analysis and had come up with a logical solution. The solution should have worked, but it didn't. Team members had put so much analytical effort and logical thought into the work that led up to this point that they were unable to think of anything else to do. Whenever they discussed the matter, they just kept coming back to the same stuck point, rejustifying their analysis, and decrying the lack of resources as the real root cause of the problem. Such stuck thinking is a common occurrence in quality improvement activities in business. Directed creativity can be used to relieve stuck thinking.

The Directed Creativity Approach. A directed creativity process for the medication error situation just described might have proceeded in the following manner.

Realize that analytical thinking has reached a "stuck point" and resolve to find a creative way beyond it. The team needed to acknowledge the constraints in the situation and adopt the attitude that "there has got to be something else we can do."

Clarify the focus or concept that requires new thinking. In this case: We need a way to remind busy people when a certain time has come.

Review the facts. We have tried to remind them with a time log, but that failed.

Look carefully at the current situation to identify elements that could be modified to yield a new approach. We have tried reminding them visually—sight is only one of our senses; hearing, touching, tasting, and smelling are others. We have used a paper time log—a large, white board or a computer screen is another option.

Restate the focus by modifying an element and looking for an association. How can busy people be reminded about time through hearing rather than sight? The mental association of the concepts of reminding, time, and hearing leads naturally to the identification of an alarm clock as a mechanism. We could go on to think of other ways to utilize other senses or modify other elements of the situation.

Develop the idea further to meet practical constraints. For example, it must not cost too much, and it must be flexible, portable, and easy to associate with individual patients. One way is to use a stick-on alarm clock, the kind that can be attached to an appliance or car dashboard and is typically available in the line at the supermarket check-out counter.

Express it, develop it, try it out, see what happens. The team went out and purchased a few of these stick-on alarm clocks, set them for the appropriate medication times, and stuck them to the appropriate patients' charts. Now, even if the nurses are very busy, when the alarm goes off someone hears it and is reminded that it is time to administer a medication. The implementation of this idea reduced the late-med rate to nearly zero, without the addition of extra staff.

These processes of directed creativity are based on modern theories of how the mind works. Furthermore, they utilize ordinary thought processes like noticing, associating, remembering, and selecting. No special genius is required. Finally, although the end product of the thinking—a new idea—is creative, the thought processes have a logic that makes them appealing even to serious, scientific people (like those who typically work in business).

Mental Processes Behind Directed Creativity. Although the thinking process outlined above is not a universal sequence that can be applied to all situations, it does illustrate the following five basic mental actions that are common to many successful endeavors involving creative thinking:

1. Clarify the focus with a broad statement.
2. Recognize the concepts in the current situation.
3. List alternatives.
4. Make mental associations.
5. Develop ideas into practical realities.

First, it is often necessary to stop and clarify the focus that requires creative thinking. By stating the focus broadly—for example, "I need a way to remind busy people when a certain time has come"—we give our minds both a fixed point from which to direct our thinking and a wide space in which to come up with alternatives.

Second, being clear about the current reality and looking carefully to notice the underlying concepts behind the common things around us is a critical element in directed creative thinking. Often, we fail to pause and consider how or why something works or fails. The medication time log was a good idea, but it failed. If we stop and think about why it failed, we might realize that an underlying assumption was that the nurses would find time to look at it. What we found, however, was that they were too busy, which of course simply brings us back to the original problem. The key insight here is to notice that the failed solution relied on the sense of sight to do the reminding.

Third, listing alternatives is also a key element in the directed creativity process in this situation. In recognition that reliance on the sense of sight had failed, directed creativity suggests that we simply list our other senses and consider them as alternative ways of reminding. Careful reflection on this list of senses would lead us to notice that, whereas it is difficult to look at something when one is busy with something else, it is easy to hear something even when one is otherwise occupied. This is not an earth shaking insight. Why didn't the team members think of it? It is because our minds tend to race quickly past it on the way to the only approach we can think of; namely, the way we remind nurses in a hospital is with a log sheet. Paradoxically, then, stuck thinking does not necessarily mean that thinking has stopped. A better metaphor is to say that our thoughts are racing toward a repeated collision with the same brick wall. Listing alternatives helps us slow down thinking, look around, and find an alternative side street to turn down before we hit that same brick wall again.

Fourth, this example also illustrates the fundamental thinking process of association. When we associate the concepts of reminding, time, and hearing, we come up with the idea of using an alarm clock. Association lies at the core of all creative thought.

Finally, this example illustrates the importance of further refining ideas in order to make them truly useful. Many good ideas are never implemented because first impressions of them make them seem unappealing. Since, by definition, a creative idea is a new idea, we cannot be sure what mental model people will conjure up when we first express it. For example, imagine a row of bedside alarm clocks with big brass bells going off at various times. This mental picture would certainly lead to immediate rejection of the alarm clock idea. Rather than prematurely rejecting the idea, however, we should consider the alarm clock suggestion merely the "seed" of an idea that must be further refined. In the creative development process, we can address practical issues such as cost, fit with the environment, need for flexibility, and so forth.

Directed Creativity Versus Stuck Thinking. Directed creativity is needed in business for the simple reason that sometimes creative thinking is useful. When we are stuck in our thinking—whether we are trying to solve a problem, redesign a process, develop a new service, or delight a customer—it may not do any good to simply think harder. If our analytical thinking has locked us into a particular approach that is unfruitful, thinking harder is analogous to driving faster into the same brick wall in hopes that we will break through it. Although there may be a slight chance of success with this brute-force approach, it would be easier to drive around the wall or construct a ramp over it. Driving around or over the walls in our thinking is the creative approach.

Reflecting on the late-meds case and other situations of stuck thinking like it, we can clearly see that there are limits to traditional analytical thinking when it comes to solving nagging problems or generating breakthrough ideas. What is needed is the ability to be analytical when the situation calls for it and creative when the situation calls for that. Both skills are critical for success in business.

Review of External Errors

Just as important as analysis of internal reports is an awareness of adverse medication events or potentially hazardous situations that have occurred or have been identified elsewhere. Focusing on the external environment is essential because, as Deming[13] proposes, systems have difficulty understanding themselves. Knowledge and understanding often come from reviewing the experience of others.

Where can such information be found? Anecdotal information on errors and prevention strategies is published in journals and professional newsletters. One source is the *ISMP Medication Safety Alert!*, whose content is derived mainly from reports submitted to the USP MERP, operated in cooperation with ISMP. The ISMP also publishes features on error prevention in the newsletters of various pharmacy and nursing organizations.

A pharmacist should be given the responsibility for reviewing these and other anecdotal reports each month and suggesting topics for the risk management agenda. Committee members should then ask whether the same error could happen at their institution. They should discuss the prevention recommendations made by the authors and determine whether changes are needed in their own system.

Whether the committee is examining an internal error or evaluating the possibility that an external error could occur at their institution, discussing errors from a systems perspective is not easy. Care must be taken to create an environment that promotes inquiry without fear of negative consequences.

Seek and Use Knowledge from the Outside

Experience has shown that a medication error reported in one institution is also likely to occur in another, given enough time. Much knowledge can be gained when institutions look outside themselves to learn from the experiences of others. Unfortunately, many do not seek and use this information. Recommendations for improvement, often made by those faced with unraveling a devastating error, go unheeded by others. Some may read about medication errors experienced by other institutions with interest, but they do not use that information to make proactive changes within their own institutions. They truly do not believe that the same errors could happen within their institutions. Still other institutions have committees addressing difficult issues, but with an internal focus only. Real knowledge about medication error prevention will not come from a committee with only an internal focus.

A system cannot understand itself. Quality guru W. Edwards Deming summarized this phenomenon by noting that organizations with an internal focus "can learn a lot about ice and know nothing about water."[13] Knowledge from the outside can provide a lens to examine what is being done, lead to suggestions for what might be done differently, and furnish a road map for improvement.[14]

In a hospital, home care company, or long-term care facility, ISMP suggests that, in order to seek and use outside knowledge about medication error prevention, a small subcommittee should be established, ideally comprising a nurse, a pharmacist, a physician, and a medical librarian. The committee should follow and routinely search both the professional literature and the news media for descriptions of medication errors (or potentially hazardous situations) that have occurred in other institutions. These errors should then be examined and any recommendations for prevention considered. The information should be brought to other internal committees so that error prevention strategies can be implemented, thus following a proactive rather than a reactive approach. In community pharmacy or in other sites where the various types of practitioners are limited, employee and management staff must work together.

The ISMP Action Agenda. One of the most important methods for preventing adverse drug events is the concept of an action agenda. ISMP recommends that a formal agenda be developed in order to best utilize outside information. This agenda should be shared with high-level management.

The concept of an action agenda can be used at any practice site, including hospital and community pharmacies, long-term care facilities, hospitals, and home care companies. This would be an effective way for accreditation agencies, state boards, and state departments of health to function. These groups could request to see the files and review the actions taken to ensure that appropriate safety measures were undertaken.

Action Agenda Items. The following items appeared in the *ISMP Medication Safety Alert!* between January and March 1998. Each item was based on errors reported to ISMP through FDA MedWatch or the USP MERP. Each item is followed by a recommendation from the reporter or from ISMP. Added to this list should be errors or risks that actually occurred at the practice site.

1. Look-alike drug names and packaging

Proscar® and Posicor®

- *Problem.* There is concern about mix-ups between these two drugs because serious drug interactions are associated with Posicor®. (Posicor® was taken off the market in 1998.)

- *Recommendations.* Input alert flags into pharmacy computer system and include drug indications with order. Have prescribers indicate the purpose of the medication in prescriptions. Do not use a trailing zero for Proscar® 5-mg doses.

Hemoccult® and eye drops

- *Problem.* Patients and nurses inadvertently mix up bottles with ophthalmic solutions.

- *Recommendations.* Keep Hemoccult® out of patients' bathrooms. Store the product by tying it to a fixture in soiled utility room where stools are tested, or keep it in a locked cabinet.

Bausch and Lomb ophthalmic products

- *Problem.* Solutions and ointments are packaged in same-size, look-alike packaging with a color-coding scheme that highlights drug names by class, so that all drugs within the same class look identical.

- *Recommendation.* Take appearance into account when choosing ophthalmic products; ISMP has asked the company to address this concern.

Brevibloc® vials (single dose) and ampuls (concentrate)

- *Problem.* Concentrate in ampul may be confused with the single-dose vial used for a loading dose. This confusion has been responsible for at least 30 accidental deaths when the drug has been injected without dilution.

- *Recommendation.* Remove ampuls from stock on patient care units, including operating rooms; the manufacturer's reminder label on the ampul neck is not an effective barrier.

Proleukin® (IL-2 or IL-II) and Neumega® (rhIL-11 or IL-11)

- *Problem.* Mix-ups are likely if synonym abbreviations are used (the eleven in the latter is misread as Roman numeral II); serious side effects can occur with even normal doses of Proleukin®.

- *Recommendation.* Do not use synonym abbreviations; order by generic or brand names.

Heparin and Hespan® premixed bags

- *Problem.* Look-alike bags may be stored near each other or accidentally placed in the wrong location.

- *Recommendations.* Store products separately. Label storage bins of Hespan® by enhancing the letter "S." Add auxiliary labeling to the outside of Hespan® bags. The manufacturer has been asked to address this issue.

Zolmitriptan and sumatriptan

- *Problem.* Telephone and written orders may be misunderstood; tablet strengths differ by a factor of 10 (25 mg and 2.5 mg), making errors more likely if the decimal point is misread. Such a mix-up could have a dangerous outcome.

- *Recommendations.* Prescribe these drugs using both the brand and generic names. Implement a computer warning for dose ceiling.

2. Ambiguity or errors in drug references

Handbook on Injectable Drugs, outdated editions

- *Problem.* Outdated editions imply the safety of diluting albumin with sterile water, regardless of volume, leading to death of patients from hemolysis and renal failure.

- *Recommendation.* Discard outdated texts or mark them with a notice such as "Expired text—for historical purposes only."

Nursing 97 Drug Handbook

- *Problem.* The monograph on pyridostigmine (page 519) contains a typographical error stating "for IM or IV use, 1/3 of oral dosage is given"; the text should state "1/30 of oral dosage is given."

- *Recommendations.* Implement computer warning of dose ceiling. Discard 1997 books and replace them with the current edition.

3. Storage and dosing problems

Roxanol® (20 mg/mL) and morphine elixir (10 mg/5 mL)

- *Problem.* Mix-ups may occur between the concentrated and standard dosage forms of morphine elixir and solution.

- *Recommendation.* Remove the concentrated solution from nursing units, if possible, and dispense only for specific patients with chronic pain.

Conventional and lipid-based products: Abelcet® (amphotericin B) and Doxil® (doxorubicin)

- *Problem.* Dosing recommendations differ between products, causing fatal overdoses when mixed up.

- *Recommendations.* Provide formulary control and education when introducing these new products. Avoid storing the products anywhere near one another. Implement warning labels and computer warnings. Refer to brand names only when prescribing lipid-based products. Eliminate nursing access to pharmacy after hours.

Dangerous chemicals in the operating room

- *Problem.* Ultra-Stop® (a lens-defogging chemical) has been injected instead of contrast media when the two products were stored next to each other in the operating room.

- *Recommendation.* Nondrug products and external medications must always be stored separately from systemic medications.

Exceeding maximum dose limits with colchicine

- *Problem.* A patient died due to a massive overdose when the drug was ordered in a dosage of 2 mg intravenously every hour "until symptoms relieved or diarrhea develops."

- *Recommendations.* Implement computer warnings for course doses exceeding 4 mg intravenously (e.g., 1 mg every 6 hours or 0.5 mg every 6 hours in 48 hours); once 4 mg is reached, give no more colchicine for 7 days by any route. Use a reduced dose for geriatric patients and patients with impaired renal or liver function, and use only when treatment fails with safer nonsteroidal anti-inflammatory drugs.

Uncontrolled dosing of topical phenylephrine

- *Problem.* A child died during adenoidectomy due to an adverse drug reaction (severe hypertension) from 0.5% phenylephrine that was applied with a noncalibrated dropper to stop bleeding. Hypertension was treated with a beta-blocker, causing bradycardia and respiratory difficulty.

- *Recommendations.* Standardize exact concentration and dose of phenylephrine (and other topical agents for bleeding) in children, using only calibrated droppers or syringes for measurement before wetting a swab and applying it to a bleeding site. Wait 15 minutes before treating a sudden hypertensive episode resulting from the application of a vasoconstrictor. Use glucagon to counteract the effects of beta-blockers used to reverse excessive phenylephrine doses.

4. Miscellaneous

Faxing orders to pharmacy

- *Problem.* Distortion of faxed orders may lead to misinterpretations.

- *Recommendation.* Fax orders from originals only, clarifying any distortions before dispensing. Provide routine maintenance of fax machines.

Preprinted order forms

- *Problem.* Orders transfer responsibility from the prescriber to others for choosing the most appropriate drug, dosage form, dose, route, frequency, and indication, or checking for allergies.

- *Recommendation.* Preprinted order forms should be developed, reviewed, and approved by all disciplines.

5. For discussion

Potassium chloride concentrate injection survey

- *Results.* Potassium chloride concentrate is not present on 75% of medical surgical units; 87% to 93% of pediatric, neonatal, and ambulatory units; 57% to 59% of emergency departments and adult intensive care units. When the drug is stored on units, most lock it in a cabinet or use special warning labels. Eighty-seven percent removed the concentrate after learning about the potential for serious error. The most frequently cited reasons for not removing the concentrate included opposition from nurses or physicians, having no problems in the past, and lack of 24-hour pharmacy services.

- *Recommendations.* Develop protocols for standardized concentrations. Remove potassium chloride from all nonessential areas and stock units with premixed small- and large-volume bags. Beware of dispensing unit doses of concentrate for individual orders and storage in automated dispensing cabinets and crash carts. JCAHO now suggests removing the concentrate from patient care areas.

Interchangeability of drug with narrow therapeutic index

- An FDA investigation revealed no problems with substituting brand-name products with generic products. Duplicative therapy is problematic (e.g., dispensing of Coumadin® and warfarin) when patient care is provided by multiple physicians, prescriptions are filled at different pharmacies, and duplication is unrecognized by the patient.

Dangerous chemicals in patient care areas

- *Problem.* Death occurred in a confused patient who drank Zenker's solution that was left at the bedside. Another patient sustained severe esophageal burns when potassium hydroxide left at the bedside was administered orally instead of potassium chloride.

- *Recommendation.* Dangerous chemicals must be not be stored in patient rooms or where medications are prepared.

The Use of Benchmarking

Benchmarking is an ongoing process that determines how other organizations have achieved optimal performance. Through the process of benchmarking, ways are suggested for adapting the best practices that result in exceptional performance. Although measurement is one of its components, effective benchmarking is a dual process that requires two products: *benchmarks* and *enablers.*[15]

Benchmarks are measures of comparative performance that answer the question: "What is your level of performance?" By itself, this information has little use in improving performance. To be effective, benchmarking must also provide a systematic method of understanding the underlying processes that determine an organization's performance. To that end, enablers must be identified. Enablers are the specific practices that lead to exemplary performance; they answer the question: "How do you do it?" Overlooking either one of these components in the benchmarking process renders it useless, even dangerous.

Although medication error rates may seem ideal for benchmarking, we must question the wisdom of applying the benchmarking concept to the medication use process when the focus is on error rates. Certainly, the confusion surrounding the term "benchmarking" perpetuates the myth that one can gauge the quality and safety of the medication use process simply by comparing error rates, both within an organization and externally. The true incidence of medication errors varies, however, depending heavily on the rigor with which the events are identified and reported.

Currently, there is no consistent process among health care organizations for detecting and reporting errors. Because many medication errors cause no harm to patients, they remain undetected or unreported. Still, organizations often depend only on spontaneous, voluntary reporting of errors to determine the rate at which errors occur. The inherent variability of determining an error rate in this way invalidates the measurement, or benchmark. A high error rate may suggest either unsafe medication practices or an organizational culture that promotes error reporting. Conversely, a low error rate may suggest either successful error prevention strategies or a punitive culture that inhibits error reporting. Moreover, the definition of a medication error may not be consistent among organizations or even between individual practitioners in the same organization. Thus, spontaneous error reporting is a poor method of gathering benchmarks; it is not designed to measure medication error rates.

Of equal concern is the mistaken belief that benchmarking is simply a process of comparing numbers.[16] Although this activity produces no meaningful information, health care organizations have embraced the practice of comparing error rates. Yet there has been little effective effort directed at identifying enablers for safe medication use to accompany this attempt at benchmarking. As a result, organizations focus undue attention on maintaining a low error rate, giving the errors themselves, rather than their correction, disproportionate importance. This promotes an unproductive cycle of underreporting errors, which results in unrecognized weaknesses in the medication use system. Thus, low error rates can result in a false sense of security and a tacit acceptance of preventable errors.

Benchmarking for the medication use process can be effective only if a system of objective measurement, which is more reliable than spontaneous error reporting alone, is used to identify best practices (such as observational methods or systematic evaluation of errors[17,18]).

In addition, the benchmarking process must include a method for accurately determining the specific processes that enable the organization to achieve an environment in which medications are safely used. Success is more likely with benchmarking projects that are focused on specific areas of drug therapy (such as insulin therapy or anticoagulant therapy) so that accurate benchmarks (performance measurements) and enablers (practices that lead to exemplary performance) can be more easily identified and implemented.

Benchmarking projects should be carefully selected. Organizations are urged to place less emphasis on error rates that are based solely on spontaneous, voluntary reporting programs. Instead, error reporting should be encouraged in order to identify and remedy problems, rather than to provide statistics for comparison.

High-Alert Drugs

One means of preventing adverse drug events is to identify drugs, drug classes, or drug delivery devices that, improperly used, have the potential to cause the greatest harm (see Chapter 5). These products can be identified through both external and internal sources. Once they have been identified, the organization should develop procedures that will prevent or minimize the potential of these products to cause harm.

One way to accomplish this is to use failure mode and effects analysis (see Chapters 3 and 4).[3,4] For example, with each high-alert drug, drug class, or device that is identified, a multidisciplinary team can examine what would happen if the drug or device were improperly used for a variety of reasons. The team can then examine the safety systems that are in place to detect the failure before the medication reaches the patient and, if necessary, devise new safety nets. Using this method for each new drug added to the formulary helps the organization make proactive attempts to reduce the likelihood of systems failures. Table 20–1 shows examples of elements commonly involved in medication errors, including common failures and examples of the errors that result.

Case Study

In 1993, mivacurium (Mivacron®) was accidentally administered instead of metronidazole to several patients at a large hospital. Three patients went into respiratory arrest, and one died. The case resulted in the termination of a pharmacist and a pharmacy technician and the suspension of several nurses.

This case study analyzes this event to determine the failure points, the root causes of the failure points, the key elements involved, and the actions that can be taken that will most likely prevent this event from recurring. The amount of information available to the committee charged with investigating this event is typical of that available in most situations of this nature.

Step 1: Identify Failure Points

Failure points are determined by reviewing the medication use process and identifying those points in the process where a problem contributing to the event occurred. No problems were identified during prescribing and order processing. Problems were found, however, in the drug dispensing activity. A review found that the technician in the intravenous-admixture room pulled foil-wrapped, premixed intravenous items from the bulk intravenous storage area and placed the labels on the foil outerwrap. The pharmacist checked the bags and the computer-printed labels that said "metronidazole." No one noticed that the foil-wrapped bags actually contained mivacurium. Points of failure identified during the drug-dispensing process included pulling the wrong medication, labeling the wrong medication, identifying the wrong medication, and failing to double-check to detect the labeling error.

The next area examined was drug administration. The nurses noted the pharmacy label for metronidazole on the outer foil wrap and verified the drug name on the label with the transcribed order on the patient's medication administration record. Believing the drug was metronidazole, the nurses administered it to the four patients. Points of failure identified during drug administration included identifying the wrong medication and failing to double-check to detect a dispensing error.

Step 2: Identify Root Causes of Failure Points

To discover the root causes of this event, the investigating team repeatedly asked "why" questions until no additional relevant questions or answers could be articulated. This process was repeated for each failure point identified. The questions focused on the system, not on individuals.

First Level of Inquiry. To find out why the dispensing error occurred, the team asked the following questions:

- Why was the wrong drug pulled from the pharmacy shelves?

- Why did the system of double-checks fail to identify the error?

The answers revealed that metronidazole and mivacurium minibags had similar foil-wrapped packaging. The name of the drug did not appear on the foil outerwrap and was not easily visible through the plastic window in the foil pouch. Metronidazole was stored next to mivacurium in the intravenous-admixture area.

Finally, before this event, metronidazole was the only foil-wrapped pre-mixed intravenous item known by the pharmacist and technician to be stocked in the pharmacy. Confirmation bias allowed the staff to believe that a foil-wrapped item could not be anything other than metronidazole.

To determine why the error in administration occurred, the team asked, "Why was the mivacurium dispensed by the pharmacy identified as metron-idazole on the nursing unit?" The nursing staff, like the pharmacy staff, believed that the only foil-wrapped, premixed medication available in the hospital was metronidazole. Thus, after receiving the foil-packed container with a pharmacy label identifying the drug as metronidazole, they under-took no additional inquiry. The inner container was never removed from the foil outerwrap to aid in further identification.

Second Level of Inquiry. The team continued to ask "why" questions related to the answers given to the previous questions. Examples included the following:

- Why was the name of the drug not visible through the plastic window?

- Why was mivacurium stored next to metronidazole?

- Why was mivacurium stocked in the pharmacy?

- Why was the staff unaware that mivacurium was stocked in the phar-macy and available for use in the hospital?

- Why was the inner container never removed from the foil outerwrap?

Answers to these and other questions revealed numerous root causes, as list-ed in Step 3.

Step 3: Identify Systems Failures

Building on the preceding steps, the team identified the following key ele-ments as involved in the systems failure:

- Packaging, labeling, nomenclature, and advertising

  — Look-alike foil packaging,

  — Drug name not printed on the outer wrap,

  — Poor visibility of the drug name on the inner container because of the foil wrapping,

  — Poor visibility of the drug name on the inner container because the crimp at the bottom of the foil bag was not high enough to prevent the container from slipping below the plastic window.

- Communication

  — Failure to communicate decisions recently made by the Pharmacy and Therapeutics Committee concerning

    – a trial of mivacurium by the anesthesiology department, and

    – the addition of mivacurium to the formulary.

  — Failure of the manufacturer and the FDA to alert health providers of a previous death resulting from a similar adverse event involving mivacurium. The manufacturer had issued a nationwide "stat gram" to provide stickers on the outside foil packages of mivacurium. The stickers were not in the form of a warning; they simply reinforced the drug name. The manufacturer's communiqué did not refer to the potential for confusing mivacurium with other foil-packaged drugs, and it did not mention the recent death.

  — Lack of clear directions. A technician was told to place the stickers on the bags, in keeping with the manufacturer's instructions. However, the technician misunderstood the directions and believed the stickers were to be affixed at the time the drugs were sent to patient care units. Therefore, the bags remained unlabeled.

- Staff education

  — Lack of education regarding previous adverse events involving mivacurium. A few months before this incident, the potential for mix-up between mivacurium and other foil-packaged drugs was reported to ISMP. Two months later, in another institution, mivacurium was accidently administered instead of Zantac®. One of the pharmacists saw an alert sent out by ISMP but did not share this information with colleagues.

  — Failure to inform staff that mivacurium had been added to the formulary.

  — Lack of staff knowledge regarding the appropriate administration technique for metronidazole. The nursing staff believed metronidazole must be hung with the outer foil wrap in place. Had the foil been removed, the dispensing error may have been detected.

- Drug storage and stocking

  — Incautious storage of mivacurium. Mivacurium was originally placed in an area reserved for anesthetic drugs. Later, a clinical supervisor moved it to the bulk intravenous storage area. The drugs in this area were arranged alphabetically, and mivacurium was placed directly beside metronidazole. The cartons of the two products looked similar. Large product codes, expiration dates, and lot numbers on the boxes made the product names less visible.

• Quality assurance and risk management

— Failure to report an earlier incident when a technician found mivacurium in the metronidazole bin.

Step 4: Identify Prevention Strategies with the Highest Leverage

Once the root causes and systems failures had been identified, staff at this hospital could have implemented numerous prevention strategies. The challenge was to identify those that would result in prevention of this specific error and others caused by similar systems failures. Following is a partial list of the prevention strategies that the team identified:

• Manufacturer packaging and labeling changes;

• Timely communication, via a report or newsletter, to all staff about decisions of the Pharmacy and Therapeutics Committee;

• Multidisciplinary review of adverse drug events reported in professional journals or newsletters;

• Changes in storage practices for metronidazole and mivacurium; and

• Promotion of reporting, communication, and correction of potentially dangerous situations and errors that never reach the patient.

As a result of this adverse drug event, several manufacturers have repackaged and relabeled their products in foil outerwraps to facilitate drug identification and to allow space for hazard warnings. Although the manufacturers' actions are important, they are not necessarily those with the highest leverage for internal change. Providing timely information about the activities of the Pharmacy and Therapeutics Committee to all involved in the medication use process is a high-leverage action, because it can help prevent not only this error but also other errors related to a systems failure with communication. A process for multidisciplinary review of external errors and proactive prevention strategies is likewise essential.

References

1. U.S. Pharmacopeial Convention. National Council focuses on coordinating error reduction efforts. *Quality Review.* 1997; 57.

2. Joint Commission on Accreditation of Healthcare Organizations. *Sentinel Event Alert.* No 3, May 1, 1998.

3. Cohen MR, Senders J, Davis NM. Failure mode and effects analysis: a novel approach to avoiding dangerous medication errors and accidents. *Hosp Pharm.* 1994; 29: 319–30.

4. Williams E, Talley T. The use of failure mode effect and criticality analysis in a medication error sub-committee. *Hosp Pharm.* 1994; 29: 331–38.

5. Leape LL. Error in medicine. *JAMA.* 1994; 272: 1851–57.

6. Leape LL, Bates DW, Cullen DJ, et al. Systems analysis of adverse drug events. *JAMA.* 1995; 274: 35–43.

7. Senge PM, Kleiner A, Roberts C, et al. *The Fifth Discipline Fieldbook: Strategies and Tools for Building a Learning Organization.* New York: Currency Doubleday; 1994: 91–94.

8. Senge, PM. *The Fifth Discipline: The Art and Practice of the Learning Organization.* New York: Currency Doubleday; 1990: 7–8, 40, 57–59.

9. Reason J. The contribution of latent human failures to the breakdown of complex systems. *Philos Trans R Soc Lond B Biol Sci.* 1990: 327, 475–84.

10. Reason J. Foreword. In: Bogner MS, ed. *Human Error in Medicine.* Hillsdale, NJ: Lawrence Erlbaum; 1994: vii–xv.

11. Smetzer JL, Cohen MR. Lesson from the Denver medication error/criminal negligence case: look beyond blaming individuals. *Hosp Pharm.* 1998; 33: 640–57.

12. Plsek PE. *Creativity, Innovation, and Quality.* Milwaukee, Wis: ASQ Quality Press; 1997. <www.DirectedCreativity.com>

13. Stevens T. Dr. Deming: management today does not know what its job is. *Industry Week.* January 1994; 17.

14. Deming WE. *The New Economics.* Cambridge, Mass: Massachusetts Institute of Technology Center for Advanced Engineering Study; 1993.

15. Dinklage K. Learning from the best: using benchmarking to improve performance. *Pharmaguide to Hospital Medicine.* 1994; 7 (3): 5–8.

16. American Society for Healthcare Risk Management. *Health Care Risk Management Benchmarking Primer.* Chicago, Ill: American Hospital Association; 1996.

17. Allen EL, Barker KN. Fundamentals of medication error research. *Am J Hosp Pharm.* 1990; 47: 555–71.

18. Lesar TS. Factors related to errors in medication prescribing. *JAMA.* 1997; 277 (4): 312–17.

19. Cohen MR. System analysis needed to prevent serious errors: blaming employees for medication errors makes no sense. *Hosp Pharm.* 1996; 31 (3): 1–4.

Index

Key to Abbreviations

cp: color plates
f: figure
t: table

fraud, possibility of, with verbal orders, 8.18

free flow, in intravenous line, protection against, 5.4, 11.13

furosemide, *xiii*

G

generic names. *See also* drug names; *specific name*
versus brand names, and order transcription, 5.6, 11.5

gentamicin, 13.9, 13.10*f*

geriatric patients
dosing of, double-checking of, 5.4, 8.14
education of, and compliance, 14.9–14.10
medication organizers for, 14.10
medication schedule for, 14.9–14.10, 14.10*t*
swallowing problems in, 14.10

Glynase Prestab, 13.17–13.18, 13.19*f*

Grabenstein, John D., 17.1

gravity control, for intravenous medications, 5.4, 11.13

Green, Laurence, 15.1

H

Haemophilus influenzae type b vaccine, 17.3–17.4, 17.6–17.7, 17.9

Handbook on Injectable Drugs, 20.24

hand washing, staff, patient education about, 14.1

handwriting
improvement of, guidelines for, 8.2
legibility of, 8.1–8.2, 14.4
poor, 1.2, 8.1–8.2, 14.4, 17.5
errors caused by, legal concerns with, 8.2–8.3, 8.3*t*

Harriet Lane Handbook, 16.7

Harvard Medical Practice Study, 2.1

Health Care Financing Administration (HCFA), 6.23–6.24

health care providers. *See also* nurses; pharmacists; pharmacy technicians; physicians
communication among, improvement of, 15.13, 15.19
disciplining of
appropriate, 19.9–19.10
as deterrent to incident reporting, 2.2–2.3, 2.8, 2.13, 6.12, 7.5, 7.7, 18.1–18.2, 19.8–19.9
education of
about immunologic drugs, 17.10–17.11
in cancer chemotherapy, 15.3–15.5, 15.18
emphasis on error-free practice during, 2.2–2.3
in error prevention, 18.16
lack of, 20.8*t*, 20.11, 20.32
failure to report errors, 7.3–7.4
hand washing by, patient education about, 14.1

implications of immunologic drug errors for, 17.12

involvement in labeling/packaging error prevention, 13.18, 13.20

needs of, for reporting system improvement, 19.15

patient interchange with, after serious event, 19.13–19.14

performance improvements, 19.2

primary goal of, 7.1

public trust in, 7.1

reactions to making errors, *xiv–xv*, 7.1–7.10

HEMEA. *See* human error mode and effects analysis

Hemoccult, 20.23

heparin, 5.4, 5.24–5.26, 16.2, 18.4
packaging/labeling of, 13.3–13.4, 13.8–13.9, 13.9*f*, 13.15–13.16, 13.16*f*, 18.4, 20.24

hepatitis A-hepatitis B vaccine, 17.4

hepatitis B vaccine, 17.6, 17.10

hepatitis B virus, 17.4, 17.10

Hespan, 13.3, 20.24

Hib vaccine. *See Haemophilus influenzae* type b vaccine

high-alert drugs, *xiv*, 5.1–5.40. *See also specific drug*
access to, limiting of, 5.8
commonly used, 5.2*t*
constraints on use of, 5.8
definition of, 5.1
differentiation of, 5.6–5.7, 9.10
dosing for, standardization of, 5.11
errors involving
consequences of, minimization of, 5.3
prevention of, 5.1–5.2
improvement in, framework for, 5.2–5.3
visibility of, 5.3
labeling of, 5.6–5.8, 9.4, 9.12–9.14, 18.14
ordering of, guidelines for, 5.7–5.8
packaging of, 5.6–5.7, 18.14
differences in, 3.6–3.7
preparation of, standardization of, 5.11
risk analysis for, 20.29
safeguarding, key change concepts for, 5.3–5.11, 5.14*t*–5.15*t*
storage of, *xiii*, 5.7
warning reminders about, 5.8, 18.14

Hismanal, 13.17, 13.19*f*

home, medication storage in, 14.5

hospital discharge, patient education at, importance of, 14.9

hospitals
complexity of, 2.12

melphalan, 15.6
Memorial Mission Hospital (Asheville, NC), 4.2
Memorial Sloan-Kettering Cancer Center, 15.10
memory, biased, 2.4
meningitis, BCG-associated, 17.7–17.8
mental association, 20.20
mental functioning
    automatic, 2.3–2.4
    and error analysis, 2.3–2.5
Merck & Co., 17.4
mesalamine, 13.11, 13.11*f*
methotrexate, 15.8, 17.8
metric system, 1.3
    versus apothecary symbols, 8.5–8.7,
        11.5–11.6, 18.14
metronidazole, 13.8, 16.5, 20.29–20.30
Micromedex, 15.5
Milazzo, Charles J., *xvi,* 19.1
milrinone, 9.11
Minnesota Board of Pharmacy, 10.10
missing doses. *See* dose omissions
mistakes, 2.4–2.5
    definition of, 9.1
    knowledge-based, 2.4
    rule-based, 2.4
mithramycin. *See* plicamycin
mitoxantrone, 13.17, 15.6
mivacurium (Mivacron), 1.2*cp*, 13.8, 13.17,
        20.29–20.33
mnemonics
    computer, for drug pairs, 9.10
    for immunologic products, 17.11
    problems caused by, 9.10
mobile cart, automated, 10.7*t*, 10.10
monoclonal antibodies, 17.4
morphine sulfate, 18.4
M-R-VAX IIV. *See* measles-rubella vaccine
MSTA. *See* mumps skin test antigen
Muller, Raymond J., 15.1
multidisciplinary process
    of error reduction, *xii–xiii, xv,* 18.16–18.20,
        20.3, 20.11, 20.22
    of error reporting, 7.7–7.8, 9.18–9.19, 19.5
    of quality improvement, for cancer chemothera-
        py, 15.13–15.14
multi-ingredient products, precautions with, 14.4
mumps-rubella vaccine, 17.5
mumps skin test antigen, 17.11
mumps vaccine (Mumpsvax), 17.11
N
Nahata, M. C., 6.17
names
    company, on labeling, 13.11–13.12

drug (*See* drug names; *specific name*)
    of patients (*See* patient identification)
    of prescriber, legibility of, 8.2
narcotics, 5.35–5.37. *See also specific drug*
nasogastric tubes
    device standards, 11.14
    medications meant to be given by, intravenous
        administration of, 11.13–11.14
National Cancer Institute, 15.5, 15.12, 15.14
National Coordinating Council for Medication Error
        Reporting and Prevention, 5.7–5.8,
        18.16–18.20, 19.3–19.4, 20.1,
        20.3
    error categorization, 18.18, 18.18*t*
    goals of, 18.17
    members of, 18.16–18.17
    prescription writing guidelines, 18.19, 18.19*t*
National Council on Patient Information and
        Education, 14.6
National Drug Code (NDC) numbers, 9.15, 13.5
National Institutes of Health, 15.6, 15.20, 17.7
National Library of Medicine, 15.5
National Patient Safety Foundation (AMA), 14.1
Navelbine. *See* vinorelbine
NCC MERP. *See* National Coordinating Council for
        Medication Error Reporting and
        Prevention
NCR (no-carbon-required) forms, 11.3–11.4
NDA. *See* New Drug Application
NDC number. *See* National Drug Code (NDC)
        number
near misses, 20.1
Neofax '95, 20.15
Neuenschwander, Mark, *xv,* 10.1
Neumega, 20.24
neuromuscular blocking agents, 5.37–5.38. *See
        also specific agent*
    packaging of, 13.17
    warning labels for, 17.9
nevirapine, 17.4
New Drug Application, 12.6
new products
    pediatric, approval of, 16.3
    screening of, 5.7, 12.6
New York State Department of Health, *xi*
NIH. *See* National Institutes of Health
nitroglycerin, 13.16
no-carbon-required (NCR) forms, 11.3–11.4
noise, errors caused by, rate of, 6.22
nomenclature. *See also* drug names; names; *specific
        drug or term*
    for cancer chemotherapy, 15.8–15.11,
        15.18–15.19
    for error reporting, standardization of,
        19.3–19.4